SECOND EDITION

Introduction to Motor Behavior
A Neuropsychological
Approach

SECOND EDITION

Introduction to Motor Behavior
A Neuropsychological
Approach

George H. Sage
University of Northern Colorado

Addison-Wesley Publishing Company
Reading, Massachusetts
Menlo Park, California · London
Amsterdam · Don Mills, Ontario · Sydney

This book is in the
ADDISON-WESLEY SERIES IN PHYSICAL EDUCATION

Dedicated to Liz

Preface

Within the past 15 years there has been a surge of interest in the psychological dimensions of human movement in several professions which deal in the development of effective and efficient motor performance. This attention has been especially prevalent in the field of physical education, but it has also been evident in fields such as special education, physical therapy, and industrial psychology.

In physical education, traditionally professional preparation programs have emphasized physiological and mechanical factors in human movement. But in recent years, with greater understanding and appreciation of the variables affecting movement activities, new subjects have been added to the curriculum. One of these new subjects deals with the psychological parameters of human movement, and courses such as "Psychology of Motor Behavior" or "Psychology of Motor Learning" have emerged. At first these courses were offered at the graduate level, but they have now become a regular part of undergraduate classes throughout the country.

This book is designed to serve as a textbook in courses concerned with the psychology of motor behavior. The purpose of the book is to describe the basic knowledge that has been accumulated in the field of motor learning and performance and to examine the relevant empirical evidence and research on this subject. This volume gives special emphasis to the important role that the nervous system and other physiological mechanisms play in motor behavior. This role has received relatively little notice in previous texts on this subject which have been written by physical educators.

I have used a neuropsychological approach in an attempt to integrate neurophysiological and behavioral information since, it seems to me, knowledge of the functioning of the nervous system is necessary if a beginning is to be made toward understanding motor behavior. This is not to imply that the neural correlates to all motor behavior are known. Of course they are not, and only a beginning has been made along these lines. But the future holds much promise, and when advances are made toward understanding motor behavior, chances are very strong that they will be made by scholars who have a thorough knowledge of neurophysiological functioning.

Only the more important information with regard to neuroanatomy and neurophysiology has been selected for use in this book; other material had to be omitted. Much of the neuroanatomical and neurophysiological literature is excellent as a source of reference, but this mass of information is too comprehensive for a text of this type.

It is difficult to bridge the gap between basic research findings and applications to teaching and coaching. I have been conscious of this so I have tried not to overstate the applications of research to teaching motor activities in a strained attempt to pretend that we know just how to apply all existing knowledge. I will admit, however, that I have occasionally taken some liberties with basic research in making generalizations or describing implication for motor skill acquisition and performance. I hope the "purists" will forgive these transgressions.

There are numerous scholars in many disciplines who have made profound and enduring contributions to our understanding of motor learning and performance. It is impossible for me to acknowledge individual indebtedness to all the writers of articles, monographs, and books which I have consulted, much as I should like to mention every author by name. I have conscientiously attempted to indicate sources of original information and ideas. Such a task is large, however, and the possibility of error is great. The references at the end of the book are a means by which I have attempted to give credit to those whose works I consulted.

The actual preparation of the book involved considerable work, and I wish to thank the various secretaries of the University of Northern Colorado who helped lighten my work in many ways, especially Harriett Amos, Shirley Dressor, and Gertrude Fillinger, who were helpful in various phases of preparing the manuscript. I am particularly grateful to Marlene Krieger for her painstaking deciphering of my handwritten drafts and her efficient typing in preparing the manuscript for publication.

The dedication of this book signifies my indebtedness to my wife, who sacrificed many weekend and evening activities while I was busy writing this volume.

Greeley, Colorado   G.H.S.
August 1976

Contents

CHAPTER 21   TRANSFER OF MOTOR LEARNING   433

CHAPTER 22   MOTIVATION: AN OVERVIEW   455

CHAPTER 23   THE AUTONOMIC NERVOUS SYSTEM   471

CHAPTER 24   AROUSAL AND MOTOR BEHAVIOR   493

1

Introduction to the Study of Motor Behavior

The study of motor behavior is specifically concerned with motor skill acquisition and performance. This subject consists of a body of knowledge, compiled by the use of the scientific method, about the psychological aspects of human motor behavior. Thus, it may be viewed as a subfield of psychology.

Most texts devoted to learning and performance emphasize the acquisition and use of verbal skills. Since verbal behavior is of great importance in human affairs, this emphasis on verbal behavior is well founded. In this text, however, our primary concern is the acquisition and performance of motor skills, or motor behavior. Of course, language itself depends on muscular movement, and the very act of talking is a very complex motor skill, but we shall not examine this type of behavior in this volume.

In order to provide the reader with an overview of the subject matter of this text, a brief explanation of the development of general psychology and the subfield of motor behavior follows. The chapter concludes with a description of neuropsychology and what a neuropsychological approach, the approach of this text, means.

THE STUDY OF PSYCHOLOGY

Psychology is the study of behavior; the majority of professional psychologists focus their attentions on human behavior but many are interested in the behavior of other species, and they are psychologists as well. For centuries men and women have speculated about the causes of human behavior and have tried to make sense of their experiences of themselves and of

1

others. But psychology, as a separate academic discipline, is a rather young science, emerging in the latter years of the 19th century. The initial impetus for separate university departments of psychology came from Europe, and Wilhelm Wundt is considered the founder of modern psychology because he opened the first formal psychological laboratory in Leipzig, Germany, in 1879, and began publishing the first journal of experimental psychology in 1881.

American universities were quick to develop psychology departments. At Johns Hopkins University, G. Stanley Hall founded the first formal psychology laboratory in 1883 and was instrumental in establishing the first American psychological journal in 1887, the *American Journal of Psychology*. In most cases, the early psychologists were actually academically trained philosophers and were members of university philosophy departments. In the transition to a separate department of psychology, many universities listed a department of "philosophy–psychology" for several years.

In the first decades of this century psychology witnessed an exciting on-rush of new theories and research. Sigmund Freud developed and published his work on psychoanalysis which has been one of the more powerful forces in psychology in the 20th century. Growing out of the work of the Russian physiologist, Ivan Pavlov, and the American psychologist, Edward Thorndike, a large group of American psychologists led initially by John B. Watson adopted "behavior" as the subject matter of this discipline during the 1920s; the emphasis of this approach was on observable phenomena instead of hypothesized or nonobservable phenomena, the "Behaviorists" rejected the notion that the introspective* study of conscious experience was the province of psychology. A third major force in psychology emerged at about the same time that Watson and his followers were advancing the cause of "Behaviorism." This approach, called Gestalt psychology, emphasized that the understanding of behavior should be the study of experience in all its complexity, rather than the molecular study of sensations and actions then common in psychological laboratories. Gestalt psychology is considered to be the forerunner of contemporary cognitive psychology; "Cognitivism" may be viewed as a variation of the Gestalt approach. These three systematic approaches to the study of human behavior have been the foundation and focus in American psychology for the past 70 years. Of course, other theoretical perspectives have vied for recognition and respect during this period and at the present time there are numerous theoretical positions which have their followers and advocates.

---

*Introspection is a word used to refer to the description of one's own conscious processes.

As the academic discipline of psychology has developed, it has come to uniquely act as a bridge between two major groups of disciplines: the biological sciences and the social sciences. On the one hand, it is allied closely to the biological sciences such as physiology, neurology, anatomy, biochemistry, and many of its findings and theories are derived from these sciences. But psychology is also closely related to such social sciences as sociology, anthropology, and history. This division results in two major approaches to psychological study. The first is aligned with the biological sciences; the second has its main affinities with the social sciences. An illustration of how the field of psychology may be viewed is shown below. This clearly demonstrates the bridgelike position of this discipline.

Psychology

Biological sciences	*Social sciences*
Physiology	Sociology
Neurology	Anthropology
Anatomy	History
Biochemistry	Social philosophy
Zoology	Social psychology

Psychology is a distinct science, even though it uses information from other fields of study. There are few, if any, disciplines which do not borrow basic content from other disciplines.

Psychology, as a scientific field of study, may be formally defined as the study of complex forms of integration or organization of behavior (Hebb, 1972). It is an attempt to learn about and understand behavior. Applied, or professional, psychology is the application of the knowledge of basic psychology in specific situations or problems. The use of psychological facts and theories, in teaching movement activities such as games, sports, and dance skills is one application of psychology.

THE STUDY OF MOTOR BEHAVIOR

As basic subject matter, the study of motor behavior is an attempt to learn more about, and understand better, all of the psychological factors that are involved in motor learning and performance, regardless of whether this behavior takes place in the gymnasium, athletic field, industrial plant, or in outer space. The primary concern of the scientist working in this subject area is with understanding and advancing knowledge about human movement. He or she may or may not also be interested in the solution of "practical" problems. Scientists of any discipline consider that any knowledge, regardless of whether it is "practical," is worthy of study. There is a fundamental difference between the scientist who discovers knowledge and the professional who applies it. In the case of physics, the physicist (the scientist) discovers the laws of mass and volume, while the engineer (the professional) applies the laws to "practical" problems, such as those of building a bridge. In another case, the bacteriologist who discovered penicillin was a scientist seeking an understanding of the world of microscopic organisms; the physician who prescribes penicillin for an ill patient is acting as a professional applying knowledge which was discovered by the scientist. No value judgment is intended as to whether one role, that of the scientist or the professional, is more worthy than the other. Indeed, both roles are essential in each field of study for the systematic advancement of that field.

Scientists studying motor behavior have a two-fold purpose in seeking to understand the behavioral dimensions of human movement. Prediction is the first purpose. As a result of understanding the subject matter, they want to be able to predict behavior. Their second purpose is behavior control. As a result of understanding and being able to predict behavior, they want to be able to control behavior. The aim of every science is understanding, prediction, and control, but the notion of control over human behavior tends to have unpleasantly authoritarian and manipulative connotations. However, the notion of "control" in the context of motor behavior is usually concerned with the improvement in the subject's (or student's) learning rate or performance. It is assumed that the subject (or student) willingly and voluntarily undertakes the task and is not coerced or forced to perform against his or her will. The so-called control, then, has an underlying humanistic foundation.

Just as with many scientific subject areas, there is a variety of applications for motor behavior knowledge and there are scholars who are doing research to advance the applied aspects of this subject. Applications of the basic subject matter of motor behavior are employed in several occupational fields. Industries frequently obtain the services of "industrial psychologists" to study the "human factors" involved in performing work tasks. This often results in the redesign of equipment and/or job tasks to make the movements more effective and efficient for workers. The military has often employed motor behavior specialists for the same purposes. In recent years the space program has made extensive use of "space psychologists" in preparing astronauts and their equipment for space flights.

Another profession that makes wide use of motor behavior subject matter is physical education. A knowledge of motor behavior is imperative for the physical educator-coach for numerous reasons. A thorough understanding of perception, learning, motivation, and other psychological factors is essential in order to predict and control the behavior of students in the gymnasium, on the playing field, in the swimming pool, or in other areas where sports, games, and dance occur. Psychological variables constitute the most obvious and modifiable types of conditions in the educational process. The effective physical educator-coach must be a skilled practitioner in the educational application of motor behavior subject matter.

In the past decade, the term "sport psychology" has been adopted by those scholars who study motor behavior in sports environments. According to one of these scholars: "Sport psychology is an area which attempts to apply psychological facts and principles to learning, performance and associated human behavior in the whole field of sports" (Lawther, 1972). The position taken in this book is that since so little of the body of knowledge on human motor behavior has been derived from research in sports settings, it is better, at least for the present, to use the more generic term of motor behavior. However, in this text, illustrations for the application of this subject matter are directed toward the physical educator and coach, since most readers of this text will probably enter these professions. Most studies, examples, and implications which are presented are related to human movements in games, sports, and dance situations.

THE NEUROPSYCHOLOGICAL APPROACH OF THIS TEXT

There are several approaches to studying human behavior. Each has its unique techniques and procedures and each has a rich heritage of research findings and theories. The basic orientation of this text is neuropsychological. In describing the neuropsychological approach, we shall contrast this perspective with two other popular approaches in psychology.

The accumulation of knowledge in the field of psychology is similar to that followed in other disciplines and research is conducted employing the variables of unique interest. In psychological research, just as with research in other disciplines, two major categories of variables are employed: Independent variables and dependent variables. Before proceeding with the discussion of approaches to studying behavior, an explanation of these two categories of variables is essential because research in which these two types of variables are employed is the foundation on which knowledge in every field of study is accumulated and advanced.

A variable is any condition in an investigation which may change in quantity and/or quality. Examples of important variables to motor behavior are sex, age, intelligence, anxiety, level of aspiration, amount of feedback given subjects, etc. One type of variable, independent variables, is controlled and manipulated by the experimenter in an experiment. The second type of variable is called the dependent variable and its changes are consequent upon changes in the independent variable. An independent variable is the presumed cause of the dependent variable, the presumed effect. In psychology, behavior, or a response of some kind, is typically the dependent variable. In an experiment, the investigator manipulates independent variables and observes the effects on dependent variables. For example, when motor behavior investigators study the effect of different feedback techniques on learning, they may manipulate feedback, the independent variable, by using different feedback methods and observe the variation in learning rate, the dependent variable, as a presumed result of variation in the independent variable. Or to take another example, if one wished to ascertain the effects of a certain drug on motor performance of some kind, the drug would be the independent variable and the performance would be the dependent variable. The most common dependent variables in motor behavior research are learning and performance.

In one approach to the study of human behavior, investigators manipulate behavior (independent variables) and study the behavioral responses (dependent variables) without any concern for the underlying neural mechanisms involved. This approach commonly goes under the rubric of "Behaviorism," which was the heir to the Stimulus-Response Connectionist approach pioneered by Pavlov and Thorndike. Behaviorism focuses on the objective and observable components of behavior—that is, the stimulus and response events. Investigators using this approach are content to assume that there must be some neurological mechanisms that are related to the organizing and information-processing events that are assumed to occur in the organism but they do not give much attention to these neural activities; they rarely consider the means of neurological representation of motor behavior or the neurophysiological processes associated with motoric activity. John B. Watson gave Behaviorism its name, but B. F. Skinner, the famous Harvard psychologist, perhaps best represents the Behaviorist tradition.

In another approach to the study of behavior, the investigators also manipulate behavior, or the environment, and study the behavioral response with little concern for the underlying neural mechanisms involved, but they are concerned primarily with explaining those higher mental processes not easily explained using the Behaviorist paradigm (research strategy). This approach is called "Cognitivism," which is a descendant of Gestalt psychology. This is an orientation characterized by a relative lack of concern with stimuli and responses as well as neural activities. The primary concern is with such topics as perception, problem solving through insight,

decision making, and "understanding." In all of these processes, cognition*
is of central importance. Wolfgang Kohler was the first of the Cognitive
psychologists while Jerome Bruner, of Harvard, is perhaps the best known of
the current "Cognitivists."

A third approach to the study of human behavior, and the approach
that will be used in this text, is a neuropsychological approach. Neuropsychology goes by several names: physiological psychology, biopsychology,
psychobiology. The basic goal is to understand human behavior and psychological processes in terms of underlying physical and biological
mechanisms, especially the brain and its functions. As a science concerned
with living individuals, psychology has close ties with biology and is therefore concerned with the bodily processes that make behavior possible; thus
some psychologists are particularly interested in the nervous system,
especially the brain which is the most complex structure of this system.
Neuropsychology is an attempt to relate neurological mechanisms to
behavior; this approach focuses on the neural basis of behavior, which
comes down to a study of the nervous system and how it functions to control
behavior. The neuropsychologist attempts to find out how the nervous system regulates and controls behavior and psychological processes. Although
neuropsychologists manifest a great deal of interest in neural structures
and functions in an effort to understand behavior, they are still concerned
with behaviors that involve the whole organism, just as other psychologists
are.

Two major strategies are employed by neuropsychologists in order to
advance our understanding of human behavior. In the first strategy, the
independent variables are physiological manipulations while the dependent
variables are behavior, such as test performance, subject report, behavioral
observation, or ratings, and so on. The major physiological techniques are
ablation, lesioning, electrical stimulation, and chemical applications.
Ablation refers to the surgical removal of a particular part of an organism's
nervous system while lesioning involves destroying a part of the nervous system. In both cases after the technique has been employed, study is made of
the resulting impairment or alteration in behavior. These techniques have
yielded important information about what parts of the nervous system are
responsible for particular kinds of behavior. They are, however, not possible
with humans, but illnesses or injuries to humans frequently destroy or
require the removal of certain structures in the nervous system. In these

---

*Cognition is a general concept embracing all forms of knowing. It includes perceiv-
ing, thinking, imagining, reasoning, and judging; it means putting things together in
relating events.

cases investigators may study the postoperative effects on the patients' behavior. Since the nervous system is essentially an electrical system, it is possible to stimulate nerve cells by an outside electrical source, and this is done in electrical stimulation research. Typically, a small electrode is inserted into a particular site in the nervous system and a weak electric current is then passed through the electrode. The investigator then observes the results. Work of this kind has provided psychologists with enormously valuable information about the nervous system function. As with all body tissue, numerous biochemical events are constantly taking place in the nervous system. Therefore, chemicals play an important role in behavior. Neuropsychologists frequently explore the effects of various chemical substances on behavior. They may administer the chemicals orally, intravenously, or via implanted electrodes and observe the behavioral effects.

In the second major strategy used by neuropsychologists, the independent variables are psychological manipulations, such as learning a task or performing a task under certain conditions, and the dependent variables are the physiological effects. Here, the investigator creates situations calling for behavior of some kind under certain conditions and then observes the effects on neural activity. These effects are often measured by the responses of the heart, blood pressure, perspiration, muscle tension, and hormonal secretions, since all of these structures or activities are under the control of the nervous system. The electrical activity of the brain itself is often assessed also. The brain is constantly active in the living organism and is therefore spontaneously emitting electric signals. This electrical activity may be monitored by placing surface electrodes on the skull and recording the signals with a special instrument called an electroencephalograph (EEG). It has been found that humans emit several very distinct electrical patterns, depending upon whether they are relaxed, excited, thinking, or sleeping.

Before concluding this discussion on the neuropsychological approach of this book, two important points need to be made. First, concepts such as Behaviorism, Cognitivism, and Neuropsychology exist only as convenient labels for classifying the focus and interest of various investigators and their work. No one approach is completely satisfactory for answering all of the questions about human behavior. And psychologists using each of the approaches mentioned above occasionally employ the theories, research strategies, and techniques of the other approaches in their quest to discover new information about human behavior. Second, there are very few studies of motor behavior in sports, games, and dance where a neuropsychological perspective has been employed. Inferences from research done in the neuropsychological laboratory must be made when attempting to employ a neuropsychological approach to motor behavior in sports, games, and the dance.

The position taken in this text is that the study of motor behavior must first focus on a study of the nervous system because this system is responsible for all human behavior. The study of behavior is certainly a complex subject but any thorough interpretation of behavior is dependent upon a basic understanding of the structures and functions of the nervous system. Every kind of behavior is the result of neural activity, and we must recognize that a study of neural structures responsible for behavior is essential to understanding an individual's activity. Thus, ours is a neuropsychological approach which emphasizes the relationship between neural structure and functions and behavior. It is an approach which seeks to ascertain how the nervous system regulates and controls behavior and psychological processes, recognizing that much is still unknown about how the nervous system functions to control behavior.

Since an understanding of neural processes requires a knowledge of the structures and basic functional activity of the nervous system, the following two chapters of this volume deal with these subjects. This content has been kept to the minimum that was considered necessary for understanding materials about neural processes which appear in later chapters of the book.

MOTOR LEARNING AND PERFORMANCE

The terms motor learning and performance are used frequently throughout this text, and, while there may be a tendency to think of them as having the same meaning, they are not synonymous. Motor learning is commonly defined as a relatively permanent modification in motor behavior which results from practice or experience, and which is not a result of maturation, motivation, or training factors (such as improvements in strength). Since learning occurs within the individual, it cannot be observed directly; it can only be inferred by observing behavior, or performance. It is presumed, of course, that any permanent modification in behavior is represented by some biochemical and/or structural change in the nervous system. Techniques for measuring motor learning will be described in Chapter 16.

Motor performance, as distinct from motor learning, is the achievement or score, on a given trial, practice period, or game. For example, the time of 10 seconds is the performance of a track sprinter during a given race. Fifteen out of 20 free throws which are shot consecutively is a basketball shooter's performance.

The term motor behavior is a generic term which is used when no distinctive importance between motor learning and performance is necessary.

2

Basic Neuroanatomy
of the
Nervous System

The primary purpose of this chapter is to supply you with a general overview of the various structures and relative locations of these structures which make up the nervous system. Only the most elementary facts about functions are introduced at this point; more detail about the functions of the specific parts of the nervous system will be provided later in the book as the need arises. This chapter, then, describes the basic anatomy of the nervous system.

Since neuroanatomists use special terminology when describing the location of structures, the first section of this chapter presents the terms and their meanings which are most frequently employed in the remainder of the chapter and throughout the book when nervous system structures are discussed. There follows a description of the structural and functional unit of the nervous system, the neuron, and finally the major structures of the nervous system are identified and briefly described.

TERMINOLOGY USED IN NEUROANATOMY

Before we begin our examination of the nervous system, it is necessary for you to have an understanding of some of the terminology which is used when describing the location of certain structures in the body. This terminology is not unique to this book; it has been adopted by anatomists to precisely describe structure position.

The terminology is all based on the human body in "anatomical position," which is a standing position, with the arms hanging at the sides and the palms facing forward. In this position, there are three primary planes:

sagittal, coronal, and horizontal. A sagittal plane divides the body into right and left parts; a sagittal plane that divides the body into right and left *halves* is called a median plane. A coronal plane (also called a frontal plane) is at right angles to the sagittal plane and divides the body into front and back parts. A horizontal plane (also called the transverse plane) divides the body into upper and lower parts, so it is at right angles to the other two planes (Fig. 2.1).

Much of the anatomical terminology comes from that used with four-footed animals. Structures located toward the front of the body are "ventral" and structures located toward the back of the body are "dorsal." While these same terms are used in reference to some human nervous structures, the more commonly used words are anterior for structures toward the front, and posterior for structures toward the back of the body. The posterior horns of the spinal cord, for example, are also called dorsal, while the anterior horns are frequently referred to as ventral horns.

The words cranial and superior are synonyms used to indicate upper structures, and caudal and inferior are used in the same way to indicate

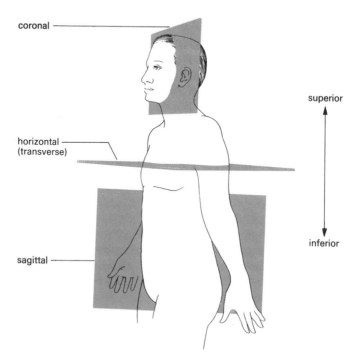

Fig. 2.1   Anatomical planes in the anatomical position. (Based on Langley *et al.* 1969.)

lower structures. The word medial means toward the middle of the body, or toward the median plane. Lateral means toward the side of the body, or away from the median plane. Peripheral means away from the center of the body. Ipsilateral means on the same side, while contralateral means on the opposite side (Fig. 2.2). These latter two terms are used when describing the initiation and termination of a set of nerve impulses. Impulses which originate and terminate on, let's say, the right side of the body are ipsilateral whereas if they originated on the right side and ended on the left side, the transmission would be considered contralateral.

term	definition
superior, cranial	toward the head
inferior, caudal	toward the feet
anterior, ventral	toward the front of the body
posterior, dorsal	toward the back of the body
medial	toward the middle of the body
lateral	toward the side of the body
peripheral	away from the center of the body
ipsilateral	on the same side of the body
contralateral	on the opposite side of the body

Fig. 2.2   Neuroanatomical terminology.

GENERAL PARTS OF THE NERVOUS SYSTEM

Like every other system in the human body, the nervous system is made up of individual cells. These cells are specialized to carry out a unique task, which is the transmission of nerve impulses from one cell to another. The nervous system is traditionally divided into two general parts, based on spatial location. One part is called the central nervous system (CNS) and is composed of those cells lying entirely within the vertebral column and skull. The major structures of the CNS are the brain, the brainstem, and the spinal cord. The second part of the nervous system is the peripheral nervous system (PNS) and consists of all the nerve cells and parts of nerve cells which enter or leave the brainstem and the spinal cord and connect them to the rest of the body. The PNS may be subdivided into a somatic nervous system and an autonomic nervous system (ANS). The former conducts impulses from sensory receptors in the skin, joints, and muscles and controls the striated, or skeletal, muscles—the so-called voluntary control muscles. The ANS sensory input is from smooth muscles, heart, and glands and it controls these same structures, the control being typically involuntary.

THE NEURON

The structural and functional unit of the nervous system is the neuron; it is the individual component of which the whole nervous system is built. Like all of the body's cells, neurons are designed in ways that are appropriate to their functions, which are primarily receiving and transmitting nerve impulses. A membrane surrounds the gelatinous protoplasm within the neuron, much like the skin surrounds a sausage. Protoplasm is a fluid substance containing a number of chemicals, granules, and other substances. The three main parts of a neuron are: (1) the cell body, (2) dendrites, and (3) axon (Fig. 2.3).

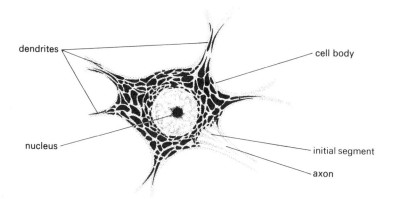

Fig. 2.3   Basic components of a typical neuron. (Based on Langley *et al.*, 1969.)

Cell body.   The cell body, also called the soma, is the metabolic center of the cell. It contains the nucleus, which is responsible for regulating the various processes of the entire cell. Extending out from the cell body are one or more fibers, some of which are microscopically short while others are over a meter in length. Neuron cell bodies are located mostly within the CNS, but some are found in ganglia (singular, ganglion), which are clusters of cell bodies outside the CNS. Clusters of cell bodies within the CNS are called nuclei.

Dendrites.   A dendrite is one type of nerve fiber extending from the cell body. A neuron may have anywhere from one to thousands of dendrites projecting outward from the cell body. These fibers typically divide like the branches of a tree into a number of small fibers before terminating. The primary function of the dendrites is to receive signals from other neurons.

Axon.   The second type of neuron fiber is called an axon, and it is attached to the cell body at a point called the initial segment. There is only one axon for each neuron, but an axon typically gives off many side branches, called collateral fibers. The end portions of an axon are called presynaptic terminals (other terms are telodendria, boutons, and knobs), and each axon may have numerous presynaptic terminals because it may have given off many collateral branches. The axon extends out like a telephone cable from the cell body and sends tiny fibers to the dendrites and cell bodies of other neurons, or to the muscles and glands in the rest of the body.

A. NEURON FUNCTION

One of the major purposes of the neuron is to pass messages, or impulses, from one part of the body to another. It does this by an electro-chemical process whereby an impulse, much like an electric current in a wire, is propagated from neuron to neuron. Nerve impulses come to a neuron by way of the many nerve fibers from other neurons making contact on the surface of the cell body and dendrites. This activity may trigger a nerve impulse in the initial segment of the neuron which is transmitted down the axon to its presynaptic terminals where it connects with another neuron. Axons typically conduct impulses away from the cell body. However, they can transmit in either direction, and in one type of neuron which has no dendrites the long axon fiber transmits impulses toward the cell body. The functional connection between one neuron and another is called a synapse. A neuron may have thousands of synapses on the surface of its dendrites and cell body so that signals from numerous other neurons impinge upon it. Presynaptic terminals also end on muscles and glands; we will have more to say about these kinds of connections at a later time.

From the above, it may be seen that a nerve impulse is transmitted from one part of the body to another by a sequence of dendrite and/or cell body to axon to dendrite and/or cell body of another neuron, linked together through many neurons. This forms the conduction pathway of the nervous system; indeed, the nervous system functions exclusively by these neuron chains.

B. CLASSIFICATION OF NEURONS

There are two methods for classifying neurons. One is based on location and function, and the other is based on structure. In the first method, neurons are classified as afferent, efferent, or interneuron. Afferent and efferent neurons lie mostly outside the CNS while interneurons lie within the CNS. Afferent neurons carry nerve impulses from the sensory receptors into the spinal cord or brain. On the other hand, efferent neurons transmit impulses

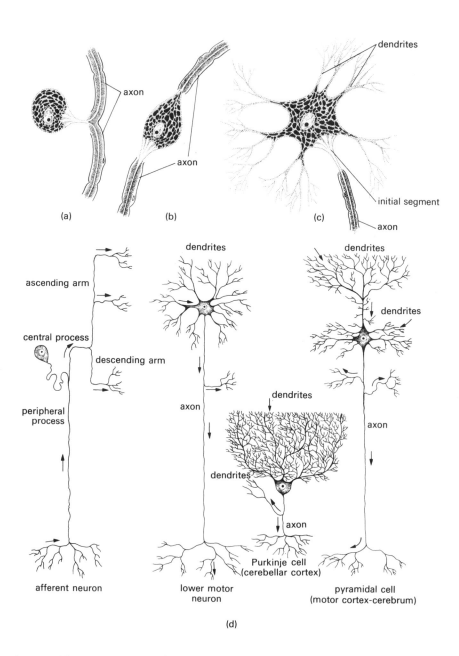

Fig. 2.4 Three main types of neurons. (a) A unipolar neuron. (b) A bipolar neuron. (c) A multipolar neuron. (d) Schematic illustration of some principal forms of neurons which are found in particular parts of the nervous system. [(a), (b) and (c) based on Langley *et al.*, 1969; (d) based on Crouch, 1965.]

from the CNS out to the effector organs—the muscles and glands. Efferent neurons which impinge on skeletal muscles are called motorneurons. The interneurons originate and terminate wholly within the CNS, and over 95 percent of all neurons of the nervous system are of this type.

Neurons are also classified by structure, specifically the number of fibers extending from the cell body. Some neurons have only one fiber process, and neurons of this type are called unipolar. In unipolar neurons, only the axon is connected to the cell body; there are no dendrites. Unipolar neurons are located in the spinal and cranial nerves and carry afferent signals from the sensory receptors. The single fiber process, the axon, divides into central and peripheral branches very close to the cell body in a T-shaped manner.

A second type of neuron has only two fiber processes, and is thus called bipolar. Bipolar neurons are rather rare, and are found only in two or three sites in the nervous system. The most common type of neuron in the human nervous system is the multipolar neuron, in which numerous dendrites and an axon extend from the cell body. Multipolar cells are found throughout the CNS and the PNS (Fig. 2.4).

C. NEUROGLIA

Within the CNS there is a special type of nonneural cell whose main role seems to be to hold the neurons together and to synthesize and store materials for use by the neurons. These cells, called neuroglia (or just glia), outnumber neurons ten to one and are in close proximity to the neurons, and they literally do glue the CNS together. A complete understanding of the functions of the neuroglia awaits resolution.

D. NERVES AND TRACTS

A nerve is a collection, or bundle, of nerve fibers, not including the cell bodies, bound together by well-organized connective tissue sheaths and lying outside the CNS. Thousands of nerve fibers are necessary to form a nerve. There are 12 pairs of cranial nerves extending from the brainstem and 31 pairs of spinal nerves projecting from the spinal cord. Nearly all nerves contain both afferent and efferent nerve fibers, so they are called "mixed nerves." Thus, within a nerve some fibers will carry impulses toward the CNS while others will carry impulses away from the CNS. Many nerves have local enlargements, called ganglia, which consist mainly of cell bodies of neurons.

Inside the CNS a bundle of nerve fibers is called a tract. The spinal cord has numerous tracts for carrying impulses from the sensory receptors to the brain and from the brain to the muscles and glands.

THE CENTRAL NERVOUS SYSTEM (CNS)

The brain, brainstem, and spinal cord make up the central nervous system. The CNS structures are protected by the skull, the spinal column (vertebrae) and its ligamentous connections, and the cerebrospinal fluid. The foramen magnum (Latin for large opening) is an opening at the base of the skull, and it is through this opening that the brain is continuous with the spinal cord (Fig. 2.5).

The structures of the CNS basically function to carry out two tasks: (1) Transmit information about the environment and the body to the brain where it is recorded, stored, and compared with other information; (2) Carry information from the brain to muscles and glands, thus producing movement or bodily adaptations to environmental demands.

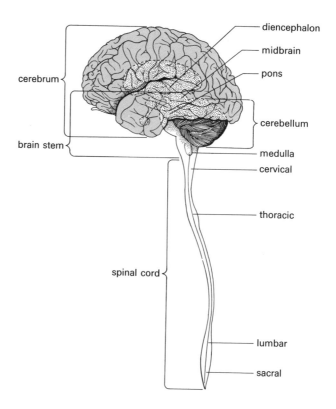

Fig. 2.5   The central nervous system (CNS) and its major parts. (Based on Langley *et al.*, 1969.)

A. THE BRAIN

John C. Eccles (1973), the Nobel laureate in neurophysiology, said that the human brain "is without any qualification the most highly organized and most complexly organized matter in the universe." It is the master control, the guiding force behind all human actions. This organ regulates heart and respiratory rates, controls body temperature, and performs numerous other duties without our really being aware of it. It also keeps us in touch with the environment by processing visual, auditory, tactile, etc. information impinging on us. For each of us, our brain is the material basis of our personal identity.

The brain was described by one writer as "two fistfuls of pinkish-gray tissue, wrinkled like a walnut and something of the consistency of porridge." It weighs about 3.5 pounds, but although it makes up only about 2.5 percent of the total body weight, it receives 15 percent of the total blood supply and uses about 25 percent of all the oxygen used by the body.

The brain uses only glucose as the food supply from which to make the energy substance adenosine triphosphate (ATP), which is the major form of biological energy. This process requires a steady supply of oxygen; therefore, if the flow of blood to the brain is interrupted for as little as 15 seconds, loss of consciousness may result; and interruption of blood flow for more than four minutes causes irreversible damage to brain cells and may cause death.

Since the early 1900s textbooks have compared the brain to a telephone switchboard; more recent books use the analogy of a computer. Both analogies are functionally useful for illustrative purposes—the brain functions as a switchboard and computer—but they are technically inaccurate. No switchboard or computer can accomplish anything like the miracles of scrutinizing, sorting, coding, and remembering performed by the brain.

The brain can be conveniently subdivided into several parts: the cerebrum, cerebellum, diencephalon, mesencephalon (or midbrain), and brainstem. The brain also contains several small cavities, called ventricles.

1. The cerebrum

This is the large umbrella-like dome of the brain which is divided into two cerebral hemispheres by the longitudinal fissure (a groove or furrow). The two hemispheres are symmetrical, one on the right and one on the left, with the fissure between them, running from front to rear. By and large, functions on the left side of the body are controlled by the right hemisphere, functions on the right side by the left hemisphere.

The cerebrum is further divided by the central fissure (also called the fissure of Rolando) which extends laterally across the midportion of each hemisphere. Another fissure, the lateral fissure (also called the fissure of

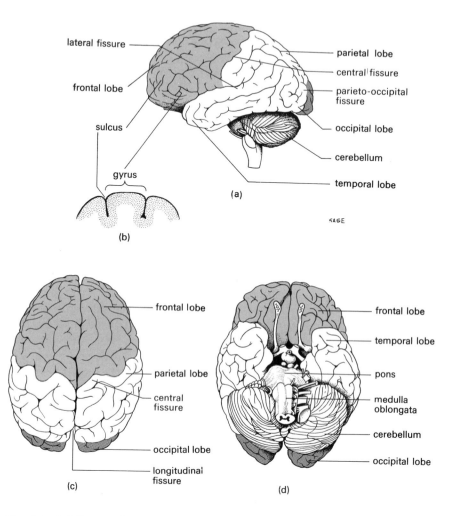

Fig. 2.6   (a) The cerebrum and its lobes. (b) Cross section of the cortex. (c) The cerebrum from above. (d) The cerebrum from below. [(a) and (b) based on Langley *et al.*, 1969; (c) and (d) based on Francis, 1964.]

Sylvius) is deep and runs laterally directly below the central fissure. The lateral and central fissures help to mark off the four major regions of each cerebral hemisphere. These regions are called lobes (Fig. 2.6).

The frontal lobe is in front of the central fissure. This area increases in size most dramatically with the ascent of the phylogenetic scale. In the cat or dog, the area forward of the central fissure is very small, but in humans the frontal lobe amounts to half the lateral area of the cerebrum. The parietal (pa-ri'-e-tal) lobe is behind the central fissure and extends back to the parieto-occipital fissure. The occipital lobe is at the very back of each cerebral hemisphere and makes up the posterior aspect of each cerebral hemisphere. The division between the parietal and occipital lobes is not clear-cut because the fissure separating the two lobes is not as large and deep as those separating the other lobes. Below the lateral fissure is the temporal lobe, which makes up the remaining portion of the lateral surface of the hemispheres.

The cerebral cortex. The outermost layer of the cerebrum is called the cerebral cortex and is composed mostly of the tightly packed cell bodies of the neurons. The cortex is only about ¼ inch thick but of the approximately 14 billion neurons in the human nervous system, 9 billion are found in the cortex.

As one ascends the phylogenetic scale, the surface of the cortex increases in area and becomes folded. Humans have a very large cortex, so large in fact that it virtually covers and encloses the other structures of the brain. In order to fit into the skull, the cortex has numerous folds, or convolutions as they are called. The "hills" or convolutions are called gyri (singular, gyrus), while depressions, or grooves, between the gyri are called sulci (singular, sulcus) or fissures if they are quite deep. If the cortex of an adult were unfolded and spread out, it would be about 20 square feet—the area of a 4′ × 5′ rug!

All sensory systems project their signals to the cortex, each to a specific region. A great deal of motor control of muscles and glands arises from other regions of the cortex. Basically there are three important aspects of behavior mediated by the cortex: (1) The reception and interpretation of sensory information; (2) the organization of complex motor behaviors; (3) the storage and utilization of learned experiences.

Cerebral pathways. The cerebral cortex and other functional components of the nervous system are linked together by an elaborate circuitry of pathways and interconnections forming a network of communication. The nerve fibers which make up these pathways extend into and out of the cortex or interconnect various parts of the cortex and can be generally divided into three categories: (1) Projection-motor fibers; (2) association fibers; (3) commissural fibers.

Projection-motor fibers stream into and out of the cortex, collecting in a relatively narrow column near the center of the brain in what is called the internal capsule. Ascending fibers transmit impulses from the thalamus, a structure deep within the brain, to the various sensory projection regions of the cortex. Descending fibers carry impulses from different regions in the cortex to lower-brain centers and to the spinal cord.

Association fibers interconnect different parts of the cortex. This fiber network is extensive and very complex, but it serves to connect each part of the cortex to every other part.

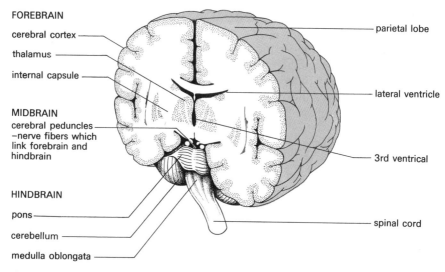

Fig. 2.7 Coronal section through brain. (Based on McNaught and Callander, 1963.)

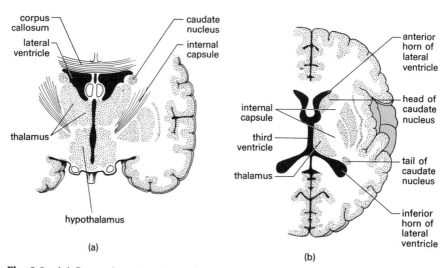

Fig. 2.8 (a) Coronal section through cerebrum. (b) Horizontal section through cerebrum. (Based on Langley et al., 1969.)

The two cerebral hemispheres are united by several commissures (sites of union of corresponding parts) of nerve fibers that cross the midline similar to the way the two halves of a walnut are connected to the middle. The most prominent is the corpus callosum, which is located at the bottom of the longitudinal fissure and consists of a broad sheet of densely packed fibers.

There are about 200 million callosal fibers in the human brain and in these fibers there is an incessant traffic. This arrangement allows the two hemispheres to "keep in touch" with each other. Thus, sensory impulses that reach one hemisphere are almost automatically transmitted on to the other and when signals are sent from one hemisphere to muscles or glands, the signals are also sent to the opposite hemisphere so as to keep it informed of the ongoing activity (Figs. 2.7 and 2.8).

Recent experiments have demonstrated that one of the functions of the corpus callosum bundle is concerned with the transfer of learning from one hemisphere to the other. In a series of "split-brain" studies over the past 20 years, Sperry and his colleagues (Sperry, 1964; Gazzaniga, 1967) have found that learning in one hemisphere is usually inaccessible to the other hemisphere if the connections between hemispheres are severed.

The basal ganglia.   The term "basal ganglia" is nonspecific; it refers to a group of nuclei (ganglia is really a misnomer) located in the inner layers of the cerebrum. There is no agreement as to what cerebral ganglia constitute the basal ganglia but the structures most frequently listed are the caudate nucleus, the lenticular nucleus, and the claustrum. Others will be identified and discussed in a later chapter (Fig. 2.9).

These structures appear to play an important but as yet poorly understood role in the control of movements. This control function will be described in a later chapter.

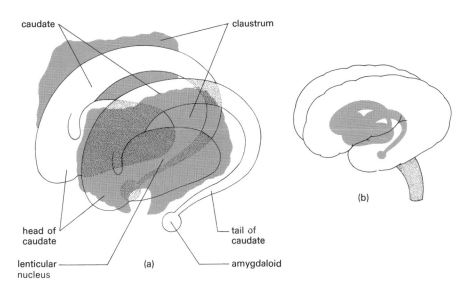

Fig. 2.9   (a) The positions of the basal ganglia. (b) Location of these structures in the cerebrum. (Based on Langley *et al.*, 1969.)

2. The cerebellum

When one views the brain the cerebrum is the dominant structure, but lying posterior and inferior to the cerebrum is another structure that looks like a small cerebrum. This structure is the cerebellum which means "little brain." It lies behind the pons and medulla (the two structures of the brainstem) and is much convoluted in appearance. It is composed of two hemispheres each of which has a cortex and a vast network of internal fiber connections. Its connections with the rest of the CNS are via three pairs of fiber tracts: inferior, middle, and superior cerebellar peduncles (Figs. 2.5 and 2.6).

Although knowledge about the precise functions of the various parts of the cerebellum is incomplete, the cerebellum seems to play an important role in coordinating and smoothing out skeletal movements. This is carried out through its connections with the cerebral cortex, other brain structures, and the spinal cord. Damage to the cerebellum tends to produce jerky, inaccurate, and/or uncoordinated movement. We shall discuss the functions of the cerebellum in more detail in a later chapter.

3. The diencephalon

From our evolutionary standpoint the oldest areas of the brain lie in its center and extend up into the cerebrum like a clenched fist, with the cerebrum enclosing these older areas. At the core of the brain is the area known as the diencephalon (di-en-sef-ah-lon) which connects the cerebral hemispheres with the mesencephalon (mes-en-sef-ah-lon), or midbrain. This area consists of a variety of structures which lie on either side of a narrow internal cavity, the third ventricle (a small cavity). For our purposes, only two of those structures need to be mentioned: (1) the thalamus; (2) the hypothalamus (Figs. 2.7, 2.8, and 2.10).

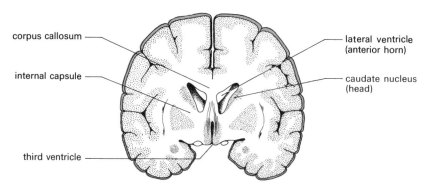

Fig. 2.10 Coronal section through the cerebrum. (Based on Noback, 1967.)

The thalamus consists of a pair of nuclei, one of which is located on each side of the third ventricle, and in general shape this structure is somewhat like two small footballs. One part of the thalamus is concerned with relaying information from the sensory systems for vision, hearing, touch, joint and muscle receptors, and perhaps pain, to the cerebral cortex. Another part of this structure does not seem to be involved in relaying specific sensory impulses but appears to play an important role in the arousal of the individual for activity. Some of the nerve fibers from the cerebral cortex and the cerebellum also terminate in the thalamus.

The hypothalamus is made up of a group of small nuclei located close to the base of the brain, close to the "master gland," the pituitary gland. In spite of its small size, the hypothalamus contains the highest integrative centers for the control of the autonomic nervous system; it is involved in such functional activities as the regulation of body temperature, endocrine gland activities, and emotional behavior in general. The hypothalamus is by far the most important center in the brain in the elicitation and coordination of motivated behavior (Fig. 2.8).

The role of both the thalamus and the hypothalamus will be discussed in later chapters in connection with their sensory and motor functions.

4. The mesencephalon (midbrain)

Below the diencephalon lies an area of the brain known as the mesencephalon or midbrain. This area constitutes the top of the brain stalk and is composed of several structures. The largest portion of its area contains the cerebral peduncles (a stemlike part), which are comprised of fibers originating in the cerebral cortex and projecting to the pons and/or the spinal cord. The median parts of the midbrain contain all the various pathways which are ascending to the thalamus. The roof of the midbrain includes two pairs of small hemispheres called the superior and inferior colliculi. The first is involved in reflex movements caused by visual stimulation and the latter is involved in reflex movements caused by auditory stimulation. This area also contains other small nuclei which have connections with the cerebellum, cerebral cortex, and several of the cranial nerves (Fig. 2.11).

5. The brainstem

The two major structures of the brainstem are the pons and the medulla. There is also a complex mixture of cell bodies, fibers, and nuclei spread throughout the brainstem which is collectively called the brainstem reticular formation (Figs. 2.5, 2.6, and 2.7).

The pons.   The word pons, meaning bridge, is derived from the thick band of transverse fibers (fibers crossing from one side of the midline to the other)

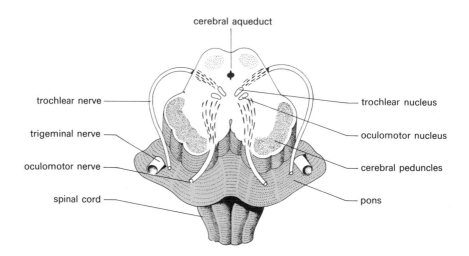

Fig. 2.11 Cross section of the mesencephalon. The cerebral aqueduct connects the third and fourth ventricles. (Based on Langley *et al.*, 1969.)

that make up its ventral portion and serve in part as a bridge between the hemispheres of the cerebellum. This ventral portion of the pons is composed of several fiber tracts and nuclei. There are, first, afferent and efferent tracts which pass parallel to the main axis of the nervous system. Some of these contain fibers which originate in the cortex and pass through the pons on their way to the spinal cord (corticospinal fibers*) and others which originate in the cortex and end in the pons (corticopontile fibers). Many of the fibers in these tracts synapse with a set of nuclei in the pons, the nuclei pontis. The fibers from these nuclei curve upward to enter the cerebellum.

The dorsal part of the pons contains the terminations of the cochlear nerve (nerve from the ear). Also, the nuclei of the vestibular nerve are found here. These later nuclei play an important role in reflex control of the head, neck, and eyes.

Together, the ventral and dorsal parts of the pons contain several nerve tracts and collections of nuclei which allow for coordination and involuntary influences on automatic movement and posture (Fig. 2.12).

---

*Fiber tracts in the CNS are named by the origin and termination of their nerve fiber transmission. Thus, the first part of the name of a tract from which the nerve fiber signals originate in the cerebral cortex is the combining form, cerebro-. A tract that originates in the cerebral cortex and ends in the spinal cord is called a cerebrospinal tract; one from which the fibers transmit signals from the spinal cord to the thalamus is called a spinothalamic tract.

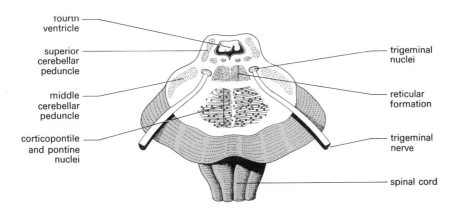

Fig. 2.12   The pons in cross section. (Based on Langley *et al.*, 1969.)

Medulla oblongata.   The medulla is the superior extension of the spinal cord and contains a number of sensory and motor tracts. For example, some sensory fibers project upward in the spinal cord and end in two groups of nuclei in the medulla, the nucleus gracilis and the nucleus cuneatus, where they connect with neurons whose fibers cross the midline and continue upward to the thalamus in a tract called the medial lemniscus. Motor fibers of the corticospinal tract merge to form one large tract on each side of the medulla, called the pyramids. To do this, the lateral corticospinal tracts decussate (cross over the midline) from one side of the medulla to the other (Fig. 2.13).

The medulla also contains a collection of neurons and nerve tracts which serve an important function of providing regulation of vital internal processes, such as respiration, blood pressure, heart rate, etc. Finally, the medulla possesses nuclei from which cranial nerves emerge. The cranial nerves carry sensory signals from sensory systems in the head and upper body and motor signals for the control of these same parts of the body.

The reticular formation.   Extending throughout the brainstem is a complex set of neurons and nuclei called the reticular formation. This network of cells receives input from all of the sensory systems, which give off collateral fibers to synapse on reticular formation neurons. Nerve fibers from the cerebral cortex also make synaptic connections here. The neurons of this structure are also sensitive to stimulation from drugs and certain endocrine products.

The two major output fiber networks of the reticular formation are directed to spinal and cranial neurons and to the cerebral cortex and other brain structures. Stimulation of descending reticular fibers may either

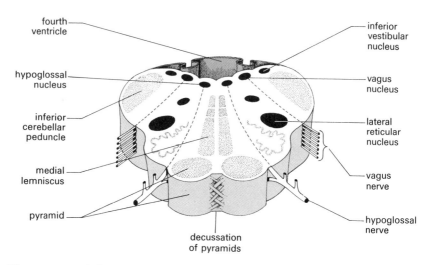

fourth ventricle · inferior vestibular nucleus · hypoglossal nucleus · vagus nucleus · inferior cerebellar peduncle · lateral reticular nucleus · medial lemniscus · vagus nerve · pyramid · hypoglossal nerve · decussation of pyramids

Fig. 2.13   Medulla oblongata in cross section. (Based on Langley *et al.*, 1969.)

cause inhibition (decrease) or facilitation (increase) in the firing of neurons controlling the skeletal muscles. The ascending reticular fibers seem to be critically involved in the control of sleeping and waking, and appear to play an important role in attention and activation of the individual for activity.

6. The ventricles

Within the brain are four hollow openings, called ventricles, which are filled with cerebrospinal fluid (this fluid will be discussed later in the chapter). There are two lateral ventricles, a third ventricle, and a fourth ventricle. The lateral ventricles lie on either side of the fissure that divides the cerebrum into two hemispheres. They are the largest of the ventricles and they run the length of the cerebrum in an outward curve, commencing near each other in the frontal lobe, and separating as they move toward the back of the brain. These lateral ventricles connect with the third ventricle via the foramen of Monro. At the lower level of the long thin third ventricle, a narrow opening called the cerebral aqueduct connects into the fourth ventricle. The fourth ventricle is located at the base of the brain. At its end, the fourth ventricle narrows and continues as the central canal of the spinal cord (Fig. 2.14).

B. THE SPINAL CORD

If the nervous system is viewed as a mechanism for information input, coordination and processing, and output, the spinal cord has an essential role in both the input and output phases. It carries up to the brain all sensory infor-

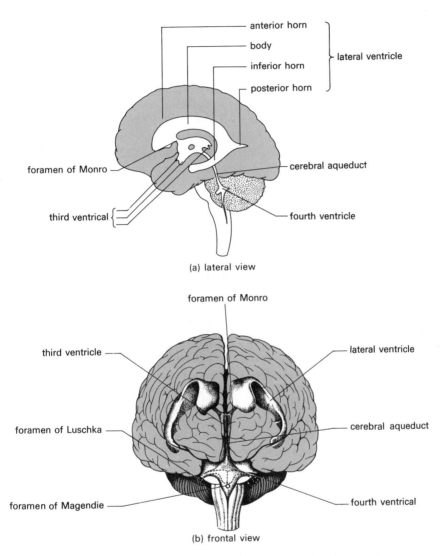

Fig. 2.14   Ventricles of the brain. (Based on Noback, 1967.)

mation from the body and all motor commands sent down from the brain to muscles and glands. It is, therefore, primarily a transmission pathway. But it also has important reflex functions as well.

The spinal cord joins the brain at the brainstem through an opening in the skull, called the foramen magnum. It occupies the vertebral canal, formed by the vertebrae, which gives protection and support to it. The cord extends from the foramen magnum to the level of the first or second lumbar

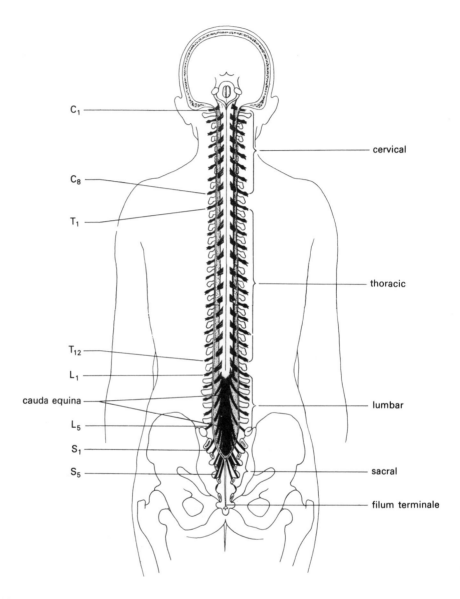

Fig. 2.15 Vertebral column in posterior view with the surface of the spinal cord exposed. (Based on Langley *et al.*, 1969.)

vertebra. Below this level, separate nerve trunks and roots of nerves continue to run through the vertebral column. This mass of nerves in the vertebral canal below the spinal cord resembles the tail of a horse, thus the anatomical name for it is *cauda equina* (Fig. 2.15).

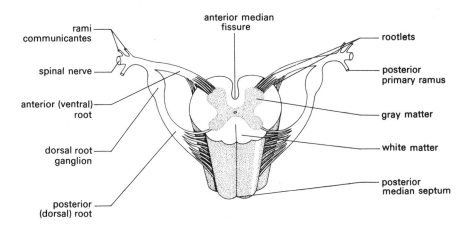

Fig. 2.16   A spinal cord segment. (Based on Langley *et al.*, 1969.)

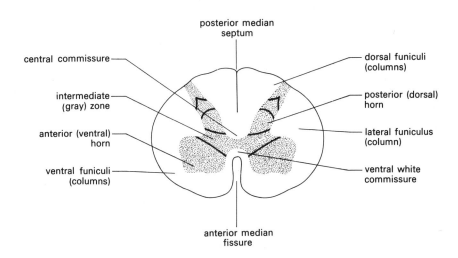

Fig. 2.17   Section through the spinal cord at the cervical level. (Based on Noback, 1967.)

In cross section, the spinal cord consists of a center portion and an outer part; the former is in the shape of a butterfly (or H) and is gray in color. This gray color is a result of tight packing of neuron cell bodies in this part of the spinal cord. The outer part of the cord surrounds the gray matter and is white in color because it is made up of nerve fibers rather than cell bodies (Figs. 2.16 and 2.17). The cord is about as thick as an adult's little finger and has the consistency of jelly.

The ventral horns of the gray matter contain cell bodies the axons of which project outward through spinal nerves to connect with muscles and glands. The dorsal horn cells receive incoming impulses from sensory receptors, transmitting them to the brain and other levels of the spinal cord. These latter, or intracord impulses, are carried over relatively short intersegmental tracts and support a variety of reflexes at the spinal level.

The upward- and downward-coursing fiber tracts which make up the white matter of the cord are called fasciculi and are organized into three columns: the dorsal, lateral, and ventral. These columns, called funiculi, are each made up of nerve fiber tracts which subserve sensory and motor functions (Fig. 2.18).

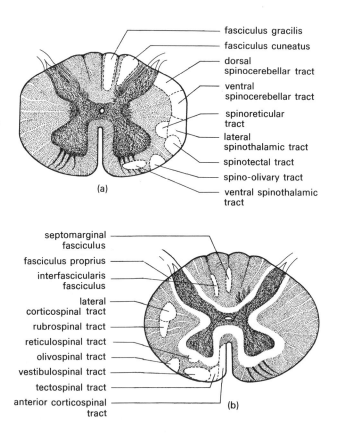

Fig. 2.18   (a) Ascending spinal fasciculi, or pathways, (b) Descending spinal fasciculi, or pathways. (Based on Woodburne, 1967.)

C. MENINGES AND CEREBROSPINAL FLUID

The brain and spinal cord are protected by layers of nonnervous tissue called meninges (singular, meninx). There is an outer layer, called the dura mater, a middle layer composed of the arachnoid membrane, and an inner layer, the pia mater, which is closest to the brain. The dura mater is a tough, fibrous membrane which lines the inner surface of the skull and vertebrae; it is, then, basically a bone lining (Figs. 2.19 and 2.20).

The innermost of the meninges is the pia mater which is a soft, tender membrane which lines the brain and spinal cord. Between the dura mater and pia mater is the arachnoid membrane.

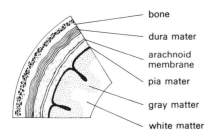

bone

dura mater

arachnoid
membrane

pia mater

gray matter

white matter

Fig. 2.19 Meninges depicted through a vertical section in the skull and brain. (Based on Langley *et al.*, 1969.)

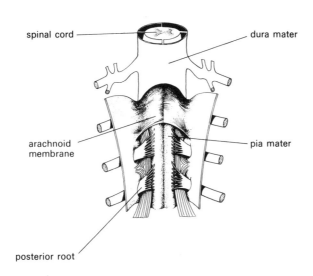

spinal cord

dura mater

arachnoid
membrane

pia mater

posterior root

Fig. 2.20 The meninges surrounding the spinal cord. (Based on Langley *et al.*, 1969.)

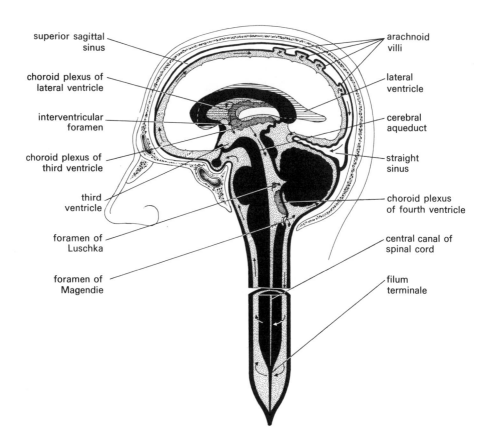

superior sagittal
sinus

arachnoid
villi

choroid plexus of
lateral ventricle

lateral
ventricle

interventricular
foramen

cerebral
aqueduct

choroid plexus of
third ventricle

straight
sinus

third
ventricle

choroid plexus
of fourth ventricle

foramen of
Luschka

central canal of
spinal cord

foramen of
Magendie

filum
terminale

Fig. 2.21   The cerebrospinal fluid and its circulation pathways. CSF circulates within the subarachnoid space and the ventricles. (Based on Langley *et al.*, 1969.)

Cerebrospinal fluid (CSF) fills the space between the arachnoid membrane and the pia mater over the entire brain and central canal of the spinal cord. The brain and spinal cord virtually float in this solution. The ventricles play an important role in the production and circulation of the CSF (Fig. 2.21).

CSF has several functions. Surrounding as it does the brain and spinal cord, it provides a protective covering for the delicate nerve cells by acting as a cushion for blows to the head and quick movements of the head. It also helps to keep the total volume of cranial contents constant. Finally, it appears to play a role in the exchange of metabolic substances between it and nerve cells, but whether it has a part in the nutrition of the CNS is as yet uncertain.

THE PERIPHERAL NERVOUS SYSTEM (PNS)

The peripheral nervous system (PNS) lies outside the bony protection of the skull and vertebral column and consists of all those nerve fibers which enter or leave the brainstem and spinal cord and innervate (supply) the sensory receptors, muscles, and glands. These fibers are enclosed in cable-like structures called nerves. The PNS is further divided into somatic and autonomic components.

The somatic peripheral system controls all the skeletal muscles—the muscles that we contract when we make voluntary movements or when involuntary adjustments in posture and other reflexes are made. The autonomic nervous system, in contrast, controls the heart, smooth muscles (blood vessels, digestive, and reproductive organs, and so on), and glands. Each system also contains sensory fibers. Sensory input to the somatic system is from skin, joint, and muscle receptors, and includes touch, pressure, temperature, joint angulation, muscle tension, etc.; sensory input from the autonomic system is from smooth muscles and glands and is generally less precise than the somatic sensory input.

Essentially the PNS represents lines of communication, whereas the CNS is the center of coordination and the place of determination of the most appropriate response to incoming impulses.

The PNS originates in 31 pairs of spinal nerves, which emerge between the spinal vertebrae, and 12 pairs of cranial nerves, which leave the brainstem.

A. SPINAL NERVES

There are 31 pairs of spinal nerves—eight cervical, twelve thoracic, five lumbar, five sacral and one coccygeal. The number and names of the spinal nerves correspond closely to that of the vertebral column. This column consists of 33 vertebrae, which are named according to the regions of the body they occupy. There are seven cervical, twelve thoracic, five lumbar, five sacral, and four coccygeal vertebrae. Spinal nerves pass through lateral openings between the vertebrae called intervertebral foramina (singular, foramen) (Fig. 2.15).

Each spinal nerve of the pair that arises from each spinal cord segment begins as a series of fibers from the dorsal and ventral parts of the spinal cord. The fibers from dorsal and ventral roots merge and pass through the intervertebral foramina. Just before the fibers unite, there is an enlargement on the dorsal root called the dorsal root ganglion. This ganglion contains the cell bodies of sensory neurons. Cell bodies of the ventral root fibers are located in the ventral horn of the gray matter of the spinal cord (Figs. 2.16 and 2.22).

The fibers of the dorsal root of spinal nerves are all sensory fibers. Thus, peripheral sensory fibers carrying nerve impulses from receptors pass through the intervertebral foramina and enter the spinal cord at the dorsal horn. Impulses then travel to the brain along tracts in the spinal cord. Impulses descending from the brain are transmitted down motor tracts in the spinal cord and synapse on motorneurons in the ventral horn of the spinal cord. Motor impulses are then transmitted to muscles and glands by means of the motorneurons.

Upon emerging from the intervertebral foramina, spinal nerves divide into a complex network of branches which then supply segments of the skin and muscles with nerve fibers. Many of the nerves form plexuses (networks or tangles of nerves), or junctions, from which peripheral nerves arise which actually supply the various skin areas and muscles.

Each spinal nerve supplies fibers to a specific segment, or region, of the body. A segment of the body that is supplied by a spinal nerve is called a dermatome. Since there are 31 pairs of spinal nerves, there should be, theoretically, 31 pairs of dermatomes. But since the first cervical nerve has no dorsal root, it does not innervate a dermatome; therefore there are actually 30 pairs of dermatomes in the body.

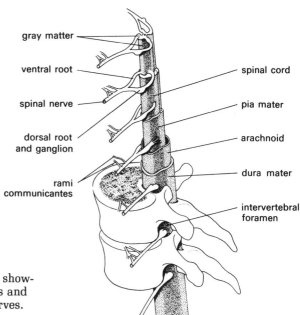

gray matter

ventral root

spinal nerve

dorsal root and ganglion

rami communicantes

spinal cord

pia mater

arachnoid

dura mater

intervertebral foramen

Fig. 2.22 The spinal cord, showing ventral and dorsal roots and the emergence of spinal nerves. (Based on Gardner, 1963.)

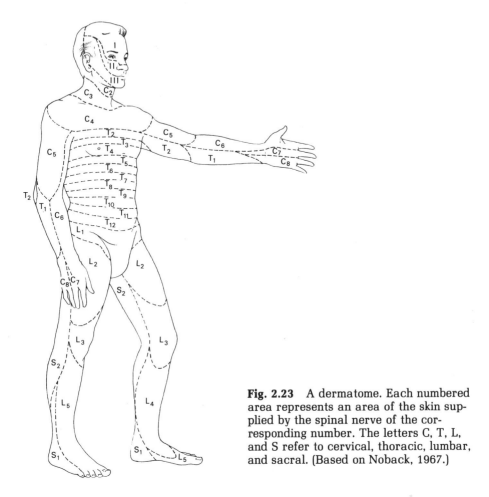

Fig. 2.23 A dermatome. Each numbered area represents an area of the skin supplied by the spinal nerve of the corresponding number. The letters C, T, L, and S refer to cervical, thoracic, lumbar, and sacral. (Based on Noback, 1967.)

On a dermatome chart, each dermatome is labeled by the spinal nerve that innervates that part of the body; i.e., dermatome L_2 means that part of the body is innervated by the second lumbar spinal nerve. There is, of course, some overlapping between contiguous dermatomes. Thus, if one spinal nerve becomes nonfunctional, the region of the body that it once innervated does not become inoperative (Fig. 2.23).

B. CRANIAL NERVES

The 12 pairs of cranial nerves arise from the lower centers of the brain, especially the brainstem. These nerves are simply numbered one to twelve in Roman numerals, according to the point of juncture with the brain, beginning at the cerebrum and ending in the medulla. Each cranial nerve also has its own proper name. The numbers and proper names of the cranial nerves are:

I. Olfactory	VII. Facial
II. Optic	VIII. Vestibulocochlear (Acoustical)
III. Oculomotor	IX. Glossopharyngeal
IV. Trochlear	X. Vagus
V. Trigeminal	XI. Spinal
VI. Abducens	XII. Hypoglossal

Generations of medical school students have memorized the following sentence using the first letter in each word to recall the names of the cranial nerves: On Old Olympus's Towering Top A Finn And German Viewed Some Hops.

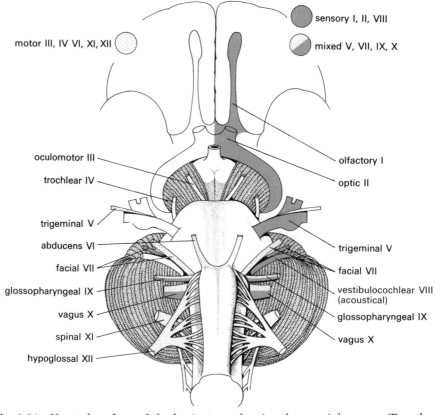

Fig. 2.24   Ventral surface of the brainstem, showing the cranial nerves. (Based on Langley *et al.*, 1969.)

The cranial nerves carry sensory information to the brain from the eyes, ears, nose, mouth, and from the same general sensory receptors found in the spinal nerves. These nerves also project motor fibers to control movements of the eyes, mouth, face, tongue, and throat, and they supply the major outflow for the control of smooth muscles and glands in the visceral regions of the body (Fig. 2.24).

3

Neural Transmission

All human behavior depends upon the biochemical and physiological processes of the nervous system and this system is made up of neurons whose purpose is to receive and send messages, in the form of nerve impulses, from one part of the body to another. The overall function of the nervous system is to integrate and control all the body's activities. In order to do this, neurons have the ability to receive and respond to stimulation; this has been called the irritability function. Neurons also have the ability to transmit signals from one neuron to another; this is their conduction function. The irritability and conduction functions allow the nervous system to exhibit these basic activities: First, afferent neurons receive and transmit information to the CNS; second, efferent neurons send specific information from various parts of the CNS to the muscles and glands; third, there is a complex network of interneurons which perform many integrative functions; fourth, a network of neurons regulates the internal structures of the body.

In Chapter 2 the basic features of a neuron were described. In this chapter we will consider how a neuron transmits a nerve impulse along its own axon and how a nerve impulse is propagated from one neuron to another. We shall also consider how nerve impulses are transmitted to muscle fibers, bringing about muscle contraction.

CONDUCTION OF NERVE IMPULSES BY AXONS

One of the unique features of a neuron is that it is designed to conduct an electric current. In order to understand how the neuron accomplishes this task, one must understand several features of electricity and nerve cells.

The functioning of a nerve cell depends upon the electric events which take place across the membrane of the cell, and the electric events occurring at the cell membrane depend upon the presence of charged particles called ions. An ion is an atom which has gained or lost one or more of its electrons. An atom consists of a minute central nucleus surrounded by electrons. In a neutral atom the surrounding negative charged electrons are equal in number to the positive charges on the nucleus (Fig. 3.1). Some atoms, however, have a tendency to lose one or more of the electrons, or they may gain one or more electrons. Since electrons carry a negative electric charge, atoms that lose electrons possess a positive charge, and are called cations; atoms that gain electrons possess a negative charge and are called anions. Atoms charged either way are called ions. When ions are placed in fluid, an electric current can be passed through the solution. Such a solution is called an electrolytic solution and is so because it contains ions. Dry table salt (NaCl) will not easily allow electricity to pass through it (conduct electricity), but when table salt is dissolved in water, it dissociates (breaks down) into Na^+ and Cl^- ions. The solution is now electrolytic.

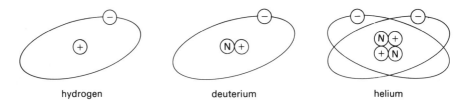

hydrogen   deuterium   helium

Fig. 3.1   Some simple atoms according to Bohr's theory of atom structure. The proportions are enormously compressed. Electrons are farther out from the nucleus than as shown.

From what was said in the paragraph above about atoms, it may be seen that there are two types of electric charges in the universe. It is customary to refer to them as "positive" and "negative" charges. Characteristic of these charges is that positive charges repel positive charges and negative charges repel negative charges, but positive and negative charges attract each other. Thus, when positive and negative charges are separated, an electric force draws the opposite charges together. Why this is so is unknown; it is a fundamental property of matter.

Now, if oppositely charged particles are allowed to come together, work will be done since a force will be exerted over distance, because Work = Force × Distance ($W = FD$). Therefore, when oppositely charged particles are separated, they have the "potential" of doing work if they are allowed to come together. The movement of electric charge is called electric current, and voltage is defined as the amount of work done by an electric charge when moving from one point in a system to another.

It may be seen, then, that the first requirement in producing an electric current is that positive and negative charges must be separated from each other. In the neuron the separation of positive and negative charges is accomplished by several mechanisms, and the net result is that an equilibrium occurs when the voltage inside the cell membrane is about − 70 millivolts (1 millivolt = 1/1000 of a volt). This is called the resting membrane potential.

A. RESTING MEMBRANE POTENTIAL

The first essential for the conduction of a nerve impulse through a neuron is the establishment of an electrical potential across the cell membrane. This is accomplished in a neuron because the membrane is semipermeable and acts as a selective barrier to ionic movement and it has an active transport mechanism which helps to maintain ionic imbalance. The result is that the inside of the membrane becomes electrically negative with respect to the outside; thus, a "potential" is established. The surface of the membrane of a neuron separates two aqueous solutions that have very different ionic concentrations. In the resting state of a neuron there are more sodium ions (Na $^+$) on the outside of the membrane than there are on the inside because they are actively transported outward through the membrane by a mechanism called the "sodium pump" and these ions are too large to pass inward through the membrane in its resting state. Inside the cell membrane various organic ions (A $^-$) are concentrated which are too large to pass out of the cell membrane. Potassium ions (K $^+$) are also highly concentrated on the inside of the membrane in its resting state because they are highly permeable to the cell membrane and are pulled to the inside by the negatively charged

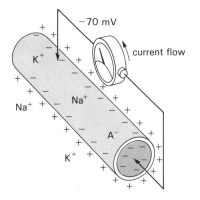

Fig. 3.2   Resting, or membrane potential. Sodium (Na $^+$) ions are in high concentration outside the membrane, while potassium (K $^+$) ions and organic anions (A $^-$) are in high concentration inside the membrane. The potential across the membrane is about − 70 millivolts. (Based on Noback, 1967.)

organic ions found there. Accumulation of potassium ions inside the cell due to the indiffusible organic ions creates a concentration gradient favoring the outward flow of potassium, even against the attraction of the organic ions. But there is a limit to this process, and an equilibrium is reached when the tendency of potassium to diffuse out is balanced by the electric pull of the organic ions. The outward movement of potassium ions does not completely neutralize the state of electronegativity on the inside of the membrane. Thus, the interior of the neuron is about − 70 millivolts (mV) in relation to the external fluid. That difference—negative potential of 70 mV— is called the resting membrane potential. In resting neurons, then, the membrane potential is not zero, but instead is a fraction of a volt; the neuron is literally a battery with its negative terminal on the inside. It now has the "potential" for performing work—in this case conducting an electric current (Fig. 3.2).

B. THE ACTION POTENTIAL IN THE AXON

We will now examine the steps in the propagation of a nerve impulse in the axon. The roles of the dendrites and cell body in the process of nerve transmission will be discussed later in this chapter.

As described above, membrane polarity is maintained by a differential balance of ions on the inside and outside of the membrane. Sodium (Na^+) concentration is much greater outside the membrane than inside, and conversely on the inside of the membrane organic ions (A^-) and potassium are more concentrated than on the outside. The membrane voltage of − 70 mV produces a strong pressure for inward flow of sodium ions and a strong outward flow of organic ions. However, the resting membrane is impermeable to these classes of ions.

If the membrane of the axon is stimulated, there is a sudden change in membrane permeability, making the membrane highly permeable to sodium. Any stimulus that suddenly increases the permeability of the axon membrane to sodium elicits a sequence of rapid changes in the membrane. If the stimulus lowers the resting potential to a critical level, called the threshold potential, which is usually around − 55 to − 60 mV, in the axon (that is, if the internal voltage of the axon changes from, say, − 70 to − 55 mV), an explosive action occurs. The increased permeability causes ions to flood in through the membrane at a rapid rate. The potential difference in the membrane is not only neutralized but is relatively reversed in less than a millisecond. The outside briefly becomes negatively charged 30 to 40 millivolts in relation to the inside of the membrane. This entire sequence of changes which the axon membrane goes through when it has been stimulated strongly enough to alter the membrane to a threshold potential is called an action potential (Fig. 3.3). The action potential occurs in two separate

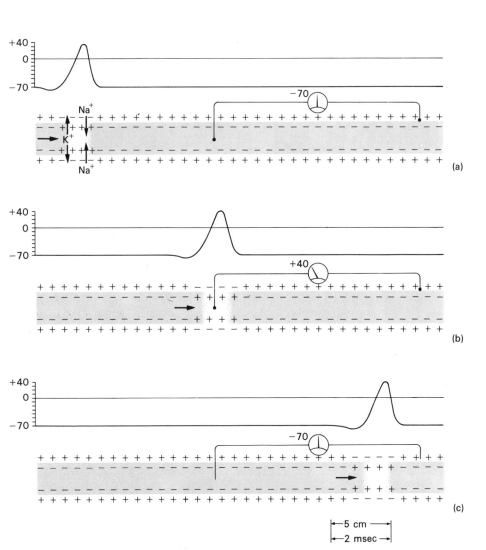

Fig. 3.3 Propagation of an action potential in the axon of an unmyelinated neuron. The arrows show the direction of transmission. In (a) sodium rushes into the axon, causing the membrane potential to be changed locally to positive. At this point, sodium is prevented from passing out of the membrane, but potassium rushes out of the axon and the normal resting potential is now restored (b) and (c). At the point of the action potential (light zone), the potential across the membrane is reversed to about + 40 millivolts as measured on a galvanometer. (Based on Noback, 1967.)

stages: depolarization and repolarization. The transmission of the action potential along an axon is actually the nerve impulse.

When the action potential begins, the axon's membrane barrier to sodium ions breaks down allowing sodium ions to rush into the axon. As they enter, they reverse the internal potential of the membrane from about -70 mV to about $+40$ mV. This process "ignites" the nerve impulse. This impulse, or spike on an oscilloscope, changes the permeability of the membrane immediately ahead of it and establishes the conditions for sodium to flow into the membrane, repeating the process in an impulse wave until the spike has reached the end of the axon. As successive portions of the membrane become depolarized these newly depolarized areas cause local circuits of current to flow still farther along the axon, which results in progressively more depolarization, and this process travels the entire length of the axon fiber, much as the fuse in a firecracker burns its way from where the match is applied on down to the firecracker itself. Thus, when depolarization takes place at one point in an axon, it acts as a stimulus for depolarization elsewhere. Although there are apparently some exceptions, when the action potential travels down the axon, it activates all the axon collateral branches. When the action potential reaches the end of the axon, a reaction is triggered which leads to the release of a transmitter substance. The transmitter substance diffuses onto the cell which is in close contact with the axon terminal and produces an electrical response in the membrane of this cell. We will describe this process more fully later in the chapter.

At the peak of the depolarization wave, there is a reduction of entry of sodium ions, and at this point the permeability of the membrane increases for potassium to a greater extent than during the resting state, allowing potassium ions to flow rapidly out of the membrane. Thus, at the peak of depolarization the membrane becomes impermeable to sodium and simultaneously highly permeable to potassium; this causes a rapid outflow of the potassium ions, thus restoring the original negative charge on the interior of the membrane, and a membrane potential develops across the membrane caused entirely by the potassium ions. The rapid outflow of potassium is more than capable of returning the membrane potential back to its resting level of -70 mV as the potassium ions move to the outside and establish electronegativity inside the membrane. This is the repolarization phase of the action potential.

The initial return of resting membrane potential is caused by diffusion of potassium ions outside through the membrane; but in order for the membrane to return to its original resting condition, with the large concentration of sodium ions outside the membrane, the sodium ions which diffused to the inside of the cell membrane during the action potential must be returned to the outside and potassium ions must be returned to the inside of the membrane. The "sodium–potassium pump" is an active transport mechanism for returning the sodium ions to the outside of the membrane and the potassium ions to the inside, thus restoring the original distribution of ions characteristic of the resting membrane potential. Very little is known about the details of how the sodium–potassium pump works.

Action potentials can occur in a neuron as often as several hundred times per second. Since quantity of sodium and potassium involved in maintaining potentials is minimal compared to the total ionic stores, over 100,000 action potentials may be produced in an axon before its ionic supplies are exhausted.

1. Refractory periods. The period immediately after the depolarization wave, when the neuron's membrane potential is returning to the – 70 mV, is called repolarization. Depolarization and repolarization occur in minute fractions of a second, and between the second of depolarization and complete repolarization the membrane experiences a period known as the refractory period, which actually consists of two brief periods (Fig. 3.4).

Immediately after a nerve impulse has been transmitted along an axon, the axon cannot transmit a second impulse regardless of the intensity of the stimulus. This is called the absolute refractory period. In firing a rifle, another shot cannot be fired until another bullet is in the chamber and the firing pin drops again. Similarly, there is a short period following one nerve impulse in which another one cannot be set off, no matter how strong the

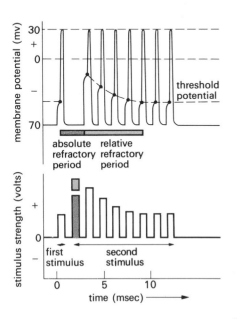

Fig. 3.4 Immediately following an action potential, the axon is absolutely refractory to all stimulus intensities and thus cannot fire another impulse. During the relative refractory period, the intensity of a second stimulus necessary to fire a second action potential must be greater than the resting threshold and decreases as the time between the first and second stimulus. (Based on Vander et al., 1970.)

stimulus. In large axons this period may last 0.5 millisecond. This continues into a second period, the relative refractory period, in which nerve impulses can be transmitted, but the stimulus must be stronger than threshold level. To illustrate, if the threshold potential for a given axon in its resting state is − 55 mV, during the relative refractory period the threshold potential may be − 45 mV; thus, a stimulus to the axon must be more intense to alter the cell's membrane potential to achieve the threshold and cause an action potential than if the axon was in a resting state. The relative refractory period varies from 4 to 8 milliseconds.

C. THE ALL-OR-NONE LAW

All that can be propagated along an axon is a response that is full-sized for the condition of that axon; the alternative is no response. If a stimulus is strong enough to initiate an action potential in the axon, it travels the entire length of the axon. This is known as the "all-or-none law," and the process may be compared to shooting a pistol. As soon as a pull on the trigger is strong enough to drop the firing pin (threshold) the pistol fires; a harder pull on the trigger will not change the velocity of the bullet because the powder charge in the bullet, and not the pull on the trigger, is responsible for the response. The amount of response an axon produces is essentially independent of the intensity of the stimulus exciting it.

A stimulus which is not strong enough to achieve threshold is said to be subthreshold, while a stimulus stronger than threshold is said to be suprathreshold. It should be noted that the threshold is not the same for all neurons. Some neurons have lower thresholds, and thus respond to weaker stimuli than other neurons. Thus, a stimulus which is suprathreshold for some neurons will be subthreshold for others. In a normal resting membrane, when the membrane potential of the initial segment of the axon (location where the cell body and axon join) depolarizes about 15 mV, to − 55 mV, the threshold for firing the axon on an all-or-none basis is achieved and an action potential begins.

Various factors may alter the normal threshold potential in a neuron. During the refractory periods the threshold is altered. Some drugs modify the ionic composition in and around the neuron and either increase or decrease threshold potential. Fatigue, stress, and disease may also modify threshold potential.

The cell body and dendrites differ somewhat in their response to stimulation. The effect of excitation in these parts of the neuron is graded, resulting in a varying electrical potential being produced as a consequence of varying stimulation. This means that a weak stimulus produces a weak effect and a strong stimulus, a strong effect. This will be described more completely below.

D. FREQUENCY CODING

Because of the all-or-none response in an axon, a single action potential cannot convey any information about the intensity of the stimulus which initiated it. If a stronger stimulus does not produce a stronger action potential response in the axon, what effect does a stronger stimulus have on axon response? The answer is deceptively simple. A stronger stimulus fires the axon more frequently (per unit of time) than a weaker stimulus. Thus, a more intense stimulus produces a greater frequency of impulses in an axon than does a less intensive one. This phenomenon occurs primarily because a more intense stimulus can excite the axon while it is still in its initial relative refractory period, while a weaker stimulus cannot. This conversion of stimulus intensity into frequency of impulses is called "frequency coding." Another term that is used for this phenomenon is "temporal summation." More will be said about this in a later chapter.

It may be seen that the transmission of impulses in an axon may be likened to the action of a machine gun. When the trigger on the machine gun is pressed very lightly, the gun fires the shells infrequently, but if the trigger is pressed hard, the gun fires bullets in rapid succession. In similar fashion, a weak stimulus fires axons at a very slow rate while an intense stimulus can cause the axon to fire hundreds of times per second.

E. IMPULSE CONDUCTION IN MYELINATED AXONS

Many axons within and outside the CNS are covered with a layer of fatty material known as myelin. Myelin is located external to the axon cell membrane and extends from just outside the cell body to near the presynaptic terminals. It is a substance that will not conduct electric current.

All axons outside the CNS, whether myelinated or not, have a thin sheath called the neurolemma which consists of a succession of flat cells (cells of Schwann) with their own nuclei. Each myelin segment is produced by a nucleated Schwann cell which winds its cytoplasm tightly around the surface of the axon, producing a spiral envelope of many turns forming a jelly-roll type of structure (Fig. 3.5c). The myelinated axons in the CNS differ from those of the PNS in the absence of neurolemma sheaths. Instead there is an investment of glia cells. It has been suggested that these glia cells may be concerned with the development of myelin sheaths.

Approximately every millimeter or two along the length of a myelinated axon, the myelin is broken by a node of Ranvier. At the nodes, regular membrane depolarization can occur, but beneath the myelin-sheath membrane depolarization cannot take place because the myelin sheath is a very effective insulator of the membrane from electrical currents (Fig. 3.5a and b). At the nodes of Ranvier, nerve fibers show action potentials just like those found in unmyelinated axons. But the myelinated sections do not give action

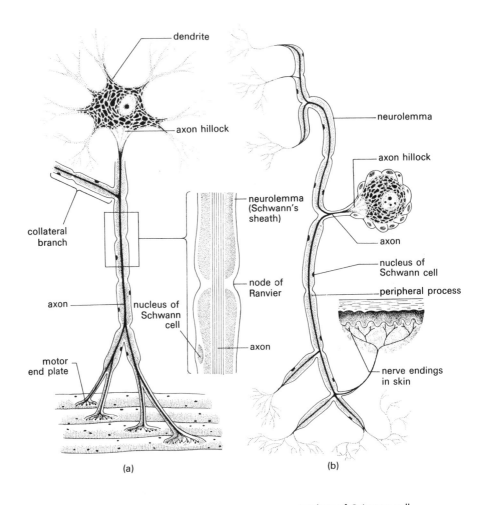

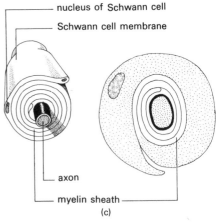

Fig. 3.5 (a) An efferent (motor) myelinated neuron. (b) An afferent (sensory) myelinated neuron. (c) Lateral view of a myelinated axon. [(a) and (b) based on Crouch, p. 495; (c) based on DeCoursey, 1968.]

potentials when depolarized. When an action potential occurs at one node the depolarization wave spreads passively along the internode regions into the next node where, if greater than threshold, it acts the same way any other depolarization would, and results in full-sized action potential. Thus, the action potential in myelinated axons moves along the fiber by passive spread in the myelinated regions and by the occurrence of action potentials at the nodes (Fig. 3.6).

This type of neural transmission is called saltatory conduction and it is valuable for two main reasons: (1) It increases the velocity of conduction along the axon; (2) It prevents the polarization of large areas of the fiber, thus preventing leakage of large quantities of sodium to the inside of the axon, thus conserving energy required by the sodium–potassium pump to expel the sodium.

Occasionally, persons will suffer a degeneration of myelin. When myelin degenerates, it causes a loss of function of the axon. This degenerative-type disease is known as multiple sclerosis, and it most frequently afflicts persons in the 20 to 40 age range. It is often a progressive disease with a proliferation of involved axons. Death is the eventual result.

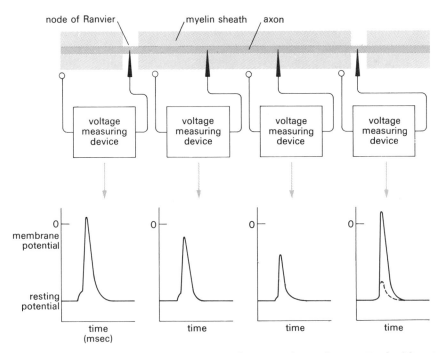

Fig. 3.6 Transmission of an action potential in a myelinated axon. Dashed line in graph on the right shows what voltage would have been at that node if the membrane at that node had not been able to produce an action potential. (Based on Stevens, 1966.)

F. SPEED AND FREQUENCY OF AXON TRANSMISSION

The speed of axon transmission is a function of the cross-section diameter and the myelination or nonmyelination of the fiber. Basically, the larger the cross-section diameter, the faster the speed of transmission; and myelinated axons conduct impulses at a faster speed than unmyelinated axons. In unmyelinated fibers from 0.2 to 1.0 microns in diameter the speed of the conduction is from 0.2 to 2.0 meters per second, depending on the size of the axon. The range in velocities for the normal range of myelinated axons with diameters ranging from 2 to 20 microns is 12 to 120 meters per second (Fig. 3.7).

It appears that axon speed is related to the urgency of the information that it is called upon to transmit. The faster conducting axons are concerned with the control of movement. At the other extreme, axons carrying visceral information are small, unmyelinated, and slow conducting. Thus, in the evolutionary design of the nervous system, it seems that axon size has developed in relation to the urgency of the information it carries for the survival of the organism.

The number of impulses which can be transmitted per unit of time is determined by the refractory periods of the axon, and this depends upon the cross-section diameter of the axon. The larger the diameter, the shorter the refractory periods. Thus, at one extreme, very large axons can transmit 2500 impulses per second and at the other extreme small axons transmit only 25 impulses per second.

type	diameter (microns)	velocity (m/sec)	function
A (alpha)	12-20	80-130	motor, proprioception
A (beta)	8-12	40-80	touch
A (gamma and delta)	1-8	5-40	pain, temperature
B	3	3-15	autonomic preganglionic
C	1 or less	0.5-2.0	autonomic postganglionic

Fig. 3.7 Some examples of the relationship of nerve fiber diameter and speed of transmission. (Based on Langley et al., 1969.)

RESPONSE OF DENDRITES AND CELL BODIES TO STIMULATION

The preceding section focused upon conduction of a nerve impulse in axons. Dendrites and cell bodies have properties of conduction different from those of the axon. The distinctive feature of the axon is an active response to above-threshold depolarization—the action potential. It appears that a large part of the dendrites and cell bodies have different properties, and that over much of their extent do not function on the all-or-none principle, except in the initial segment of the axon (the region of the cell body from which the axon arises). Thus, dendrites and cell bodies do not respond to depolarization, as does the axon of the neuron, by producing action potentials, but instead show only passive responses to stimuli of all magnitudes. This means that when a dendrite or cell body is stimulated depolarization occurs at that point and neighboring regions are simultaneously depolarized as well, but the effect decreases with distance from the stimulus, just as the displacement of water diminishes with distance away from where a rock was dropped into the water. Thus, if a dendrite or cell body is depolarized 10 millivolts at one point, half a millimeter away it might be depolarized by five millivolts. Therefore, for large as well as small dendrites and cell bodies, their response to a stimulus is approximately proportional to the strength of the stimulus. Moreover conduction may be decremental; that is, a dendrite may be activated at some distance from the cell body and not excite the latter because the electrochemical disturbance in the dendrite may decrease with the distance it travels toward the cell body.

TYPES OF STIMULI THAT EXCITE THE NEURON

Various types of stimuli can initiate a nerve impulse. Basically, anything that causes sodium ions to begin to diffuse into the cell membrane in sufficient numbers will set off the automatic "activation" mechanism. Most neurons are especially sensitive to certain kinds of energy, which serve as a stimulus; e.g., the sensory neurons in the eye (rods and cones) are especially responsive to light energy. But many neurons can be activated by various kinds of energy—electrical, chemical, mechanical, sound, etc.

Nerve impulses are transmitted from neuron to neuron primarily by chemical means. The axon terminal of the first neuron secretes a chemical substance that stimulates the cell body or dendrite with which it makes contact.

SYNAPTIC TRANSMISSION

We have examined the electrical process of the nerve impulse and how it travels along the axon. Now we may ask, "What happens to the nerve impulse once it reaches the end of the axon?" Although all of the details of this question cannot be answered, there is a rather good understanding of this process.

As an axon approaches another cell, it decreases in size and forms a small terminal called a presynaptic terminal (also called by various other names such as telodendria, knobs, boutons). At the site at which the presynaptic terminal connects with another neuron there is a submicroscopic gap between the individual cells called the synapse. When two neurons make contact with each other, we say that they "synapse with each other."

The synapse is a specialized junction between two neurons; it is here that the electrical activity of one neuron influences the activity of the second, producing either excitation and perhaps the firing of an impulse in the second, or inhibition and an inability to fire an impulse in the second. It is at the synapse that the interactions and modifications of nerve impulses that are responsible for determining an organism's behavior take place.

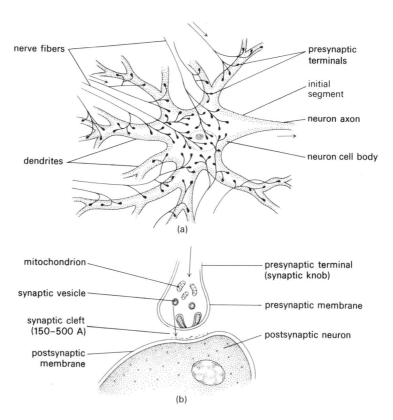

Fig. 3.8 The synapse. (a) Presynaptic terminals impinging upon the cell body and dendrites of a neuron. (b) Microscopic view of a single synapse. [(a) Based on Eccles, 1965; (b) based on DeCoursey, 1968.]

A single axon may have synapses with only a few cells or, since axons typically give off many collateral fibers each of which ends with a presynaptic terminal, it may have synapses with up to several thousand neurons. At the same time, any given neuron may have hundreds or thousands of synaptic contacts on its cell body or dendrites. It has been discovered in recent years that virtually all of the surface of a neuron's cell body and dendrites have presynaptic terminals from other neurons impinging on it. Notice that presynaptic terminals make contact only on the cell body and dendrites of other neurons (Fig. 3.8a).

The submicroscopic space which completely separates the presynaptic terminal and the postsynaptic neuron is called the synaptic cleft; the distance between the cell membranes at this point is about 200 angstroms (approximately 1/50,000 millimeter) (Fig. 3.8b). When a nerve impulse arrives at the presynaptic terminal, certain chemicals are released from the presynaptic terminal and diffuse across the cleft separating the two neurons at the synapse and interact with the outer surface of the membrane of the postsynaptic cell. This interaction leads to a change in the permeability of the membrane to certain ions. The resultive reaction in the postsynaptic neuron may then cause it to fire a nerve impulse. This series of events at the synapse occurs within a millisecond or so. The more that a presynaptic terminal fires, the more transmitter substance that is released into the synaptic cleft and the more likely the postsynaptic neuron will be triggered into firing.

The presynaptic terminal contains a number of circular structures, or tiny sacs, called vesicles. The vesicles are believed to contain a substance that serves as a chemical transmitter of the nerve impulse. Apparently when a nerve impulse arrives at the presynaptic terminal it releases a small quantity of this substance which then crosses the cleft and thereby delivers a signal that excites or inhibits that cell. The vesicles return to the interior of the presynaptic terminal for refilling.

When a nerve impulse arrives at a synapse there is a release of chemical transmitter substance which alters the resting membrane potential of the postsynaptic cell. This change in the postsynaptic neuron is called a postsynaptic potential (PSP). There are two different types of synapses, classified by their effect on the postsynaptic neuron: Excitatory synapses and inhibitory synapses. Some presynaptic terminals secrete an excitatory transmitter substance and when they are active they are said to produce an excitatory postsynaptic potential (EPSP). Other presynaptic terminals secrete an inhibitory transmitter substance and therefore produce an inhibitory postsynaptic potential (IPSP) when they are firing.

An excitatory transmitter substance increases the permeability of the postsynaptic cell at the point of the synapse. This allows sodium ions to flow rapidly to the inside of the cell and the intense ionic movement across the postsynaptic membrane causes some depolarization to occur. As a result, the resting potential of the cell membrane decreases. This does not mean that the second neuron fires off a nerve impulse when it receives transmitter substances from a presynaptic terminal. It merely means that its resting state has been altered. This will be further explained below. The inhibitory transmitter substance has the opposite effect of the excitatory transmitter. Instead of increasing the permeability of the postsynaptic neuron's membrane, the inhibitory transmitter hyperpolarizes the membrane, which tends to prevent the generation of a nerve impulse in the postsynaptic neuron. Both types of PSP will be discussed in more detail below.

A. TRANSMITTER SUBSTANCES

The chemical transmitter substances at excitatory and inhibitory synapses are still largely unknown. One excitatory substance in the brain and at the neuromuscular junction (site where axon presynaptic terminals and muscle fibers connect) is acetylcholine, but glutamate and several other compounds appear to be involved. In the case of acetylcholine, it is injected into the synaptic cleft to act on the postsynaptic neuron membrane. Then within 1 to 2 milliseconds it is destroyed by a hydrolizing enzyme, cholinesterase. After acetylcholine is broken down by cholinesterase the choline is recycled by hydrolysis. It diffuses back into the presynaptic terminal and choline acetyl transferase combines it with acetic acid to re-form acetylcholine in the cytoplasm. Pumping into the synaptic vesicles replenishes their acetylcholine supply and so completes the cycle. The other transmitters undergo a similar process.

The inhibitory transmitter in the spinal cord is glycine while at the supraspinal level, the higher level of the brain, gamma amino butyric acid (GABA) is prominent. These transmitters, like the excitatory transmitters, are packaged in the synaptic vesicles and liberated into the synaptic cleft in a quantal manner.

Other compounds that are reasonably well established as being neurotransmitters are serotonin, epinepherine, norepinepherine, and dopamine. They exist in the presynaptic terminals of neurons located at various sites in the nervous system.

All the presynaptic terminals of a single neuron secrete the same transmitter substance. For example, all synapses made by a neuron which secrete acetylcholine will secrete the same substance despite great differences in the location of the cells on which it synapses. If the effect of a given neuron is to be excitatory on one neuron and inhibitory on another, as in reciprocal innervation of antagonistic muscles, an additional (inhibitory) neuron is interpolated between the first neuron and the one that is to be inhibited.

B. EXCITATORY POSTSYNAPTIC POTENTIAL (EPSP)

As noted above, there are two different types of synapses. An excitatory synapse, when functioning, increases the likelihood that the postsynaptic neuron will reach threshold and fire an impulse. An inhibitory synapse, when firing, produces changes in the postsynaptic cell which lessen the likelihood that the cell will fire an impulse. A neuron is controlled, as it were, by two opposing operations: Excitation and inhibition.

The EPSP will now be described in more detail. A presynaptic terminal that is firing frequently will release a large amount of transmitter substance across the synaptic cleft to the postsynaptic neuron. An infrequent firing terminal, however, will produce a small amount of transmitter across the synaptic cleft. Thus a frequent-firing nerve impulse will liberate more chemicals to cross the synapse than will an infrequent-firing impulse. The more frequent the nerve impulse, the greater the amount of transmitter liberated by the presynaptic terminal. Moreover, presynaptic terminals vary in size; and the larger the terminal, the larger the quantity of transmitter secreted. If the excitatory transmitter is able to alter the resting state of the neuron at the initial segment of the axon to its threshold potential, which in most cells is 10 to 15 millivolts less than the resting membrane potential, it will trigger an action potential in the postsynaptic neuron. If the transmitter is not able to alter the resting state of the neuron enough to achieve the threshold potential, the nerve impulse simply is not transmitted on.

A nerve impulse coming to any one synapse does not usually excite the discharge of a nerve impulse by the postsynaptic neuron; it gives only a certain influence which, if there is enough, perhaps one hundred or more impulses on an area of a neuron, causes the firing of the postsynaptic neuron. If two presynaptic terminals release their substances at once, twice as much sodium enters the cell body and twice as much excitatory postsynaptic potential develops (Fig. 3.9).

The effect of each presynaptic impulse lasts about 15 milliseconds on the postsynaptic neuron. The closer together the impulses, the greater the amount of summation that will occur.

The size of the postsynaptic potential (EPSP) is proportional to the amount of transmitter which is released by the presynaptic terminal, or terminals, firing at a given time. Furthermore, since the response of dendrites and cell bodies to a stimulus is proportional to the intensity of the stimulus and conduction is decremental, the effects of the EPSP diminishes with distance from the synapse. Thus, when a cell body or dendrite receives a transmitter substance at one of its synapses, the EPSP created by that transmitter is reduced as it moves away from synapse. If the EPSP does not reach the threshold potential at the initial segment of the axon, no nerve impulse is fired.

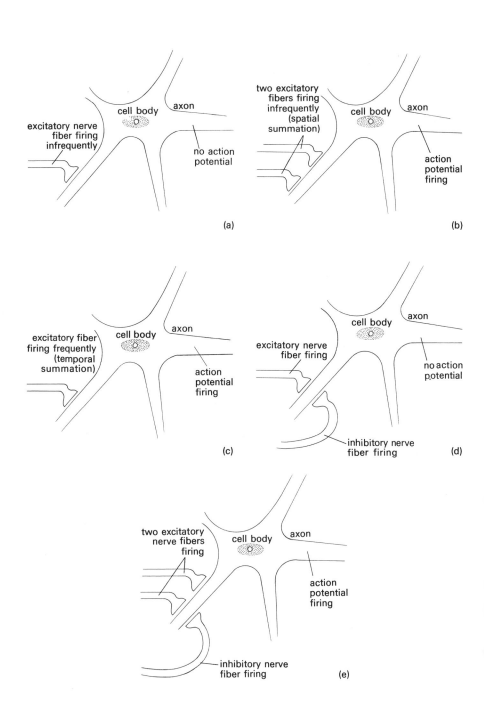

When excitatory presynaptic terminals secrete their transmitter onto the postsynaptic neuron but fail to cause an action potential in the axon of the postsynaptic cell, the neuron still becomes what is called "facilitated." That is, it becomes more capable of being fired with just a little additional stimulation. A neuron in a facilitated condition needs only a little additional excitatory transmitter secreted upon it to raise the EPSP to the threshold. If this occurs, the axon will begin to transmit nerve impulses and will continue to do so as long as the stimulus remains above the threshold. If the EPSP rises higher than just threshold, the axon will fire more rapidly.

Excitatory synaptic transmission may be viewed as following a specific sequence:

1. Arrival of nerve impulses at the presynaptic terminals.
2. EPSP in the postsynaptic neuron.
3. Summation of separate EPSPs by the postsynaptic neuron.
4. If the summated EPSPs reach the threshold level at the initial segment of the axon of the neuron, an action potential is propagated along the axon in an all-or-none fashion.

C. INHIBITORY POSTSYNAPTIC POTENTIAL (IPSP)

Another important activity which occurs at the synapse is inhibition. Inhibition at the synaptic junctions plays a critical role in the CNS, for if it were not for inhibition, excitation would spread throughout the neurons of the CNS causing a continuous state of convulsive activity in the organism.

Some presynaptic terminals secrete an inhibitory transmitter instead of an excitatory transmitter. Inhibitory synapses achieve their effectiveness by generating the inhibitory postsynaptic potential (IPSP) that directly counteracts the depolarizing action of the EPSP. The effect of an inhibitory presynaptic terminal is to hyperpolarize the membrane of the nerve cell with which it has contact, which means that inhibition opposes excitatory synaptic activity by increasing the membrane potential and thus making the generation of an action potential in the postsynaptic neuron more difficult. The resting membrane potential of -70 millivolts, under the influence of inhibition, may become -80 millivolts or more and thus more difficult to fire.

Fig. 3.9   Excitation and inhibition in a neuron are brought about by the nerve fibers which form synapses with it. (a) The stimulus of the excitatory fiber is not intense enough to cause the postsynaptic neuron to fire. (b) The impulses from a second excitatory fiber provide enough added stimulus to cause postsynaptic firing. (c) The presynaptic fiber, since it is firing frequently, provides enough stimulus to fire the postsynaptic neuron. (d) The firing of both excitatory and inhibitory nerve fibers offsets the effect of each upon the other. (e) Since there is greater excitatory stimulation, the postsynaptic fiber fires.

The sequence of events for inhibitory transmission is very similar to the sequence in excitatory transmission. The inhibitory sequence is as follows:

1. All-or-none action potentials end at the presynaptic terminals.
2. The presynaptic terminals release inhibitory transmitter into the synapse.
3. The inhibitory transmitter acts on the postsynaptic neuron to hyperpolarize the membrane.

Since the effects of EPSPs are counterbalanced by IPSPs, the state of a neuron at any moment, that is, how close the cell is to the threshold, is the resultant of all of the synaptic activity affecting the neuron at that time. Since numerous presynaptic terminals synapse upon one neuron, its firing pattern represents the integrated summation of all the excitatory and inhibitory activity impinging upon it at a given time.

D. ADDITIONAL FEATURES OF SYNAPTIC TRANSMISSION

The conduction of a nerve impulse along an axon is essentially electrical while across a synapse it is essentially chemical. It is important to note that the transmission of an impulse across a synapse takes longer than conduction over the same distance of an axon. The shift from electrical to chemical and back to electrical transmission is the reason for the delay. Thus, there is a slight delay between the time of the arrival of an impulse at a presynaptic terminal and the beginning of a postsynaptic potential. This is called synaptic delay and is probably caused mainly by the liberation and diffusion of the transmitter substance to the postsynaptic membrane.

Synaptic transmission has additional unique features. First, there is only one-way conduction at the synapse. Impulses crossing the synapse cannot be transmitted backward through the synapse into the presynaptic terminals of the first neuron. Second, the synapse is more susceptible to fatigue, anesthetics, and stimulants than the cell itself. Hypnotics, anesthetics, and acidosis all have the effect of depressing the transmission of impulses at the synapse. It is at this point that the so-called nerve gases act by obstructing chemical transmission.

THE NEUROMUSCULAR JUNCTION

All movements, every action carried out by the body, are a result of impulse transmission from neurons to muscle fibers. Motorneurons located in the cranial nerves and anterior horns of the spinal cord send out their axons to innervate muscle fibers at a site called the neuromuscular junction, which is

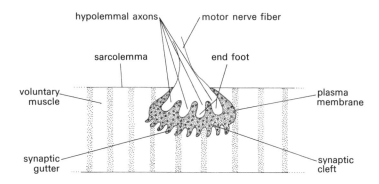

Fig. 3.10 A neuromuscular junction, or motor end plate.

a special type of synapse. The neuromuscular junction (also called a motor end plate) is the connection between a presynaptic terminal of a nerve fiber and a skeletal muscle fiber (Fig. 3.10). This junction functions to transmit nerve impulses from nerve fibers to muscles for the contraction of muscles. Each motorneuron axon branches into several hundred presynaptic terminals and each terminal innervates a muscle fiber, thus each motorneuron may innervate several hundred individual muscle fibers.

A. THE MOTOR UNIT

A motorneuron and all the muscle fibers innervated by it are called a motor unit because all the muscle fibers contract as a unit when adequately stimulated by the motorneuron (Fig. 3.11). Muscles of the eye, which perform very delicate movements, may have a single motorneuron supplying a single muscle fiber whereas the larger muscles which do not require delicacy in movement may have one motorneuron innervating hundreds of muscle fibers. In the postural muscles the ratio of muscle fibers to motorneurons is about 150: 1. Here, each motor unit consists of about 150 muscle fibers.

The amount of work produced by a single motor unit is quite small and is usually insufficient to produce any observable movement of a joint spanned by the whole muscle of which it is a part. Even in small joints, such as those of the thumb, at least two or three motor units are necessary to make a visible movement.

Normally, small motor units are recruited early when movement is produced and, as the force is automatically or consciously increased, larger motor units are recruited, and at the same time all the motor units also increase their frequency of firing. There is no single set frequency. That is, individual motor units can fire very slowly and will increase their frequency on demand.

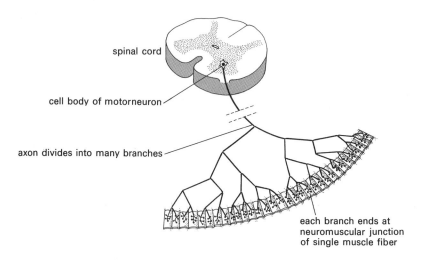

spinal cord

cell body of motorneuron

axon divides into many branches

each branch ends at
neuromuscular junction
of single muscle fiber

Fig. 3.11   A motor unit. The motorneuron with the group of muscle
fibers which it supplies. (Based on McNaught and Callander, 1963.)

B. NEUROMUSCULAR TRANSMISSION

The events occurring at the neuromuscular junction are similar to those
occurring at a synapse between two neurons. Each of the presynaptic terminals of a motorneuron passes beneath the muscle membrane. Between the
terminal and the plasma membrane of the muscle there is a synapse somewhat like that found between neurons. When a nerve impulse arrives at the
neuromuscular junction, the terminals secrete a transmitter substance into
the cleft between the presynaptic terminal and the plasma membrane.

NEURONAL CIRCUITS

Nerve transmission normally involves many neurons. In fact, from the time a
stimulus is received until behavior is exhibited in response to the stimulus
hundreds or even millions of neurons may be involved. The CNS is organized
into many different parts and it is through the functional synaptic link-ups in
various parts of the body that neurons from one part of the body, when
stimulated, can influence neurons in another part of the body. These link-
ups of many accumulations of neurons are called neuronal circuits. The neurophysiological knowledge about principles of organization of neuronal circuits is very incomplete. Indeed, there is no complete and detailed understanding of any single neuronal circuit's overall functioning, in terms of
properties of the constituent neurons and all of their interconnections.

4

Sensory Integration

Our sensory systems play a crucial role in motor learning and performance. Our simplest movements, the reflexes, are initiated by the senses; complex movements are often responses to sensory input, and ongoing sensory information is important for control and regulation while movements are underway.

The energy which impinges upon one's sensory receptors provides the raw data out of which "meanings" arise. Sensation may be viewed as the first stage in a multistage process of bringing order and organization out of the kaleidoscopic environment. For vision, this enables us to see people, trees, and houses; for audition we hear a song being sung, the cry of an infant, the ticking of a clock. This process by which sensory input is organized and interpreted is called perception.

The focus of this chapter is on the ways in which sensory information is received by receptors, transmitted to the brain, and integrated with stored information to form perceptions. This sensory integration process precipitates the responses which the individual might then make.

SENSORY FUNCTIONS

All of our ongoing daily activities are responses to environmental and internal stimuli. In order for our behavior to be effectively directed toward these stimuli, we are equipped with neural mechanisms for sensing stimuli, coding them into electrical impulses, and transmitting these impulses through neural pathways to specific areas of the brain. The various neural mechanisms which are responsible for these functions make up our sensory systems.

Although there is some difference among these sensory mechanisms, their basic functional properties are similar. The sensory receptors first respond to a stimulus, which is in the form of energy, e.g., mechanical, light, sound. At the receptor, the various forms of energy are transduced (converted from one form of energy to another) into an electrical potential which gives rise to nerve impulses which are then conducted by sensory neuron (also called afferent neuron) axons into the CNS. In the CNS, the impulses are transmitted into various lower-brain centers; then for most of the senses the impulses are projected into the cerebral cortex.

Throughout the transmission network the neural impulses are recoded because of the complex synaptic connections; thus, coding and recoding of sensory information occurs at all levels of the sensory systems, from the receptors to the cortex. Sensory systems, therefore, should be considered not only as structures activated by various forms of stimuli but as systems capable of presenting a detailed report of patterns of stimuli received from the environment.

Another important function of sensory input is the maintenance and modification of arousal, alertness, and attention levels of the individual. Most of the sensory systems project input into specific areas of the cerebral cortex. However, as these impulses ascend to the cortex, collateral axons send off impulses into a lower brain structure called the reticular formation, which is made up of numerous neurons whose cell bodies lie throughout the brainstem and thalamus. These neurons in turn send a profusion of axons throughout the brain, and when the reticular formation is activated, it enhances arousal by facilitating or even firing neurons in the cortex and other parts of the brain. So varying levels of behavioral arousal, from hyper-excitement to sleep, are partially mediated by the senses.

The sensory systems also have feedback mechanisms through connections with the motor system which control responses contributing to the reception of stimuli, e.g., visual regions of the brain control eye movements for altering the pattern of light on the visual receptors. Thus, by specific adjustive responses the brain can select its own input and only a portion of the total stimuli impinging on an individual at one time is perceived and attended to. Without mechanisms for selective attention we would respond to all stimuli impinging on the body at one time, causing disorganization of behavior.

Normally, more than one sense is used at a time in our interactions with the environment. The senses typically cooperate with and supplement one another. Each sense modality (modality means kind of sensation, e.g., visual, auditory, etc.) contributes its own unique version of an occurrence in the physical world which is usually blended into a coherent and unified single impression. When we are introduced to a strange object, we may use our hands to gain information about its size, weight, temperature, and texture; but we also obtain much valuable information about its properties by seeing it. The famous story of the three blind men who touched different parts of an elephant and described what they thought it was illustrates the importance of multisensory information. Sensory data gained simultaneously through the various senses are one means by which we build up an enriched storehouse of perceptions about our environment.

SENSORY LIMITS

As species rise from lower to higher evolutionary levels, there is an increasing dominance of sensory organs for vision and hearing over the other sensory receptors. This greatly enriches the quality and quantity of sensory experience. In humans, the sensory systems include a greater number of differentiations than those of any other species. But even with the amazing variety of stimuli to which we can respond, our senses provide us with only an incomplete pattern of information about our environment because our receptors cannot detect certain levels of physical stimuli. We cannot detect, and consequently obtain no information from, sound waves below 20 cycles per second or above 20,000 cycles per second. In between is the whole spectrum of hearing, both tone and loudness. Light rays in the form of radiant energy travel much faster than sound waves and they supply light for seeing. But there are many frequencies of radiant energy which human receptors do not detect. Radio and radar waves have frequencies of radiant energy that are too slow for the human eye to detect, while X-rays and gamma rays have frequencies that are too fast to stimulate the human eye.

Other species are not sensitive to the same levels of stimuli, or limited to the same degrees of sensitivity, as humans. Dogs have the ability to hear high pitches far beyond the range of the human ear, and the dog whistle is based on this fact. Dogs are also noted for their very sensitive noses; they smell stimuli to which humans are insensitive. Bats locate objects not with their eyes but by echoes from high-frequency sound waves which they emit. The list could go on, but suffice to say that sensory sensitivity is species specific.

THE SENSORY RECEPTORS

The sensory receptors are the windows of the nervous system. The only way that the nervous system is in contact with the environment is through the receptors.

The actual structure of sensory receptors varies considerably. Some receptors are the specialized terminations of sensory neurons, while others are separate cells which are connected to the sensory neuron endings. Moreover, some receptors have accessory structures such as the lens of the eye or the membranes in the ear which act to focus, alter, amplify, or localize a particular type of stimulus.

Sensory receptors are generally specialized to respond to a specific type of stimulus, such as light, temperature, mechanical stimulation, sound, etc. However, most of them can be stimulated by various forms of energy. For example, the visual receptors (rods and cones) normally respond to light energy, but they can be stimulated by intense mechanical stimuli such as pressure on the eyeball. The type of stimulus that a given receptor-type is most sensitive to is referred to as its adequate stimulus.

A. RECEPTION OF STIMULI

When a stimulus impinges upon a receptor, it brings about an alteration in the resting membrane potential of that structure which is graded according to certain characteristics of the stimulus, such as intensity, and which is confined to the region of the receptor. This receptor action is analogous to the chemical excitability of dendrites, and the altered membrane potential of a receptor resulting from a stimulus is called a "generator potential."

A generator potential is the graded electrical potential that triggers the all-or-none response of the initial segment of a sensory neuron, and it always precedes the firing of a nerve impulse from the sensory neuron. It should be noted that sensory neurons tend to be unipolar and bipolar type neurons. Therefore, the initial segment of these neurons is not located near the cell body but instead is located near the terminal of the axon, and impulses in these neurons typically originate at the terminal and are transmitted towards the cell body and then onward over the other fiber or fibers of the cell. Sensory neuron terminals in the skin, for example, have their cell bodies in the dorsal root ganglion near the spinal cord. The other terminal endings of these neurons project into the spinal cord.

A nerve impulse results when the generator potential achieves the threshold of that sensory neuron. If a subthreshold stimulus is applied to a receptor, a small generator potential develops. If a more intense, but still subthreshold, stimulus is applied, the generator potential will be correspondingly greater. Two subthreshold stimuli applied closely together will summate, and the generator potential they produce will be correspondingly greater. If the combined generator potential is great enough to achieve the threshold potential at the initial segment of a sensory neuron, it fires off. It may be seen that the initiation of afferent impulses is a two-stage process: the physical stimulus causes a depolarization of the receptor membrane, the generator potential, and, if the stimulus is strong enough, the generator potential initiates an action potential in the sensory neuron which propagates along its axon.

B. SENSORY ADAPTATION

Many sensory receptors respond strongly to the onset of a stimulus but either completely cease to respond to a steady stimulus after a brief time or respond at a much reduced rate; this phenomenon is called adaptation. Sensory adaptation does not occur because of fatigue at the receptors because if the stimulus is even momentarily stopped and then reapplied, an initial burst of impulse activity recurs and the process is repeated. This would not occur if the receptors were indeed fatigued.

C. DISCRIMINATION OF INTENSITY OF STIMULI

Essential to the perception of sensory data is the discrimination of intensity of stimulation. In interpreting sensory information, the nervous system estimates the intensity of sensory data. This interpretation function allows us to tell differences in degrees of cold or warmth, brightness of light, loudness of sound, intensity of pain, etc.

Information about stimulus strength is relayed to the brain in two basic ways. First, an increase in stimulus strength produces a higher frequency of nerve impulse firing in a sensory neuron; this is called temporal summation. Second, similar receptors of other sensory neurons in the immediate area of the stimulus are also activated as stimulus strength increases because stronger stimuli typically affect a larger area. For example, touching a surface lightly with a finger brings only a small area of the skin in contact with the surface, and only receptors in that area of the skin are stimulated. But pressing the finger down firmly against the surface increases the area of the skin which is stimulated, thus stimulating additional receptors. This is called spatial summation.

All sensory systems, then, have two methods of coding intensity of stimuli: Increased stimulus strength is signaled by an increased firing rate of nerve impulses in a single sensory neuron and by recruitment of receptors on other sensory neurons in the neighboring area.

TRANSMISSION OF IMPULSES TO THE BRAIN

Impulses traveling over a sensory neuron pass along nerve transmission pathways that are specific to a certain sensory system. Sensory systems may be generally classified as the special senses, somatic senses, and the

visceral senses. The special senses are served by cranial nerves and include
vision, audition, taste, and olfaction. The somatic sensations are touch-
pressure, temperature, proprioception, and pain. Branches of spinal nerves
and certain cranial nerves serve these sensations. Visceral sensations, such
as hunger, nausea, and visceral pain are served by sensory neurons which
are part of the autonomic nervous system.

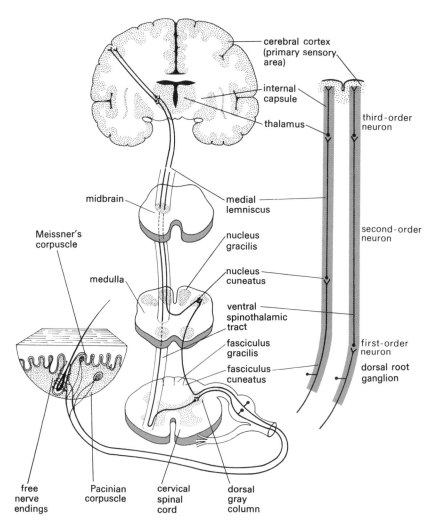

Fig. 4.1 Sensory pathways for touch and pressure. The fasciculus cuneatus or
gracilis and the ventral spinothalamic tracts. (Based on Langley *et al.*, 1969.)

Basically, the transmission network of sensory impulses from the receptor to the brain is similar for all of the sensory systems. Three orders of neurons typically make up the sensory chain: The sensory neuron which transmits the impulse from the receptor into the CNS and on to the first synapse is considered the first-order neuron. The neuron that transmits the impulse up to the thalamus is the second-order neuron. Impulses conveyed from the thalamus to the cerebral cortex travel over the third-order neuron.

A. SOMATIC SYSTEM TRANSMISSION

In the case of the somatic system (touch-pressure, temperature, proprioceptors, and pain), there are actually two transmission pathways but the three-order chain of neurons is maintained in both (Fig. 4.1). In the first, impulses from the receptors located in the skin, muscles, and joints, travel through the spinal nerves and enter the dorsal roots of the spinal cord via the sensory neuron. These impulses continue upward in the white matter of the spinal cord (you will recall from Chapter 2 that the white matter is made up of bundles of nerve fibers called tracts) where they synapse in two nuclei of the medulla, the nucleus gracilis and nucleus cuneatus. This constitutes the first-order transmission in this pathway. The second-order neuron axon decussates (crosses the midline) in the medulla and proceeds upward through the medulla, pons, and midbrain in the medial lemniscus tract and ends in the thalamus, where it synapses with the third-order neuron. The axon of the third-order neuron originates in the thalamus and projects through the internal capsule to the somatic projection area of the cortex.

The second pathway of the somatic system is used especially by temperature and pain sensations but is used by other somatic sensations as well. Sensory impulses of first-order neurons, soon after entering the spinal cord, make synaptic connections with the neurons of the second-order neuron. The axon of the second-order neuron crosses the spinal cord commissure and ascends the cord, passing directly through the brainstem and midbrain and ending in the thalamus. As with the other transmission network, the third-order neuron conveys the impulse from the thalamus to the cortex.

B. SPECIAL SENSES TRANSMISSION

Although the details of sensory transmission differ for each of the special senses, and of course differ from the somatic system, the general features of the transmission network are similar. In the case of vision, the receptors in the eye constitute the first-order neurons which synapse directly on second-order neurons which leave the eye and form the optic tract. These optic nerve fibers from each eye project backward to the optic chiasm, where about 50 percent cross the midline and extend backward to a special location in the thalamus, the lateral geniculate body. From there the third-order axon takes the impulses to the visual projection area of the cortex.

The actual transmission networks of these sensory systems are more complex than they have been described, but the details of the various sensory pathways need not concern us here, since they will be more fully discussed in chapters dealing with the sensory and perceptual aspects of specific sensory systems.

Other sensory systems are not as important to motor behavior as the ones discussed above so they will not be covered in this text.

C. THE THALAMUS AND SENSORY TRANSMISSION

All sensory impulses (except those of olfaction) pass through the thalamus, synapsing there before ascending to the cerebral cortex. The thalamus may appropriately be called the port of entry to the cortex.

Shaped like two small footballs and lying just above the midbrain in each cerebral hemisphere, the thalamus is actually a series of nuclei serving sensory as well as motor functions. Some thalamic nuclei receive direct sensory input, others project motor fibers to lower centers of the brain and spinal cord, and still others have direct cortical connections.

Many of the sensory pathways interact with one another at several levels of the nervous system, and especially at the thalamus. Thus, the thalamus is an important level for sensory integration because many of the nuclei are the final processing centers of sensory systems which project to the cortex. It is in this structure where the conscious awareness of crude sensation, such as touch, pressure, and pain, are realized. Finer sensory discriminations, which are elevated to the conscious sphere in the cortex, require the input of the information processed in the thalamic nuclei for their final resolution.

One set of neurons in the thalamus does not seem to be involved in relaying specific sensory or motor information but plays an important role in the control of such processes as sleep, wakefulness, and arousal. This part of the thalamus is called the diffuse thalamic reticular formation and will be discussed in a later section of this chapter.

D. THE RETICULAR FORMATION AND SENSORY TRANSMISSION

Before following the sensory transmission network to the cerebral cortex, it is important to consider another important subcortical structure in the sensory transmission system—the reticular formation. This structure plays a key role in sensory integration as well as making significant contributions to the motor aspects of neural function. Numerous studies have indicated the reticular formation to be of paramount importance in arousal. This structure seems to be involved in sleeping, wakefulness, and in fine gradations in attention.

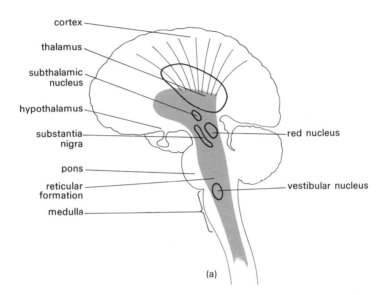

(a)

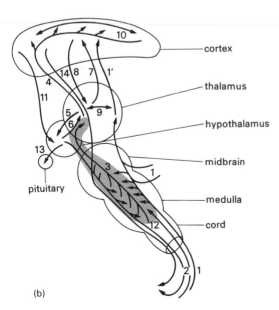

(b)

Fig. 4.2 (a) The reticular formation and nuclei which are associated with it. (Based on Guyton, 1966.) (b) A schematic diagram of the input and output transmission of the reticular formation. The cross-hatched area represents the location of the reticular formation. (Based on Lindsley, 1951.)

The reticular formation consists of a netlike mass of interwoven neurons that extends from the brainstem up to the thalamus (Fig. 4.2). All sensory systems (the special senses as well as the somatic senses) give off collateral axons on their way to the cortex which innervate reticular formation neurons. This system of neurons may actually be divided into two functional systems: first, the brainstem reticular formation system; second, the diffuse thalamic reticular system. The cell bodies of the brainstem reticular formation neurons are located at the levels of the medulla, pons, midbrain, and hypothalamus. The posterior hypothalamus is anatomically the upper part of the brainstem reticular system. The diffuse thalamic reticular system consists of cells spread through various nuclei of the thalamus.

All sensory systems supply a profusion of collateral axons to both the brainstem and thalamic reticular systems. Thus, both somatic and special sensory stimuli are able to stimulate both components of the reticular formation. It may be seen, then, that almost any kind of sensory signal can stimulate the neurons of this system. For example, signals from the muscles, pressure impulses from the skin, visual signals from the eyes, auditory impulses from the ear, can all cause activation of this mechanism. Furthermore, one important hormone of the body, epinephrine (adrenalin) also has a powerful effect in stimulating the reticular formation. All of these input sources have the effect of stimulating reticular neurons which send out axons throughout the CNS.

Not only do the sensory systems and hormones provide input to the reticular formation neurons, another source of reticular activation is found in direct projections from cortical areas to the reticular formation. Actually there is a vast network of cortical axons to both systems of the reticular formation and cortical input to the reticular systems is more widespread than of any sensory mode. However, the cortical axons to the reticular systems arise only in limited regions of the frontal, parietal, and temporal lobes.

Reticular formation axons may be classified as either ascending or descending axons. The ascending axons project into subcortical structures but especially into most of the cerebral cortex. One primary function of these reticular formation axons is to facilitate these higher brain center neurons. When they are transmitting impulses, they are said to have an "activating" effect on cortical neurons. For this reason, the ascending axon network of the reticular formation is called the "Reticular Activating System" (RAS). Like the bell on a telephone, the RAS acts as an alerting center for the rest of the brain (Fig. 4.3). Descending axons of the reticular formation project into the lower brainstem and spinal cord. Some of these axons have a facilitating effect on spinal motorneurons, while others have an inhibitory effect.

To return to the cortical connections with reticular neurons, these connections serve a critical function, for they provide a means by which cortical areas can indirectly influence cortical cells as well as lower nervous

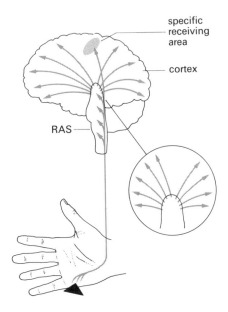

specific
receiving
area

cortex

RAS

Fig. 4.3   Schematic drawing showing how a touch stimulus to the hand is relayed
to a specific receiving area in the cerebral cortex. The sensory channel also
sends collateral branches into the reticular activating system (RAS), which in turn
projects alerting stimulation to many areas of the cerebral cortex. The inset
shows the cortical projections arising from the forward end (thalamic section) of
the reticular formation. (Based on Kimble, 1963.)

system neurons. Excitatory cortical neurons stimulate reticular formation
neurons while inhibitory cortical neurons inhibit the reticular formation.

From this description of the input and output sources of the reticular
formation, it may be seen that various feedback loops contribute to its functioning. For example, impulses from the sensory receptors feed through the
reticular systems which then send impulses to the cerebral cortex to increase its excitation; then the cortex sends back impulses to the reticular
systems stimulating these systems to feed back impulses to the cortex for
further excitation. A second feedback loop exists whereby the reticular formation sends impulses to the spinal cord to increase muscle tone; in turn, the
increased tone excites receptors in muscles and joints that send impulses
back to the reticular formation. The feedback loop can also be initiated at
the cortical level: cortical activity in the way of thoughts can produce collateral cortical impulses going to the reticular formation, stimulating neurons in this structure. The reticular neurons then feed back to the cortical
neurons stimulating them, and they feed back further stimulation to the reticular formation. Thus, thoughts can produce arousal, and excitement.

It seems that the actual activation of some cortical cells requires that they be facilitated by the reticular formation, that the signals coming from the sensory systems cannot, by themselves, supply enough stimulation to fire cortical neurons. They seem to need first to be "readied" by the reticular formation.

It also appears that the reticular formation is important in selective attention. Signals from some sensory systems appear to suppress those from others via the reticular formation, by inhibiting reticular formation activity from some sensory systems. Also the cortex may influence reticular formation activity by directing inhibition to some reticular formation neurons while at the same time exciting others.

One of the most striking differences between the RAS and the diffuse thalamic reticular system is in the arousal response itself. When stimulated, the RAS produces a general facilitation of the cortex which is manifested in a long-lasting alertness or arousal. Although high intensity stimulation of the thalamic reticular system can produce similar results, the effects of this system are more typically phasic and delicate in nature and appear to be capable of facilitating localized regions of the cortex with some selectivity.

Now this localized, phasic action of the diffuse thalamic system is blocked, or overshadowed, by the action of the RAS. The exact functional significance of this phenomenon has not been ascertained, but this overshadowing of the differential functions of the thalamic system by the RAS may be the cause of failures of discrimination which occur during periods of intense emotion.

E. THE PRIMARY CORTEX AREAS

We have seen that stimuli impinging upon sensory receptors are transduced into nerve impulses which are then transmitted into the CNS, where they ascend to the thalamus, giving off to the reticular formation collateral impulses on their way. This transmission represents the first two orders of the three-order transmission network for sensory impulses. The third-order neurons are located in the thalamus and project their axons into the cerebral cortex. All sensory systems project to the cortex, each to a specific region; the cortex is the last or highest region in the brain where sensory information from the senses is represented.

The regions of the cerebral cortex to which the third-order neurons of a sensory system project are quite circumscribed and are called primary cortex areas (also called primary projection areas). The primary somatic cortex area is located in the parietal lobe, just behind the central fissure; the primary visual area is found in the occipital lobes; the primary auditory area in the temporal lobe (Fig. 4.4). The fact that the various sensory systems have their own primary cortex area helps to explain how the brain is capable of

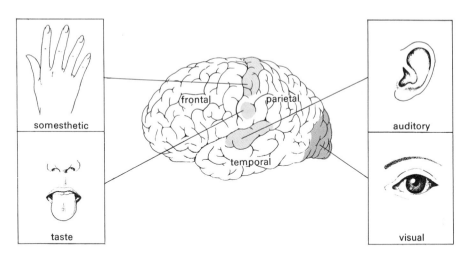

Fig. 4.4 Primary cortex areas for the various sense modalities. (Based on Kimble, 1963.)

differentiating between impulses from somatic receptors and impulses from visual receptors.

The primary cortex areas have certain functions in common. Basically they analyze the simple aspects of sensations, such as spatial localization of impulses from the receptors and generalized detection of the individual elements of the stimuli. For example, electrical stimulation in the somatic cortex evokes a generalized tingling in the skin, mild degrees of heat or cold, or numbness in a localized part of the body, such as the hand. Electrical stimulation of the primary visual cortex evokes flashes of light, colors, or moving lights; these, too, are localized to specific areas of the visual fields in accordance with the part of the primary visual cortex stimulated.

The localization of sensation in the primary cortex areas is possible because each primary area is mapped out in such a way that stimulation of different regions of the receptor surface leads to stimulation of differing groups of neurons in these primary cortex areas. This produces a coding of location of objects impinging upon the receptors. Moreover, that aspect of sensory experience which has the greatest functional significance to us, such as the center of gaze for vision and fingertips for touch, has relatively more cortical representation.

The complete analysis of interpretation of complex patterns of sensory information necessitates many other areas of the brain working in association with the various "primary" areas. This does not mean that the primary cortex areas play an insignificant part in sensory interpretation. Indeed, they have a critical function because when one of these areas is destroyed the ability to utilize sensory data in that sensory system is diminished drastically. For example, the destruction of the primary visual cortex in humans causes total blindness. Loss of the primary auditory cortex results in virtually total deafness.

INTERPRETATION OF SENSATIONS

The pathways of neural activity beyond the primary cortex areas are obscure. There are large areas in the frontal, occipital, temporal, and parietal areas of the cortex from which direct sensory information is not received or from which cortical stimulation elicits very little movement. Indeed, the primary cortex and the motor areas of the cerebral cortex occupy less than one-half of the overall cortical area in humans. Impulses from the primary cortex areas are transmitted to other areas in the cortex and even to subcortical areas for further processing so that "meaning" can be made from the sensory signals.

A. THE ASSOCIATION AREAS

The areas of the cerebral cortex which do not have direct sensory or motor functions are collectively called the association areas (Fig. 4.5). These regions of the cortex receive input from the primary cortex areas via the association fibers. Between all of the various areas of the cortex there are billions of neurons and connecting pathways. This profusion of neurons and their fibers connects every part of the cortex with every other part. In addition to the intracortical connections, the interior of the cerebral hemispheres between the cortical layers and the subcortical structures is permeated by a complex network of connecting fiber pathways. This vast network serves as the structural basis for the association activity of the brain.

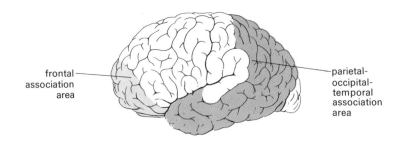

frontal association area

parietal- occipital- temporal association area

Fig. 4.5   Association areas of the cerebral cortex. (Based on Kimble, 1963.)

Sensory impulses from the skin, eyes, and ears are all transmitted into the small circumscribed primary areas in the cortex, and from each primary area the impulses go to the association areas. Although it is not possible to elucidate the specific roles performed by the association areas, it appears that a major function of these areas is to enable the individual to deal effectively with the environment by translating sensory data into information about the environment, combining it with appropriate stored information (memories), and organizing muscular movements into combinations that will produce specific and effective results.

Somatic impulses pass from the somatic primary cortex into association areas in the parietal lobes where the impulses are interpreted into the "meaning" of the sensations. The qualities of shape, form, roughness, smoothness, size, and texture of an object are ascertained. Quantities such as weight, temperature, and the degree of pressure are also interpreted. Here also is where the awareness of location of body parts, one to the other, and of one's self is perceived. Destruction of association areas in the parietal lobe produces deficits in the sphere of somatic perception.

The individual deprived of the parietal association area, if blindfolded and given a pencil to hold, does not recognize the object as a pencil. If the somatic primary cortex is functional the individual can tell that the pencil is round, smooth, light in weight. Recognition of position sense and discrimination are not impaired, but the individual is unable to integrate the bits of information into the concept of a pencil. Large-scale destruction of the parietal association area results in failure to recognize the body scheme. The recognition of self is impaired. Thus, a man with such a condition may be unaware that his leg is his leg. The recognition of an object through the somatic senses requires an intact parietal association area, whereas the awareness of simple aspects of somatic sensation, such as localization, can be brought into the conscious sphere through subcortical and primary cortex functions.

In the case of vision, objects "seen" by the primary visual cortex are processed and made meaningful by the neighboring association areas. Persons whose primary visual cortex has been destroyed are blind; if they encounter a table, they will not see it. In contrast, one who has a functional primary visual cortex but has no visual association areas sees the table, but is not able to say that it is a table or explain its function. Thus, an individual has difficulty in determining the function or appreciating the significance of objects from cues without intact visual association areas.

For hearing, the primary auditory area impulses pass into the surrounding association areas which interpret the meaning of the sounds. It seems that one part of this association area ascertains whether the sound is noise, music, or speech, while other parts interpret the meaning conveyed by the sound.

By association areas, in each of these cases, we are referring to areas adjacent to the primary cortex area but we are also referring to association areas throughout the cerebral cortex. That is, visual information probably activates association areas in the frontal lobes as well as those in the occipital-parietal-temporal lobes. Association areas do not necessarily perform functions associated with a particular sensory system. These areas receive sensory information from many different senses. Furthermore, part of the association areas of the brain are located in subcortical regions, such as the thalamus and basal ganglia, and these regions are intimately associated with cortical association areas.

B. INTEGRATIVE ACTIVITY IN THE BRAIN

How impulses to the various association areas are integrated into a meaningful thought or a coordinated movement is one of the mysteries still to be unraveled by science. Most of this work is still in a theoretical stage. It is believed by some neuroscientists that there is a "common integrative area" located in the brain at a point where the lateral fissure and the parietal lobe of the brain meet. They believe that all of the thoughts from the different sensory areas are correlated and weighed against each other here for a recognition of the meaning and a decision as to appropriate behavior.

Wilder Penfield (1958) found that electrical stimulation in various parts of this area on the conscious patient caused highly complex thoughts, including memories of visual scenes or auditory hallucinations, such as specific musical pieces or a discourse by a specific person. He states:

At operation when the posterior portion of the superior convolution of the right temporal lobe was stimulated she [the patient] gave a little exclamation...and said, "I hear people coming in." Then she added "I hear music now, a funny little piece."

For this reason, Penfield believed that complicated memory patterns are stored in the temporal lobes and angular gyrus. On the basis of electrical-stimulation experiments on hundreds of patients, Penfield found that from these areas, and from nowhere else in the brain, stimulation produced physical responses which he divided into experiential responses and interpretive responses. By experiential responses he meant that electrical stimulation in this temporal area caused the patient to be aware of some previous experience. Interpretive responses mean that, upon stimulation, the patient discovered she had changed her own interpretation of what she was seeing, hearing, or thinking at the moment. Penfield concluded that this area of the cortex makes some functional contribution to reflex comparison of the present with related past experiences and contributes to interpretation or perception of the present.

The notion of a "localization" of integration of sensations is completely rejected by other neuroscientists (Luria, 1966; Konorski, 1967). Several have found that a lesion of a narrow area of the cortex practically never leads to the loss of any single isolated function, but always to the disturbance of a large group of mental processes, forming a "symptom-complex" or syndrome. They claim that the factual evidence of clinical neurology contradicts the notion of the direct localization of interpretation and integration of sensations to circumscribed areas of the brain. There is no evidence, they say, for isolated cerebral "centers" for any of the complex forms of mental activity. Their evidence suggests that both the concept of functions and the simplified ideas of direct localization in circumscribed areas of the brain require serious revision.

Regardless of the position one might take on how the integrative activity of the brain functions, we have every reason to suppose that thought and voluntary movement is in fact the result of the combined activity of the whole brain. This does not mean, though, that all parts of the brain are equally important in these particular activities. Each segment of the brain plays its own part in the integration of sensations and the organization of voluntary movement and thought, so that the disturbance of thought and voluntary movement caused by a lesion of each of these links of the functional system will be distinct in character and easily differentiated. One fact is clear: An accurate description of the complex integration activity of the brain will not be an easy task, nor is it likely to occur in the near future.

HEMISPHERIC DOMINANCE IN THE BRAIN

It appears that the two hemispheres of the brain do not contribute equally to the integration and interpretation of sensory data. The left hemisphere seems to be predominately involved with analytic thinking, especially language and logic. It appears that this hemisphere processes information sequentially, which is necessary for logical thought, since logic depends upon sequence and order. On the other hand, the right hemisphere seems to be primarily responsible for our orientation in space, artistic talents, and body awareness. It appears to process information in a simultaneous, rather than linear, fashion.

Persons who have had damage to the left hemisphere often suffer loss of language ability. Such persons talk with difficulty and occasionally they cannot talk at all. Conversely, damage to the right hemisphere often does not interfere with language ability at all, but often causes severe deficits in spatial awareness, musical ability, and in the recognition of other persons, especially of their faces.

Neuroscientists have tended to label the left hemisphere the "dominant" hemisphere because of its primary role in language. Our culture emphasizes verbal and intellectual abilities, thus the bias that the left hemisphere is "dominant." The left hemisphere has been shown to be the functional hemisphere controlling language and verbal tasks in over nine-tenths of all people, but extreme preponderance of the left hemisphere has nothing, as a rule, to do with handedness. Most left-handed people have speech in the left hemisphere; however, a few have a complete reversal of hemisphere function, and others show a mixed pattern, e.g., both hemispheres having language function.

The notion that the two hemispheres have specialized functions does not imply that one hemisphere normally functions autonomously from the other. Since the brain's two hemispheres are connected by commissures, there is a close functional relationship; the activities of two hemispheres are not exclusive of each other.

Although the two hemispheres normally function in a coordinated, but specialized manner, if all of the commissural connections are cut, the separated halves behave as independent brains. Each has its own independent perceptual, learning, memory, and other higher functions, and neither half is aware of what is experienced by the other. Sperry (1964) and his colleagues (Gazzaniga, 1967) have conducted research on "split brain" animals and humans for the past 20 years. Their technique involves surgically separating the two hemispheres and then testing the subjects postoperatively.

CONTROL OF SENSORY TRANSMISSION BY THE BRAIN

It has been found that the brain itself by means of descending pathways can control to some extent the incoming sensory data that ultimately reach the cortex. Nerve fibers project down from the higher regions of the brain to brainstem and spinal cord synapses to exert direct control over the progression of sensory impulses. Impulses from these cortical fibers can alter the nature of sensory information that reaches the cortex by exciting or inhibiting neurons in the ascending sensory pathways.

The significance of the descending pathways is not fully known, but since the amount and kind of incoming sensory data can be controlled or "gated" at the lower levels of sensory transmission, the sensory information may be inhibited or facilitated as it proceeds to the cortex. Thus, some sensory data might be prevented from reaching the cortex. It may be seen, then, that some aspects of selective attention, where we attend to one type of sensory input and exclude others, may involve this descending pathway mechanism.

5

The Somatosensory System

The term "somatosensory" refers to sensations from the body, and somatic sensory receptors are located in the skin, muscles, tendons, joints, and the vestibular apparatus of the internal ear. Collectively, the receptors of this system are sensitive to stimuli of various kinds that impinge on the exterior surface of the body and to stimuli arising from various structures within the body.

There is actually a variety of receptor end organs which comprise the somatosensory system, and basically each receptor is most sensitive to a particular form of stimulus. To organize these various receptors into some form of meaningful groups, neuroanatomists have divided them into two general categories: (1) Cutaneous receptors and (2) proprioceptors. The cutaneous receptors are found near the skin and stimulation of them gives rise to impulses for four sensations—touch-pressure, heat, cold, and pain. Receptors in the muscles, tendons, joints, and vestibular apparatus are collectively called proprioceptors; the impressions obtained from these receptors are known as kinesthetic perceptions. This chapter will examine the role of each of these somatosensory groups.

CUTANEOUS RECEPTORS

With the exception of the distance receptors (visual, auditory, olfactory), most of our sensory receptors which are responsive to changes in the outside world are located in our skin. There is a series of somatosensory receptors closely associated together just under the skin in what is called the epidermis and in deeper layers under the skin, the dermis. These are called cutaneous receptors, meaning receptors of sensations from the skin. They provide information about stimulation of the skin and deep-lying tissue and structures within the body. Although there is some ambiguity in the literature concerning the number and nomenclature of the cutaneous receptors, touch-pressure, warmth, cold, and pain are commonly identified as the cutaneous sensory modalities.

A. TOUCH AND PRESSURE SENSATIONS

Touch and pressure are mediated by four different receptors: Meissner's corpuscles, Merkel's disks, free nerve endings, and Pacinian corpuscles (Fig. 5.1). On the hairless parts of the body, such as the lips, palms of the hands, and undersides of the feet, the Meissner's corpuscles and Merkel's disks are very profuse. The Meissner's corpuscle is an encapsulated central core of nerve fiber. Merkel's disks are disk-shaped expansions, with nerve fibers emerging from the middle of the base. These appear to be receptors for light touch, but they also react to bending of hair or pressure on the skin.

On the hairy parts of the body, free nerve endings wind themselves around the bulbous base of the hair follicles to form nerve baskets, and any deflection of the hair gives rise to a touch sensation. Furthermore, free endings exist in all parts of the skin and are activated by touch sensation and probably by thermal and pain stimuli.

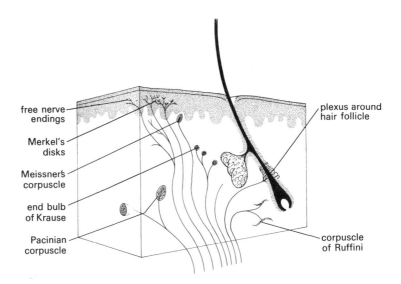

Fig. 5.1   Sensory receptors in the skin. (Based on Noback, 1967.)

Pacinian corpuscles are located deep in the dermis and are stimulated by deep compression of the skin, so they are considered the primary receptors for touch or pressure. They are very large relative to the other cutaneous receptors, each one being about a millimeter long and having an oval shape. Structurally, the Pacinian corpuscle has an inner core of bare nerve filament surrounded by successive layers of tissue, giving it the appearance somewhat like that of a cross section of an onion. It responds to mechanical stimulation, but its fiber sends impulses only at the onset and offset of stimulation and not during periods of prolonged skin displacement.

B. WARMTH AND COLD SENSATIONS

The sensations for warmth and cold are believed to be mediated by two receptors: the Ruffini organ and the Krause end bulb. The Ruffini organ is an encapsulated receptor; it is a tough connective-tissue sheath inside of which the nerve fibers end in small free knobs. The Ruffini organs are considered to be the heat receptors. The Krause end bulb is another encapsulated receptor with intertwined nerve fibers occupying most of the interior. The end bulbs are believed to be receptors for cold.

Some neurologists report a good histologic relationship between the warm and cold spots, experimentally determined, and the depth below the skin surface and the distribution of Krause and Ruffini organs. Others report that there are no morphologically specialized receptors for thermal sensations.

C. PAIN SENSATION

Pain is probably the most important cutaneous sensation because it is a protective mechanism which helps to protect the body from damage. Pain may be aroused in a variety of ways. Severe mechanical, chemical, thermal, or electrical stimuli on the body will arouse pain; exaggerated arterial dilation and arterial constriction causing ischemia (lack of blood) may produce pain; distention of visceral organs may cause pain; finally, tissue inflammation lowers pain threshold.

Although pain is an important sensation, the neurophysiology of pain is poorly understood, and there is a great deal of controversy about the mechanisms underlying this modality of sensation. The primary pain receptor, according to the older neurophysiological literature, is the free nerve ending, but more recent evidence suggests that this sensation may actually have no specialized sensory ending.

The exact manner in which pain is mediated is unknown. Some investigators believe that the excitation of pain fibers is chemically mediated, and some chemicals have been identified. Several investigators have found that histamine injected into the skin caused pain; others have found that histamine is liberated at nerve endings by scraping the skin. Acetylcholine and serotonin have also been found to produce pain when applied to an area exposed by removal of blistered skin.

Overstimulation of most cutaneous receptors elicits pain. Investigations have consistently shown that the adequate stimulus for pain in the skin is either actually causing skin damage or is potentially apt to cause tissue damage. Thermal radiation threshold for pain is at a skin temperature around 45 degrees centigrade, and below 17 degrees centigrade. These temperatures are at the threshold range for tissue damage. Similarly, a needle prick at pain threshold will produce skin damage as shown by redness later. There are rare cases of pain analgesia, meaning relative insensibility to pain and some dissociation between it and touch. Pain is felt, but the aversive reaction to it is lost. The individual may even seek painful stimuli.

Although pain is perceived by all normal persons at about the same degree of tissue damage, not all people react similarly to pain. The possible reasons for this fact and other dimensions of pain tolerance will be examined more fully in Chapter 15, "Pain Perception and Motor Behavior."

D. DISTRIBUTION OF CUTANEOUS RECEPTORS

Investigations of cutaneous sensitivity have shown that each kind of cutaneous receptor is not uniformly distributed over the body surface. Density of touch receptors varies from an extremely high density in the fingertips to a low density in the back and thigh. The density of cold receptors varies from a high number on the upper lip to a minimum on the palm of the hand. The other cutaneous receptors have their unique distributions as well.

E. SENSORY RECEPTOR SPECIFICITY

Although the emphasis of cutaneous sensitivity has been on each type of nerve ending mediating a specific sensory quality, this specificity of function is far from perfect. Recent investigations demonstrate that there is not a simple one-to-one relationship between cutaneous stimulation and activation of specific receptors. For example, in some hairy parts of the body in which touch sensitivity is high there are no Meissner's corpuscles nor Pacinian corpuscles. It is believed that free nerve endings probably mediate the sense of touch in these regions of the body. It has also been found that, while Krause end bulbs seem to mediate cold and Ruffini endings seem to mediate warmth, there are some skin areas which are sensitive to cold and warmth which do not seem to contain these structures. Again, there is good evidence that free nerve endings may, in some way, mediate these sensations. On the basis of these rather puzzling findings about the relationships between functions of the cutaneous receptors, some investigators believe that there are no modality-specific cutaneous receptors; instead various sensory qualities emerge from different patterns of excitation of the various endings. On the other hand, other investigators are convinced that some cutaneous fibers are modality specific. In short, there is considerable controversy about the subject of cutaneous receptor specificity.

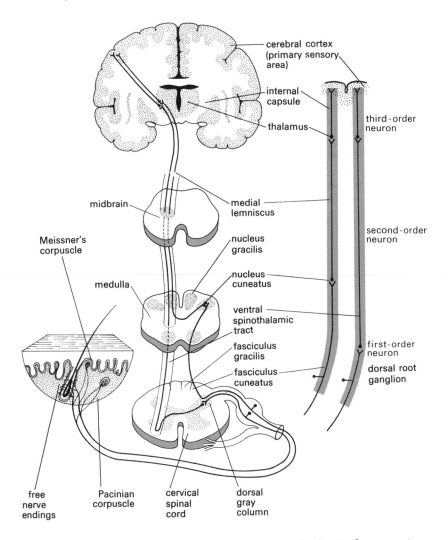

Fig. 5.2 Sensory pathways for touch and pressure. The fasciculus cuneatus or gracilis and the ventral spinothalamic tracts. (Based on Langley *et al.*, 1969.)

F. TRANSMISSION OF CUTANEOUS INFORMATION TO THE BRAIN

Impulses which have been triggered by stimuli impinging on the cutaneous receptors travel over afferent axons (also called fibers) in the peripheral nerves, enter the spinal cord, or brainstem in the case of cranial nerve transmission, and are transmitted by sensory (afferent) pathways to the brain. Most of the cutaneous sensory pathways terminate in the thalamus and cerebral cortex, which are the conscious centers for interpretation and perception of the sensations.

Upon entering the spinal cord, the fibers of cutaneous sensory neurons form two basic pathways to the brain: They ascend in the ipsilateral column of the cord to the medulla, without synaptic interruption; or they synapse with a neuron whose axon crosses the spinal cord and ascends in the contralateral portion of the cord. Three neurons typically make up the basic sensory chain: The sensory neuron which transmits the impulse from the receptor to the spinal cord and on to the first synapse is called the first-order neuron. The neuron that transmits the impulse up to the thalamus is the second-order neuron. Impulses conveyed from the thalamus to the cerebral cortex travel over the third-order neuron (Fig. 5.2). Of course, this is only the barest outline of the sensory transmission network. Each neuron gives off many collateral axons and receives synaptic connects from many other neurons.

G. THE SOMATOSENSORY CORTEX

Cutaneous sensory impulses are projected out of the thalamus into the somatosensory cortex in an orderly manner so that the topographic organization in the thalamus is preserved in the somatic cortex. The somatic cor-

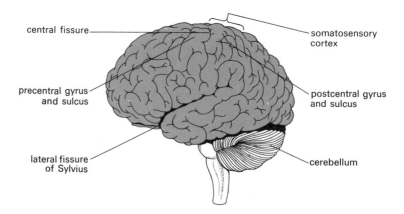

central fissure

somatosensory cortex

precentral gyrus and sulcus

postcentral gyrus and sulcus

lateral fissure of Sylvius

cerebellum

Fig. 5.3 Lateral surface of the brain showing the somatosensory cortex. (Based on Noback, 1967.)

tex is that portion of the cerebral cortex to which all of the cutaneous and proprioceptors send their sensory messages. It is located in the postcentral gyrus of the parietal lobe and extends from the longitudinal fissure into the lateral fissure (fissure of Sylvius) (Fig. 5.3). The precentral gyrus, or motor cortex, also receives some somatic projections; indeed, it seems likely that all parts of the cerebral cortex receive some somatosensory projections.

The somatic cortex is mapped out in topographical manner, and the amount of this area of the cortex devoted to a given region of the body surface is directly proportional to the use and sensitivity of that region. In other words, the sizes of the various somatic cortex areas are proportional to the number of specialized nerve endings in each peripheral area of the body. Thus, the lips, tongue, and thumb have a relatively large representation in the somatic cortex (Fig. 5.4).

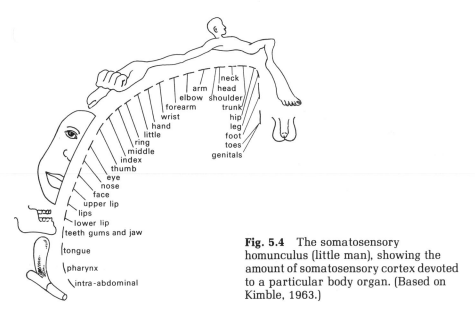

Fig. 5.4 The somatosensory homunculus (little man), showing the amount of somatosensory cortex devoted to a particular body organ. (Based on Kimble, 1963.)

The thalamus relays sensory signals into the somatic cortex where a better spatial representation is available; the somatic cortex is not primarily concerned with discriminating modalities of sensation. Instead, its function is almost entirely to determine from which area of the body a sensation originates. Thus dull and poorly localized pain and intense temperature stimuli can be perceived even when fiber tracts from the thalamus to the cortex are cut. Of course, exact localization or precise discrimination depends upon functional cortical mechanisms.

This localization ability of the somatic cortex is possible because of organization of nerve fibers throughout the nervous system. The nerve fibers are spatially oriented in the nerve trunks, in the spinal cord, in the thalamus, and in the cerebral cortex. Indeed, all the different nerve tracts of the CNS are spatially organized. In the dorsal columns of the spinal cord the sensory fibers from the feet lie toward the lateral side of the dorsal columns. This spatial organization is maintained with precision throughout the sensory pathway all the way from the receptor to the somatic cortex. Because of this organization, we can tell the difference between a song, a colorful sunset, or a slug on the arm only on the basis of the particular terminals in our brains to which the incoming nerve fibers are connected.

Electrical stimulation of cutaneous receptors evokes sensory effects mostly on the contralateral side of the cortex; in other words, receptors in the left side of the body send impulses primarily to the somatic cortex in the right side of the brain, while receptors in the right side of the body send their messages to the left somatic cortex. Tingling, numbness, a feeling of electricity or a sense of movement may result, but the sensation is perceived as an unusual rather than a normal experience. Penfield (1958) reported that the most frequently occurring sensations described by his patients when he electrically stimulated their somatic cortex during surgery were "a tingling or numbness or sense of movement."

The fibers of the somatic cortex and motor cortex are so intermingled that they may almost be considered a single mechanism. For example, electrical stimulation in the motor cortex has been found to elicit sensations as well as movement. On the other hand, stimulation of the somatic cortex may cause movements, as well as somatic sensations. The somatic cortex gives off fibers to motorneurons for cortical control of movement. At the same time, motor cortex fibers are known to project to subcortical somatic nuclei, so impulses from the motor cortex can modify electrical activity in these structures. This suggests that motor tracts may serve either a facilitative or inhibition function for transmission of information through subcortical somatic nuclei, thus altering the input into the cortex.

THE PROPRIOCEPTORS

In order to behave effectively, individuals must be able to monitor their own movements by knowing the relative position of the different parts of the body and by being able to maintain a particular orientation toward gravity. These functions are performed by complex sensory receptors called proprioceptors which are located in muscles, tendons, joints, and labyrinth of the inner ear. The proprioceptors keep the brain apprised of the physical state of the body at all times. The proprioceptors are usually considered together with the cutaneous senses because many of the receptors in the muscles, tendons, and joints look and function like those in the skin and because both groups travel to the brain through the same spinal and brainstem routes.

Sherrington (1906) introduced the word "proprioception" to include all those sensory systems which respond to stimuli arising in muscles, tendons, joints, and vestibular apparatus. The immediate stimuli arise from changes in length and from tension, compression, and shear forces arising from the effects of gravity, from movement of parts of the body, and from muscular contraction. The receptor cells in these mechanisms require mechanical deformation for their activation.

A. THE MUSCLE SPINDLE

The proprioceptor mechanism in skeletal muscles is the muscle spindle which consists of a fluid-filled capsule tapering at both ends 2 to 20 millimeters long. A spindle contains both sensory receptors and specialized muscle fibers. The capsule of the spindle lies in parallel with the main muscle fibers and is continuous at its two tapered ends with the connective tissue surrounding the regular muscle fibers. Muscle spindles are made up of from 4 to 12 specialized muscle fibers, with sensory receptors wrapped around a short noncontractible region near the middle of the spindle (Fig. 5.5). The stimulus that excites the muscle spindle receptors is the stretching of this specialized sensory region.

With the exception of a few muscles innervated by cranial nerves, muscle spindles are interspersed in all the skeletal muscles of the body. They are found in both flexors and extensors of every joint. The number of spindles in different muscle groups varies with their size, but more important than muscle size in the distribution of spindles is the degree of fine movement subserved by a muscle. The density of spindles tends to be particularly high in small muscles producing fine movements, such as those of the hand or the deep muscles of the neck.

1. Two types of muscle fibers and two types of motorneurons

Since the muscle spindle contains a unique type of muscle fiber, the *intrafusal* muscle, to avoid confusion it will be necessary to refer to the main skeletal muscles as *extrafusal* muscles. Moreover, the intrafusal muscle fibers of the spindle are supplied by a separate motor nerve supply from that of the extrafusal muscles, and the motorneurons which supply the intrafusal and extrafusal fibers have different names. Since the motorneuron axons that supply the intrafusal muscles have diameters of 2-8 millimicrons and transmit impulses at velocities of 10-50 m/sec., they have been labeled *gamma*

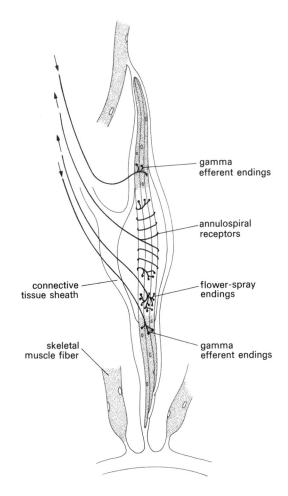

gamma
efferent endings

annulospiral
receptors

connective
tissue sheath

flower-spray
endings

skeletal
muscle fiber

gamma
efferent endings

Fig. 5.5 A muscle spindle. Three intrafusal muscle fibers are shown inside the connective tissue sheath. Arrows indicate direction of impulse transmission. (Based on Gardner, 1963.)

motorneurons. (Some authors use the term fusimotor neurons.) The motorneurons that innervate the extrafusal muscle fibers have diameters of 8-20 millimicrons and conduct at 50-120 m/sec.; they are called *alpha* motorneurons. In most spinal nerves, there is a complete deficiency of motor fibers of a size in between that of the alpha and gamma fibers. Therefore, motor fibers may be divided into large alpha fibers which supply ordinary extrafusal muscle fibers and smaller gamma fibers which supply exclusively the muscle spindle.

The essential feature of the muscle spindle is that it contains sensory receptors *and* muscle fibers; it, therefore, has both sensory and motor functions. Its structure and functions are complex. Therefore, since our focus in this chapter is on somatosensory structures and functions, the sensory aspects of the muscle spindle will be emphasized. In Chapter 8 its motor control functions will be examined.

2. Muscle spindle receptors and their stimulation.

As previously noted, the muscle spindle lies in parallel with the extrafusal muscles, with its ends attached to the sheaths of the extrafusal muscle fibers, so that its length varies in accord with those of the main muscle. The intrafusal muscle fibers of the spindle extend along its entire length but the contractile elements are absent near the middle of the spindle where the sensory receptors are located. The contractile portions of the intrafusal muscles occupy the end or polar regions of the muscle spindle and are supplied with motor nerve innervation by the gamma motorneuron fibers.

There are two types of sensory receptors in the muscle spindle. The primary receptor is called the annulospiral ending and it is located centrally within the spindle capsule. It is derived from a large medullated afferent fiber which subdivides and sends spirals round each of the intrafusal muscle fibers. The secondary sense receptors are located on either side of the central region of the spindle and they attach to the intrafusal fibers from small afferent fibers; they are called flower-spray endings. In general, the annulospiral endings are part of large, low-threshold, fast-conducting afferent neurons while the afferent neurons of the flower-spray endings tend to be small, high-threshold, and slow-conducting.

Both of these receptor groups are stimulated when the central region of the spindle is stretched, causing a mechanical deformation of the sense endings. The receptors may be stretched in three different ways: (1) By application of an external force that lengthens the whole extrafusal muscle; (2) by contraction of intrafusal muscle fibers; (3) by reduction in the firing of extrafusal fibers (so that they relax). When any of these events occurs, the intrafusal fibers are displaced, the sense endings are stretched, and nerve impulses are discharged toward the CNS. We shall examine the effects of these impulses and then return for a fuller description of the methods for stimulating the spindle receptors.

Impulses from the annulospiral receptors are transmitted over the afferent neuron and enter the spinal cord (or brainstem if they are from cranial nerves) where they synapse on alpha motorneurons which supply the extrafusal muscles in which the spindle is located. Impulses traveling over the alpha motorneurons produce contraction in the extrafusal muscle fibers. Collateral fibers from the spindle afferents ascend the CNS pathways to end in the cerebellum and somatosensory cortex.

We may now return to a fuller discussion of methods by which the spindle afferents may be stimulated. As noted above, one means by which the spindle receptors may be stimulated is the application of an external force that lengthens the whole muscle. Since the spindles are arranged in parallel with the extrafusal muscles, when the extrafusal muscles are stretched, such as when an external force is applied, this causes a stretch on the intrafusal fibers of the muscle spindle, which displaces the spindle receptors, causing them to fire off. This afferent discharge stimulates the alpha motorneurons to produce contraction in the extrafusal fibers of that muscle, which takes off the stretch on the intrafusal muscle fibers and the spindle afferents are silenced (Fig. 5.6). The knee jerk is an example of this particular phenomenon. When the patellar tendon is struck, the muscles in the thigh are stretched, including the muscle spindles; the spindle afferents fire off and transmit their impulses to the spinal cord where they synapse on alpha motorneurons supplying the anterior thigh muscles. The alpha motor-neurons cause contraction of this muscle group, and lower-leg extension is the result.

Spindle afferents can be fired a second way and can indirectly control extrafusal muscle contraction without stretch stimuli being externally supplied. This is called the "gamma loop" and works in this way: Impulses transmitted over the gamma motorneurons, the cell bodies of which lie in the

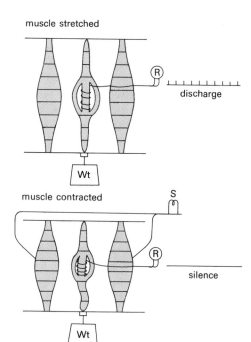

muscle stretched

discharge

Wt

muscle contracted

S

silence

Wt

Fig. 5.6 Muscle spindle is arranged in parallel to muscle fibers. Thus muscle contraction slackens tension on the spindle. (Based on T.C. Ruch and J.F. Fulton, 1960.)

spinal cord (or brainstem) produce intrafusal muscle contraction which stimulates the spindle afferents which in turn sends impulses back to the spinal cord. These impulses synapse on alpha motorneurons which then send signals to the extrafusal fibers in the same muscles, producing extrafusal muscle contraction.

A third method for spindle afferent stimulation occurs through the coordination of both alpha and gamma motorneurons. As previously noted, alpha motorneuron discharge causes the extrafusal muscle fibers to contract and tension is taken off the muscle spindle that is in parallel with it, and the spindle afferents will reduce or cease firing. However, if the gamma motorneurons cause intrafusal muscle contraction at the same time as the alpha motorneurons, the intrafusal muscle fibers will contract and therefore "take up the slack" in the intrafusal fibers so that now if there is a reduction in the firing of the extrafusal fibers, so that they begin to relax or lengthen, the spindle afferents are stimulated since the intrafusal fibers are stretched by the lengthening of the extrafusal fibers (Fig. 5.7).

This complex network of sensory and motor innervation between the muscle spindle and the extrafusal fibers serves important motor control functions. We shall take up these motor control functions in Chapter 8. For the present, we will concentrate on the CNS afferent transmission of muscle spindle signals.

3. Muscle spindle afferent transmission in the CNS

For the past 70 years there has been a great deal of controversy about spindle afferent transmission within the CNS. While the transmission from spindle afferent to alpha motorneurons for the production of reflex actions has been well documented for many years, this clearly is only a part of its central function. But whether the spindle afferent transmission also projects to higher centers has been unclear until rather recently.

Research over the past decade suggests that muscle afferents *do* project to the somatosensory cortex of the cerebrum via the dorsal column system (Oscarsson and Rosen, 1963; Eccles, 1973). However, the fact that spindle afferent impulses project to the somatic cortex does not in itself indicate that the sensory information is consciously perceived. Indeed, there is considerable information suggesting that projections from muscle receptors do not subserve conscious awareness of position or movement to muscle. Instead, they are generally viewed as being used in the control of movement and posture without producing any conscious sensation, in spite of projecting to the cerebral cortex. Matthews (1972) succinctly summarizes the current belief of neurophysiologists with regard to the role of spindle transmission to muscle perception.

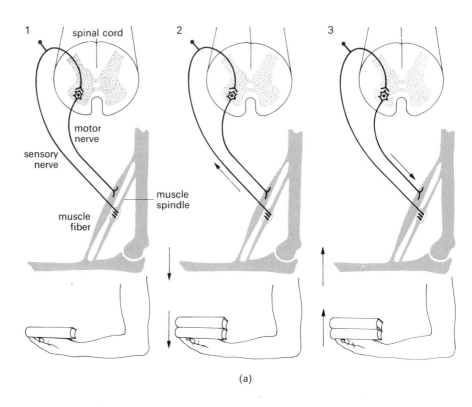

(a)

Fig. 5.7 In (a) the schematic illustration shows how the stretch reflex is mediated. A muscle is under the influence of the stretch reflex when it is engaged in a steady contraction of a voluntary nature, such as when a person's elbow is flexed steadily against a load (1). A sudden unexpected increase in the load (2) stretches the muscle, causing the sensory receptors in the muscle spindle to send nerve impulses to the spinal cord (upward arrow), where they impinge on an alpha motorneuron at a synapse and excite it. As a result, motor impulses are sent to the extrafusal muscle (downward arrow), where they cause it to contract (3). More complicated nervous pathways than the one shown may also be involved in the stretch reflex. Any real muscle is, of course, supplied with many motorneuron fibers and spindles.

In (b) the servomechanism involved in the control of voluntary muscle contractions is shown. The basic diagram (1) is the same as it is in the illustration of the stretch reflex, but with provision made for impulses from the brain to cause the intrafusal muscle fibers to contract by way of the gamma motorneurons. When a signal is transmitted along gamma motor fibers (2), the intrafusal muscle fibers contract, exciting the spindle sensory ending, just as if the spindle had been stretched. Consequently a contraction of the main muscle is excited by way of the gamma-loop (3, 4). In a real muscle this is further complicated by the existence of a direct pathway from the brain to the alpha motorneurons. (Based on Merton, 1972.)

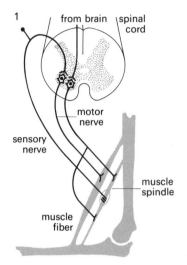

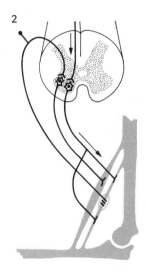

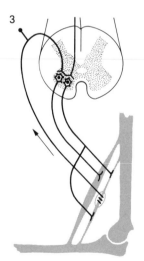

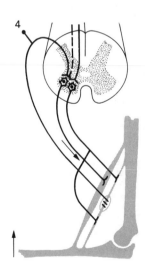

(b)

Thus, whatever else they may do, muscle spindles...would appear to have no part to play in the development of our immediate conscious awareness of the position of different parts of our body. This is not to deny, however, that they may play some part in the development of yet more elaborate perceptions.

Muscle spindle afferent transmission to the cerebellum is carried over many fibers via the spinocerebellar tracts in the spinal cord and over cranial nerves which synapse in the pons for spindle afferents from the head

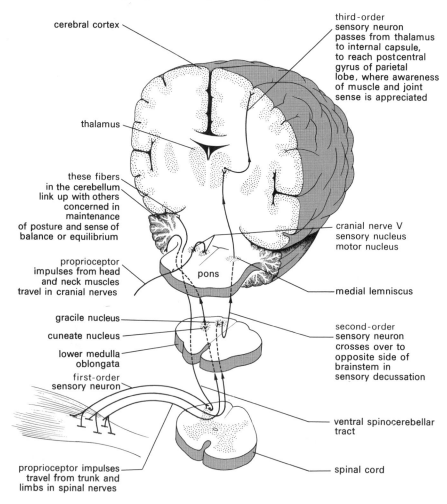

Fig. 5.8 Proprioceptive pathways to the brain. (Based on McNaught and Callander, 1963.)

and neck muscles (Fig. 5.8). It has long been accepted that the cerebellum uses the muscle afferent information in regulating muscle contraction, since the effects of cerebellar damage show the great importance of this structure in motor regulation. However, precisely what it does and how it does it remain mostly unknown. Thus, knowledge is almost totally lacking about the use to which the cerebellum puts the input it receives from the muscle afferents.

B. THE GOLGI TENDON ORGAN

The sensory receptor which is responsible for detection of tension on a tendon and the extent of muscle contraction is called the Golgi tendon organ. Its location is in the tendon near the ends of muscle fibers. Tendon organs usually lie at the musculotendinous junction rather than in the tendon proper; they occur at the origin and insertion of a muscle (Fig. 5.9).

The tendon organ is generally supplied by a single medullated nerve fiber of relatively large size (8–12 millimicrons). The main nerve fiber of the tendon organ breaks up into a series of nonmedullated sprays and each ending is enclosed in a delicate capsule which is closely applied to the surface of the tendon. In general, 3–25 muscle fibers insert on each tendon organ. When a muscle contracts, it develops forces which are applied to tendon organs, causing them to discharge.

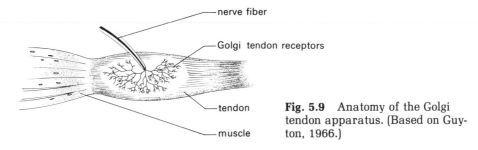

Fig. 5.9 Anatomy of the Golgi tendon apparatus. (Based on Guyton, 1966.)

1. Golgi tendon organ stimulation and functions

The classical notion of Golgi tendon function is that it serves as a reflex mechanism to protect muscles and tendons when tension produced by muscle contraction becomes too great. When tendon organ receptors are stimulated, impulses are sent to the spinal cord where they synapse on inhibitory interneurons which in turn synapse on alpha motorneurons serving the extrafusal muscles to which the tendon organ is attached. The result is that the alpha motorneuron stops firing and the muscle stops contracting. Thus, tension is taken off the tendon. This is the so-called clasp-knife reflex.

Recent research suggests that it is unlikely that tendon organs function in a purely protective capacity. It is true that simple passive stretch of a non-contracting muscle stimulates tendon organs only when quite a large tension has been built up, and the muscle stretched beyond its normal length. The knowledge about such activity in the tendon organs is what led to the belief that tendon organs were only high threshold receptors with their function only to reflexively shut off the alpha motorneurons when the tension in a muscle became dangerously high. However, recent studies have indicated that the threshold of tendon organs is considerably lower for active muscle contraction than for passive stretch; that is, tendon receptors have a low threshold for their preferred stimulus, which is tension produced by muscle contraction (Houk and Hennemon, 1967).

Tendon organs are now viewed as sensory receptors with a low threshold for their appropriate stimulus and as supplying the CNS with a signal which is suitable for helping continuously to regulate the strength of muscle contraction (Matthews, 1972). Jansen and Rudjord (1964) suggest that the tendon organ "continuously provides information about the degree of active contraction in the muscle." And Houk and Henneman (1967) note that "tendon organs continuously transmit to the spinal cord a filtered sample of the active forces being produced in the muscle."

This recently discovered function of the Golgi tendon organs does not imply that the clasp-knife reflex function is no longer present. On the contrary, this safety mechanism for protection of muscles and tendons is still considered to be a valuable function for tendon organs when extreme tension is built up on a tendon. It prevents tearing of the muscles or tendons from their attachments. As the tension within the tendon mounts, the tendon organ increases the rate of discharge which in turn increases the rate of discharge of inhibitory stimuli into the alpha motorneurons. When tension becomes dangerous, the inhibitory transmission to the alpha motorneurons tends to inhibit their firing.

2. Golgi tendon organ transmission in the CNS

Golgi tendon fibers send impulses into the CNS to produce the activity which has been described above. They also give off collateral fibers which ascend the spinal cord and enter the brain. They have a fairly direct route via the spinocerebellar tract to the cerebellum, but they do not reach the cerebral cortex in any direct manner. Thus, the tendon organs, like the muscle afferents, appear not to have any part in the development of our immediate consciousness of the position of the different parts of our body, but it is possible that they also may play some part in more elaborate perceptions, just as with the muscle afferents.

C. JOINT RECEPTORS

In the joints throughout the body are found receptors which are stimulated when the bones which come together at a joint are moved in any direction. Some authors call these kinesthetic receptors, but others refer to them as joint receptors. We shall use the latter term.

1. Joint receptor types and stimulation

There are actually three structurally different types of receptor groups located in the tissue around joints. The "spray-type" of Ruffini endings which resemble those found in the skin are by far the most common. Typically, an afferent axon of 5–10 millimicron diameter divides once or twice and then each branch divides into a series of fine sprays, and each set of sprays is enclosed in a capsule. From the functional standpoint, the entire collection of sprays supplied by a single axon comprises a sensory unit. These endings are arranged in three dimensions in the connective tissue capsule of the joints, but not in the synovial lining membrane. This location makes them

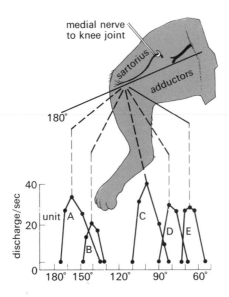

Fig. 5.10 Joint receptor discharge patterns. Five joint receptor units were isolated from the medial nerve to the knee joint of a cat. Each unit fired only over a restricted range of knee positions and had a maximum at one fairly sharply defined point. The discharge was constant at a stable position of the joint, but became elevated during movements within the response range for that unit. (Based on Skoglund, 1956.)

well suited to signal the rate, direction, and extent of joint movement as well as the steady position of the joint.

A second joint receptor resembles the Golgi tendon organ and like those found in the tendon is supplied by a large medullated afferent nerve fiber. It is located in the ligaments of the joint and is never found in unsupported areas of the capsule. This type of receptor is much less numerous than the Ruffini-type receptor. Modified Pacinian corpuscles form a third type of joint receptor. They are less numerous than either of the other types of receptors.

Several investigators have found that as a joint is moved steadily, joint receptors begin firing at a certain angle and fire gradually more rapidly for the next 10–15 degrees and then will slow down and stop as the angle of peak stimulation for those particular receptors is passed (Fig. 5.10). Since different receptors discharge at different angles, the entire movement of that joint is covered by a series of receptors, each firing during part of the range of movement. If movement is stopped at a certain joint angle, the receptors that normally fire at that angle adapt slightly within a few seconds, and then maintain discharging indefinitely. In addition to being sensitive to the absolute value of the angle of the joint position, the receptors appear to also be sensitive to the angular velocity of movement, because the firing rate increases for movements toward the angle of maximum excitation and decreases for movement away from it, regardless of the actual direction of movement.

2. Joint transmission in the CNS

The joint afferent fibers enter the CNS and ascend to the brain in a manner similar to the muscle spindles and Golgi tendon organs. In addition to projecting into the cerebellum, the joint receptors also send impulses to the thalamus and on to the somatic cortex.

3. Joint function in movement perception

The functions of the joint receptors which were described above have been the basis for the notion that the joint receptors subserve our perception of body position and body movement, since these impulses are known to project to the somatosensory cortex. But a recent report by Burgess and Clark (1969) places the traditional notion of the joint receptors function in jeopardy. They found a completely insignificant proportion of joint receptors to be maximally activated at some intermediate joint angle. They showed that virtually all endings had optimal angles for firing at the extremes of movement, and that there were practically none with preferred angles in between. Moreover, the majority of the receptors were completely silent when the joint was held anywhere between the two extremes, so that no nerve impulses appeared to be transmitted to the CNS from the joint. Finally, many of the receptors fired equally well at full extension and at full flexion so their signals would appear to be irrelevant in helping the CNS decide between those two contrasting positions.

The implications of these findings are significant but further research is needed to confirm their validity. In the meantime, it seems clear that joint receptors do provide accurate proprioceptive information over a wide range of joint angles because it has been consistently demonstrated that rate of firing following passive movement in afferent fibers serving the joint is a linear function of joint angle.

D. THE VESTIBULAR APPARATUS

One important part of the proprioceptive sense is not obtained from muscle or joint action but arises in the vestibular apparatus, located adjacent to the inner ear. The vestibular apparatus is sensitive to two kinds of information: First, it is sensitive to the position of the head in space; i.e., it signals whether the head is upright, upside down, or in some other position; second, it is sensitive to sudden changes in direction of movement of the body. The vestibular system is sometimes classified as part of the visual system because one of its functions is to assist in visual fixation during head and body movements, and some texts classify it with the auditory system, presumably because it is in close proximity to the auditory system and both systems are connected to the CNS by the same cranial nerve. However, since the underlying function of the vestibular apparatus is to maintain equilibrium and to preserve a constant plane of head position primarily by modifying muscle tone, in addition to its role in directing the gaze of the eyes, we have followed the example of most texts in placing this mechanism with the proprioceptors.

The vestibular apparatus is a part of the membranous labyrinth inside the temporal lobe in the inner ear area. One part of the bony membranous labyrinth is concerned with hearing. This part is contained in the cochlea. The other part of this structure makes up the five parts of the vestibular apparatus: three semicircular canals; the utricle; and the saccule. These structures contain a sensory epithelium (thin covering) with sensitive hair cells which produce neural impulses when displaced. The internal cavities of these structures are linked together and contain fluid endolymph (thick fluid) (Fig. 5.11).

1. The semicircular canals

The semicircular canals may be viewed as angular accelerometers because they lie in planes at right angles to each other and are stimulated by rota-

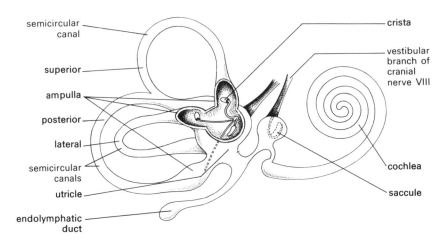

semicircular canal

crista

vestibular branch of cranial nerve VIII

superior

ampulla

posterior

lateral

cochlea

semicircular canals

utricle

saccule

endolymphatic duct

Fig. 5.11   The right bony labyrinth showing the structure of the vestibular apparatus. (Based on McNaught and Callander, 1963.)

tions of the head or body in any one of three planes or in any combination of the three. Each canal is filled with fluid endolymph and the sense endings are in the enlarged end of each canal, the ampulla, near its junction with the utricle. In each ampulla there is a ridge of epithelium, the crista ampullaris, in which are embedded numerous hair cells which project finger-like processes upward into a semigelatinous material known as the cupula. The processes embedded in the cupula constitute the sense endings in the vestibular apparatus; the hair cells are the afferent neurons. The cupula, which is shaped like an upside-down thimble, encloses the finger-like extensions of the hair cells and extends up into the ampulla. This arrangement of sensory receptors in the semicircular canals functions so that whenever the head undergoes angular or rotatory acceleration or deceleration the sense endings are mechanically displaced, and the hair cells to which they are attached transduce movement of the fluid into nerve impulses (Fig. 5.12).

If the head is moved, the inertia of the fluid in the canal causes the fluid to move in a direction opposite to that of the movement. When the cupula bends to one side or the other it excites the hair cells to initiate sensory impulses. If the movement stops, the fluid continues to flow momentarily and the cupula is bent in the opposite direction. It can be seen, then, that the maximal stimulation of the hair cells occurs when the inertia is greatest, i.e., when motion is starting or ending. If motion is continued at a steady rate in the same direction, such as while riding in an automobile, then very little semicircular sensation occurs (Fig. 5.13).

Excitation of the semicircular canals occurs primarily from acceleration or deceleration and change of direction. Thus, these structures apprise the nervous system of sudden changes in movement. This information allows

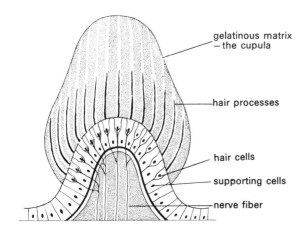

gelatinous matrix
— the cupula

hair processes

hair cells

supporting cells

nerve fiber

Fig. 5.12 The crista ampullaris and the cupula in which the hair processes are embedded. (Based on Woodburne, 1967.)

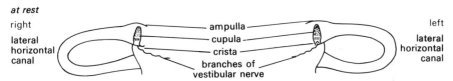

at rest

right
lateral
horizontal
canal

ampulla
cupula
crista
branches of
vestibular nerve

left
lateral
horizontal
canal

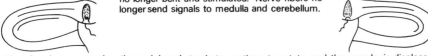

When **head starts to rotate** (e.g., to the right) the endolymph in the semicircular canals which lie at right angles to the axis of rotation tends to lag behind the movement of the head and the cupula is displaced, hair cells are stimulated and ingoing impulses form afferent pathways for reflexes leading to alteration in tone of muscles in neck, trunk, and limbs to avoid body losing balance.

After **the initial inertia is overcome** the endolymph no longer lags behind the movement of the head and the cupula is no longer displaced, hair cells are no longer bent and stimulated. Nerve fibers no longer send signals to medulla and cerebellum.

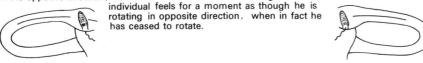

When **head stops rotating** the endolymph tends to continue to rotate and the cupula is displaced in the opposite direction, hair cells are bent, nerve fibers signal rotation of head to left, individual feels for a moment as though he is rotating in opposite direction, when in fact he has ceased to rotate.

Fig. 5.13 Diagram of how movement stimulates receptors in the semicircular canals. (Based on McNaught and Callander, 1963.)

certain brain centers to make necessary balance adjustments, sometimes even before imbalance occurs. These kinds of adjustments are essential in sports where directions change and movements occur so rapidly.

One final point in regard to the semicircular canals needs to be made. Since they achieve maximal sensitivity for rotary acceleration and deceleration, they sacrifice sensitivity to linear acceleration and deceleration. Thus, other parts of the vestibular apparatus are maximally activated by linear movements.

2. The utricles and saccule

The utricles and saccule operate differently and give different kinds of information from the semicircular canals, although the receptor cells of these structures are very similar to those in the semicircular canals. The information signaled by these structures is mainly concerned with body position in relation to the force of gravity; they respond to linear acceleration, i.e., movement of the head in a straight line, that is, forward, backward, upward, downward, or tilting of the head. Thus, regardless of the position of the body in space, the utricle and saccule provide information about body position with reference to the force of gravity; they do this by responding to changes in the position of the head in space.

The utricle and saccule are located in the upper-posterior part of the vestibule (Fig. 5.14). On the wall of these structures there is a thickening where the epithelium contains hair cells. This thickened structure is called the macula, and it contains sensory cells in its base which project finger-like hairs up into a gelatinous membrane, the otolith organ, in which many small calcium carbonate crystals, known as otoconia, are embedded. Since the density of the otolith organ is about three times that of the canal fluid, when the head is suddenly changed, the otoconia, which have greater inertia than the fluid in the canal, bend the hair tufts to one side, which motion is then transduced into nerve impulses by the hair cells.

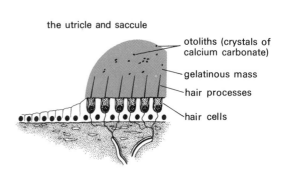

the utricle and saccule

otoliths (crystals of calcium carbonate)

gelatinous mass

hair processes

hair cells

Fig. 5.14   The utricle and saccule structure. (Based on McNaught and Callander, 1963.)

The hair cells of the utricle are set in a horizontal plane whereas those of the saccule lie in the vertical plane. The utricle, then, is maximally stimulated when the head is bent either forward or backward, and is minimally excited when the head is erect. The saccule appears to be maximally stimulated when the head is bent to the side. Thus, it is believed that the utricle supplies information about disturbances to equilibrium by shifting forward and back, while the saccule supplies data about disturbances to equilibrium by tilting laterally.

Sensory information relayed to the CNS from the utricle and saccule causes rapid adjustments of the body to a more stable position. Our upright posture and rapid adjustments to acceleration or deceleration are primarily controlled by these receptors. Although rotatory motion will of course move the otolithic organs in these structures, the semicircular canals have the advantage for this kind of motion sensitivity. The utricle and saccule are very close to the center of the head and are therefore not subject to much centrifugal force in normal head movements.

3. Vestibular transmission in the CNS

Vestibular transmission is complex and ubiquitous. The hair cells are the sensory organs for the vestibular nerve which projects via the eighth cranial nerve into the CNS. Since the vestibular apparatus is the most highly specialized part of the proprioceptive senses, it is connected very closely with the body musculature to carry out the adjustments mentioned above. Some of these connections are made directly down the spinal cord via the vestibulospinal tract. However, the major transmission network for the equilibrium is mediated through the cerebellum. This structure coordinates most of the movements involved in orientation of the body in space.

First-order fibers leading from the hair cells of the semicircular canals, utricle, and saccule have their cell bodies in the vestibular ganglion located near the vestibular apparatus. The nerve fibers of these cells project into the medulla as the vestibular branch of the eighth cranial nerve just below the pons. The vestibular nerve on each side passes to four vestibular nuclei in the medulla and pons of the brainstem. The names of the four vestibular nuclei are superior, medial, lateral, and spinal vestibular nuclei. With one exception, the first-order fibers from the vestibular ganglion synapse in one of these four nuclei. The exception is that some first-order neurons fibers from the vestibular ganglion lead directly to the cerebellum (Fig. 5.15).

After synapsing in the vestibular nuclei, the second-order neurons proceed in the following pathways: second-order neurons from the superior vestibular nucleus, which is found entirely within the pons, ascend mainly contralaterally and synapse in various nuclei for eye muscle movement. These oculomotor centers mediate the vestibular nystagmus reflex which is eli-

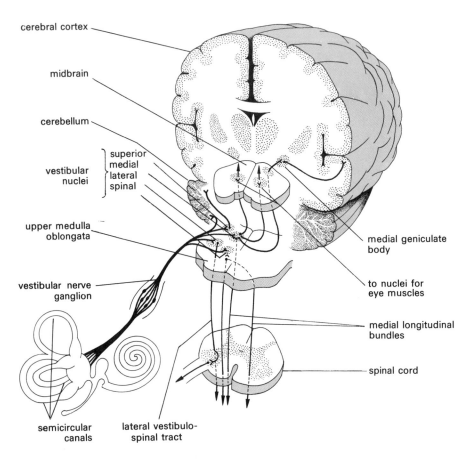

cerebral cortex

midbrain

cerebellum

vestibular nuclei

⎱ superior
⎰ medial
⎱ lateral
⎰ spinal

upper medulla oblongata

vestibular nerve ganglion

semicircular canals

lateral vestibulo-spinal tract

medial geniculate body

to nuclei for eye muscles

medial longitudinal bundles

spinal cord

Fig. 5.15   The vestibular pathways of impulse transmission. (Based on McNaught and Callander, 1963.)

cited when a person rotates about the body axis. The eyes perform a series of slow movements in a direction opposite to the rotation, with alternating quick return sweeps. The slow phase serves to retain a stationary image on the retina. The quick phase occurs when it becomes no longer possible to fixate on an object because of the rotation and the eyes sweep forward to fixate on a new object. However, this reflex does occur in dark and is therefore not dependent on vision.

Fibers in the cells of the lateral vestibular nucleus proceed down on the same side and form the lateral vestibulospinal tract. This tract runs down the spinal cord and makes possible reflex adjustment of bodily orientation and position to vestibular stimulation. It seems that this is the only direct connection between vestibular nuclei and the alpha motorneurons of the spinal cord for movements of trunk and limbs.

The spinal vestibular nucleus is limited to the medulla. The second-order fibers of this nucleus cross contralaterally and descend to lower parts of the medulla to innervate nuclei to cause reflex coordination of eyes, neck-muscle movement, and cerebellar adjustment of equilibrium.

The medial vestibular nucleus is considered the principal nucleus because it is the largest in size. It has two celled divisions. From its large-celled division second-order fibers cross the midline and divide, some ascending and some descending. These fibers make connections with eye nuclei and with the cervical cord for neck and shoulder movement. The fibers of the small-celled division form the major pathway for reflex visceral responses to vestibular stimulation. This series of nervous pathways makes possible the reflexes of vomiting and facial pallor which occur from excessive vestibular stimulation. The medial vestibular nucleus sends a profusion of fibers into the cerebellum, just as do most of the other vestibular nuclei. Collectively, then, vestibular innervation with the cerebellum is quite widespread.

At the present, it does not appear that vestibular pathways mediate directly with the thalamus for cortical projection. There is evidence, though, that vestibular impulses do arrive indirectly in a limited area of the cerebral cortex that is contiguous with the somatosensory cortex. In contrast to the visual and auditory systems, the vestibular system does not appear to fit the scheme of sensory modality specificity because in the vestibular cortex some 80 percent of the neurons are also influenced by muscle spindle and joint afferents in monkeys (Schwarz and Fredrickson, 1971). Thus, central convergence of these two modalities of proprioceptive afferents is apparently essential not only for lower reflex mechanisms but also for the conscious perception of position and movement.

4. Vestibular function

Most vestibular apparatus impulses are used for reflex purposes. In most cases, it is limited to reflex movements of the head and neck in coordination with eye-muscle movements. The impulses from the vestibular apparatus do, however, play a critical part in the maintenance of our upright posture and equilibrium. Impulses from the vestibulospinal tract exert a strong tonic effect on the antigravity muscles. If damage or severance occurs to fiber tracts above the vestibular nuclei, this has the effect of eliminating the central inhibitory control, which is normally maintained by cortical and subcortical mechanisms above the level of the vestibular nuclei. The result is an exaggerated extensor thrust (contraction of postural muscles) and the individual becomes rigid all over. This is called decerebrate rigidity.

Righting reflexes are primarily mediated by the vestibular apparatus. These righting reflexes are primary over other sensory and motor systems and they are a powerful force in bringing the body back to an upright position. The head takes the lead in the righting reflex. Once the head orientation occurs, the reflexes for orienting neck, shoulders, and body follow in sequential order. The righting reflexes will be discussed in more detail in Chapter 8.

5. Coordination of other proprioceptors with the vestibular apparatus

The detection of the position of the body in space is not just a function of the vestibular apparatus. Certainly, one of the most important information mechanisms necessary for the maintenance of equilibrium is that derived from joint and muscle spindle receptors in the neck. These proprioceptors in the neck apprise the CNS of the orientation of the head with respect to the body. When the head is bent forward or backward, the vestibular system sends information on the position of the head. Simultaneously, proprioceptors in the neck send information that the head is angulating in relation to the rest of the body. The information is processed by the higher brain centers and necessary muscular adjustments are made, after coordination of the two sets of data. Thus, while the vestibular apparatus detects head position, additional information is required because the relationship of the head to the body must be known. Proprioceptors in the neck supply this essential information and are therefore as necessary for regulating equilibrium as are the reflexes initiated in the vestibular apparatus. Of course, vision, and pressure sensations from the footpads, also play an important role in the orientation of the body in space, but the vestibular apparatus and other proprioceptors will bring about righting reflexes even if the visual receptors, or pressure receptors in the feet, are damaged or destroyed.

All of the proprioceptors provide sensory data which when organized and combined with information mainly from the cerebellum (for equilibrium) provide the basis for movement patterns, muscle tone, and the stimulation of muscles for upright bodily posture.

6

The Visual System

We live primarily in a visual world. Vision dominates our lives and, of all the senses, vision is the richest source of information about our environment. During motor behavior humans depend especially heavily on the visual system; it is an important source of information about appropriate movements for performing a particular task—indeed the observation of others performing a task usually precedes our own efforts to perform. Vision is one of the primary monitors of movement—during the performance of a task, if it is done slowly enough, vision may be used to make movement corrections to bring the performance to the intended goal. Finally, the consequences of employing a certain movement pattern is conveyed via the visual system—we see what we have done.

In order to understand how light energy in our environment can be detected and processed into meaningful perceptual information for the guidance and control of motor behavior, we must first examine how light energy from stimulus objects enters the eye and is focused so as to cast an image on visual receptors which, when stimulated, transmit impulses to central processing centers where visual perception occurs. In this chapter our concern will be with the basic structure and function of the visual system. In a later chapter we will examine visual perception and motor behavior.

RADIANT ENERGY

The light that stimulates the eye is a form of electromagnetic radiation. It belongs in the same class of phenomena as radio waves, heat waves, X-rays, and cosmic rays. Light waves travel through free space with a velocity of about 186,000 miles per second, and light waves, like ocean waves, may have peaks which are very close to one another or widely separated from each other. The distance between the peaks of two light waves is called wavelength, and wavelength is the only basic feature of visible light (that which the human eye can process) which differentiates it from X-rays, ultraviolet waves, and radio waves. A second physical aspect of radiant energy is its quantity. The quantity of radiant energy in light that falls on a unit area of the visual receptors in a defined unit of time can be specified in terms of the height or amplitude of the wave and is subjectively interpreted in some degree of brightness (Fig. 6.1).

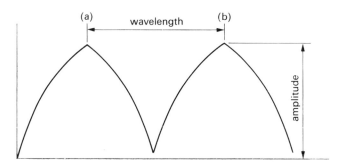

Fig. 6.1   The distance between a and b is wavelength. The visible spectrum is between the wavelengths of 400 and 750 nanometers.

Visible light is a very small region of the total electromagnetic spectrum, or range, of wavelengths. Wavelengths extend from radio waves, with wavelengths of many miles, to cosmic rays, with wavelengths of 0.00005 nanometers (one nanometer = one-billionth of a meter). The wavelength limits of the light visible to humans extend from about 400 nanometers, which are perceived as violet light, to about 750 nanometers, which are perceived as red light. This part of the electromagnetic spectrum that humans can actually see is called the visible spectrum. The eye can be excited only by wavelengths of light that fall within the visible spectrum; radiations of wavelengths beyond these limits are not visible and, therefore, are not considered to be light (Fig. 6.2). It may be seen, then, that the various wavelengths are the basis of color discrimination, and the colors of the visible spectrum are the subjective interpretation of certain wavelengths.

Light waves are produced by objects that give off radiant energy. A light bulb, the sun, a match, are examples of stimulus objects that emit radiant energy. Some stimulus objects do not produce radiant energy, but rather they reflect radiant energy. For example, a light bulb in a room pro-

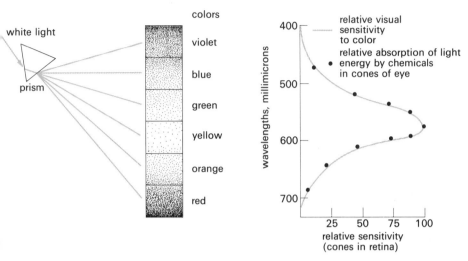

Fig. 6.2   The visible colors of light and their wavelengths. The chart shows the relative sensitivity of the human eye to color. The eye is most sensitive to green-ish-yellow. The dots on the curve indicate relative absorption of light energy by chemicals in the cones of the eye.

duces radiant energy that strikes the wall. That radiant energy is then re-flected from the wall to the individual's receptors in the eye. A desk or chair are other examples of objects that reflect, rather than emit, radiant energy. The human eye can, of course, be excited by light waves that are radiant or reflected.

ANATOMY OF THE EYE

The visual process consists of five basic components: (1) The refraction of light rays and the focusing of images on the sensory receptors of the eye. (2) The transduction of light energy by photochemical activity into nerve im-pulses. (3) The processing of neural activity at the receptors and the trans-mission of impulses through the optic nerve. (4) The processing in the brain culminating in perception. (5) The reflexes associated with the visual system.

   To carry out the eye's mechanical tasks, several structures exist in the eyeball. The light first passes through the cornea, the pupil, and lens, and then finally falls on the retina of the eye. At the retina, light is transduced into nerve impulses which are then projected into the cortex where visual perception occurs (Fig. 6.3).

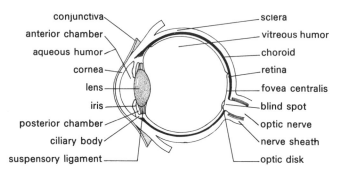

conjunctiva

anterior chamber

aqueous humor

cornea

lens

iris

posterior chamber

ciliary body

suspensory ligament

sclera

vitreous humor

choroid

retina

fovea centralis

blind spot

optic nerve

nerve sheath

optic disk

Fig. 6.3 Anatomy of the eye. (Based on DeCoursey, 1968.)

A. THE CORNEA AND SCLERA

The cornea is a transparent structure forming the anterior one-sixth of the fibrous tunic of the eye. It is an important part of the refractory system of the eye. The sclera is the white coat of the eye which makes up the posterior five-sixths of the eyeball and contains a hard, unyielding membrane which serves to maintain the form of the eyeball. At the posterior of the eyeball, the sclera is punctured by the fibers of the optic nerve.

B. THE PUPIL AND IRIS

The pupil is the black circle that you see when you look into a person's eye. It is simply an opening which changes in size to admit smaller or larger amounts of light. The size of the pupil is controlled by a special set of muscles, and it opens and closes as these muscles contract and relax. This control of the amount of light entering the eye is exercised at the pupil by both circular and radial muscle fibers (pupillary muscles) in the iris, which is a delicate, colored (commonly brown or blue), fibrous structure which lies just in front of the lens. When the circular fibers of the iris contract, the pupil becomes smaller; when the radial fibers contract, the pupil enlarges. When too much light enters the eye, the circular fibers of the iris contract, reducing the size of the pupil. This mechanism of the pupillary reaction is triggered by the reflex reactions to visual sensory input.

C. THE LENS

The lens is a clear transparent tissue which lies just behind the iris and has a convex shape. This structure is held in place by suspensory ligaments and is innervated by the ciliary muscle. The suspensory ligaments ordinarily are tight and keep the lens flattened, but when the ciliary muscle contracts it pulls the ends of the suspensory ligaments forward causing the lens to assume a more convex shape. As these muscle fibers contract and relax, the lens changes in shape, and by changing its shape the lens assures that a sharp image of the stimulus object falls on the sensory receptors at the back of the eyeball.

As the distance of objects changes, the muscles of the lens contract and relax. These variations in the shape of the lens produce a sharp image of the object on the sensory receptors. This adjustment in focusing power which enables the eye to focus on objects at various distance is called accommodation. Without this lens-accommodation mechanism, visual stimuli would be fuzzy and unclear rather than sharp and clear. This action of accommodation produced by contraction or relaxation of the ciliary muscle is, of course, a reflex response to nerve impulses which are triggered by the excitation of visual receptors.

D. CHAMBERS OF THE EYE

Structurally, the eyeball may be divided into two chambers, with the lens separating the chambers. Both chambers are filled with fluids which serve to maintain the shape of the eyeball and support structures within the eyeball. The anterior chamber is filled with aqueous humor; and the large chamber posterior to the lens is filled with vitreous humor.

E. THE RETINA

The retina is complex structure consisting of the photosensitive receptors and other layers of cells which give support to the receptors or assist in the transmission of impulses. This structure lines about 180 degrees of the eyeball on its inner posterior surface. It is here that light energy is transduced into nerve impulses.

Although the retina is very thin, ten distinct layers of cells may be differentiated (Fig. 6.4). At the back of the retina is a dark vascular coat which lines the inner part of the eyeball called the choriod. Associated with the choriod is a black pigment layer of cells which darkens the interior of the eye and absorbs the light rays which were not successful in activating the photopigments in the visual receptors. If excess light were not absorbed, it would be reflected and activate photoreceptors throughout the retina, and thus blur sharp resolution.

1. The visual receptors

The next layer of cells in the retina contains the visual receptor cells which are sensitive to light, the rods and cones. The rods and cones make synaptic connections with bipolar cells, which form the middle cellular lamina in the retina and serve mainly to relay stimulus information from the rods and cones to the final major retinal layer where ganglion cells are located. The ganglion cells give rise to the nerve fibers forming the optic nerve.

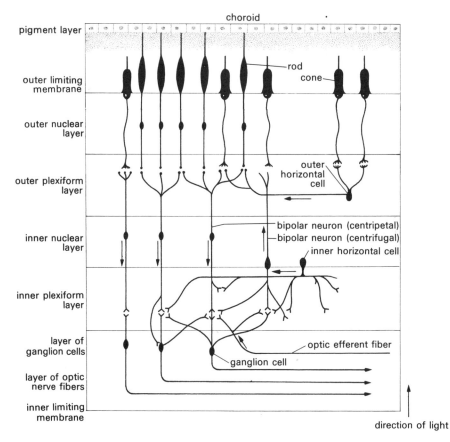

Fig. 6.4   The retina and the cells of the eye structure. (Based on Noback, 1967.)

Although the rods and cones are the photosensitive sense organs for vision, they are located, paradoxically, in the back portion of the retina and actually face away from the front of the eye. Thus, light must travel through all of the layers of the retina before reaching the visual receptors. The anatomical reason for this is that during embryonic maturation the optic vesicle projects outward from the brain and then folds back to form the optic cup.

Rods and cones are excited by light energy, and they transduce light energy into nerve impulses. They actually comprise about 70 percent of all of the sensory receptors of the entire body, so perhaps it is understandable why we depend so much upon vision. These visual receptor cells are so named because of their shape, the rods being long and narrow while the cones are slightly shorter and have a bulblike appearance (Fig. 6.5).

In addition to being different in appearance, the rods and cones are responsible for different kinds of vision. Rods are the photoreceptors most

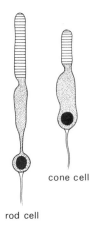

cone cell

rod cell

Fig. 6.5 Sensory receptor cells of the retina. On the left, a rod cell; on the right, a cone cell. (Based on DeCoursey, 1968.)

sensitive to light and are, therefore, the primary receptors for night vision. Rod vision, at threshold, is about 1000 times more sensitive than cone vision. Rods are used primarily in "black-white" vision so they are called achromatic (absence of color vision). Conversely, cones function best at a high intensity of illumination, so they are considered the day photoreceptors. In addition, cones contain special photochemicals which enable us to have color vision.

There are about 120 million rods and 6 million cones in the human retina, but only about one million ganglion cells whose nerve fibers form the optic nerve. Thus, single ganglion cells connect, by way of bipolar cells, to numerous receptor cells. There are three major types of connections between the ganglion cells and the rods and cones. The first and most direct transmission network is found only among some cones in the fovea (this part of the eyeball will be described in the next section) and consists of a single ganglion cell. A second transmission network consists of several rods or several cones which feed into a common bipolar cell, which then connects with a ganglion cell. Third, there are transmission systems in which rods and cones share a common bipolar cell.

In addition to the synaptic connections described above between the rods and cones, bipolar cells, and ganglion cells, there is another important type of synaptic connection in the retina which allows for impulses to be carried laterally within the retina itself. There are horizontal cells located between the receptor cell and bipolar cell levels and amacrine cells between the bipolar and ganglion cell levels, and the axons of both of these types of cells are oriented parallel to the retinal surface and at right angles to the axis of the other axons of the retina. These laterally oriented cells carry information across the retina at two distinct levels to relate activity in different parts of the visual field. They may well serve for facilitation, inhibition, and other neuronal associations within the retina.

2. The fovea

In the center of the posterior part of the eyeball is a small depression, about the size of the head of a pin, in which the retinal layers are exceedingly thin and in which only cone cells are located. This area of the retina is called the fovea centralis, or just fovea. It is the portion of the retina on which the objects of attention are focused by the refactory and directional mechanisms of the eye (Fig. 6.6).

Covering approximately 2 degrees of the central visual field, the fovea is the region of greatest visual acuity (clearness of vision), since the cones in this area of the retina are packed closely together and have a one-to-one connection with bipolar and ganglion cells. This favorable ratio of receptors to ganglion cells is evident only in the fovea and in the case of cones only. Moving outward from the fovea, there is a rapid decrease in the density of cones and a rapid increase in the number of rods. At the periphery of the retina there are very few cones. A pure cone fovea, such as humans have, is characteristic of all animals with a high degree of visual acuity.

Light rays which arise from objects and impinge on the eye are refracted by the cornea and lens to form a fairly accurate spatial representation of

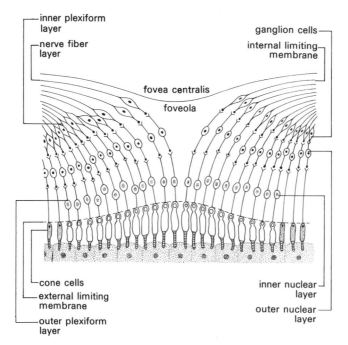

inner plexiform layer
nerve fiber layer
ganglion cells
internal limiting membrane
fovea centralis
foveola
cone cells
external limiting membrane
outer plexiform layer
inner nuclear layer
outer nuclear layer

Fig. 6.6 Fovea of the retina in a horizontal view. (Based on DeCoursey, 1968.)

the visual world on the retina. While this process of image formation is similar to that in a camera, the transformation from patterns of light and shadow on the retina into neural impulses is much more complex than a photographic film and the central pathways do not transmit a simple pictorial representation to the brain.

F. THE OPTIC DISK

The axons of the ganglion neurons follow a course parallel to the surface of the retina and merge to the nasal side of the fovea where they exit the eye at the optic disk, become myelinated, and form the optic nerve. The ganglion cells are comparable to the ascending spinothalamic tracts in the spinal cord.

The optic disk is also called the blind spot since this part of the retina has no rods or cones. Under normal viewing conditions we are not aware of the blind spot because our brain perceptually "fills in" the empty spot in our visual world.

Before examining the transmission network from the retina to the cerebral cortex, it is necessary to examine the process by which light energy is converted to nerve impulses. Light energy cannot be transmitted over nerve cells, so the light energy must be transduced to nerve impulses.

TRANSDUCTION OF LIGHT ENERGY IN THE RETINA

The functional activities of the photoreceptive rods and cones are the transduction and the genesis of the generator potential. These receptors respond to stimulation with slow, graded potentials; they do not have all-or-none action potentials. Light energy impinging on a rod or a cone initiates a series of processes that are responsible for the generation of a generator potential in these receptors. Thus, it is the rods and cones which convert light energy to an electrical-chemical current. The first step in the process of excitation of the rods and cones is the conversion of light energy into electrical energy by photosensitive substances which are located in the outer segments of the rod and cone cells.

A. THE PHOTOSENSITIVE PIGMENTS

Within the outermost segment of the rods and cones are photosensitive pigments, rhodopsin in the case of rods and three kinds of iodopsin in the case of cones, which are responsible for the transduction of light energy into neural activity. Electron micrographs show that the outer end of both rods and cones is packed with thin membranous sacs in which are found the light-absorbing pigments. Exposure of the pigments to light causes some kind of change in the receptor membrane, and this change gives rise to a generator current.

Light energy reaching rods is absorbed by rhodopsin which is bleached in the process. It is first converted into a substance called lumi-rhodopsin, but the energy absorbed from the light gives the lumi-rhodopsin a large amount of free energy. This is a very unstable compound and decays almost immediately into meta-rhodopsin, which is also an unstable compound, so it splits rapidly into two additional substances, retinene and a protein opsin called scotopsin. During this decomposition of rhodopsin, the rod generates a generator potential that triggers nerve impulses in the neurons that synapse with the rods. The exact process by which the nerve impulse is generated by these chemical processes is unknown (Fig. 6.7).

After rhodopsin has been decomposed in the process of converting light energy into an electric current, the two substances which remain are resynthesized into rhodopsin, with vitamin A playing an important role in the reconversion. It may be seen that there is a continuous cycle with rhodopsin being broken down by light energy and re-formed again by chemical synthesis.

The velocity at which this photochemical process takes place is proportional to the intensity of light and the concentration of rhodopsin. Only small amounts of the total supply of rhodopsin are bleached when exposed to light, so the mechanism of excitation is normally extraordinarily sensitive. Recent investigations have shown that one to three quanta of light reaching rods are sufficient for excitation and it is possible that one quantum can activate a single rod.

In the case of the cones of the retina, there are three types of pigment, each of which contains specific pigments that absorb light maximally at different wavelengths. As noted previously, various wavelengths are the basis of color discrimination, and the colors of the visible spectrum are the subjective interpretation of certain wavelengths.

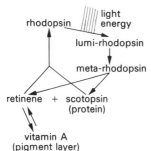

Fig. 6.7   The chemical sequence in rod function which is responsible for light sensitivity of rods. (Based on Guyton, 1964.)

One type of cone pigment is sensitive to wavelengths around 400 to 450 nanometers and gives rise to the color sensation of blue, a second type of cone pigment is sensitive to light around 500 to 550 nanometers and gives rise to the color sensation of green, while a third type cone is sensitive to wavelengths around 700 nanometers which are interpreted as red. Other colors are perceived as a result of the blending of impulses from the three cone types. All colors of the visible spectrum, then, can be formed from three basic colors, i.e., red, green, and blue. Color vision is said to be trichromatic because only three variables are needed to produce all color sensations.

The chemical process of converting light energy into a generator potential in the cones is very similar to that of the rods, except the three types of pigment, the iodopsins, in the cones are different from the rhodopsin of the rods.

OPTIC TRANSMISSION

The photochemical events which occur at the rods and cones in response to light energy become translated into action potentials at the ganglion cells of the retina. Ganglion cells receive their input from bipolar cells and amacrine cells and project their output to the midbrain and thalamus.

The axons of the ganglion cells merge at the optic disk, which is slightly medial to the fovea in each eye, and form the optic nerve as they leave the eyeball. These optic nerves from the two eyes pass backward to unite in an X-shaped structure, the optic chiasm. Here the nerve fibers from the nasal portions of each retina, about 50 percent of all optic nerve fibers in humans, cross over to intermingle with the uncrossed fibers from the temporal portion of the opposite eye. From the optic chiasm, the optic nerves separate and project posteriorly as the optic tracts.

As a consequence of the crossing of fibers at the optic chiasm, the fibers from the nasal half of the retina in one eye and those from the temporal half of the other eye proceed together in the optic tracts. Therefore, objects in the left half of the visual field are represented by impulses projecting to the right hemisphere, and those in the right visual field are sent to the left hemisphere (Fig. 6.8). The optic nerves and tracts are the photoconductive counterparts of sensory tracts within the spinal cord and lemnisci of the brainstem; the bipolar cells of the retina are the first-order neuron and the ganglion cells are the second-order neuron.

Optic tract fibers make synaptic connections with several structures in the subcortical areas of the brain. About 70 to 80 percent of the fibers terminate in a part of the thalamus called the lateral geniculate bodies; the remainder terminate mainly in a midbrain structure, the superior colliculus.

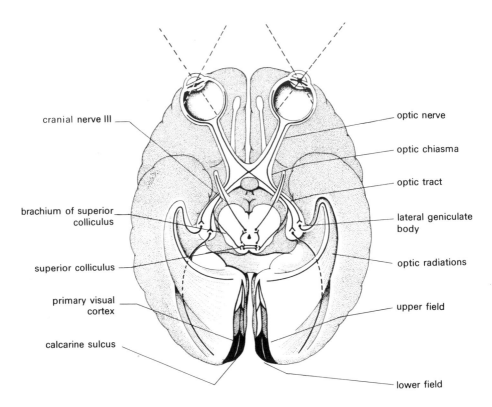

cranial nerve III

optic nerve

optic chiasma

optic tract

brachium of superior colliculus

lateral geniculate body

superior colliculus

optic radiations

primary visual cortex

upper field

calcarine sulcus

lower field

Fig. 6.8 Visual pathways from the retina. The partial crossing of nerve fibers at the optic chiasm may be noted. The upper half of the visual field projects to the primary visual cortex below the calcarine sulcus while the lower half projects to the primary visual cortex above the calcarine sulcus. (Based on Noback, 1967.)

The cells of each lateral geniculate body project their axons to the primary visual cortex (also called the striate cortex) in the occipital lobes, just as the sensory fibers from other sense modalities project to other primary cortex areas. It may be seen that there are three orders of neurons from the eye to the cortex—the retinal transmission, the optic nerve and tract to the thalamus, and the thalamus to the cortex (Fig. 6.8).

The primary visual cortex records light and darkness and simple patterns such as lines, dots, and circles. Moreover, it detects the orientation of lines or borders. Finally, sudden changes in light intensity, movement of an image across the retina, and detection of color are all important functions of this area of the cortex. Blindness results from destruction of the primary visual cortex.

From the primary visual cortex, visual impulses are transmitted anteriorly and laterally to various association areas of the brain where a perceptual interpretation of the impulses is made. Recent electrophysiological and clinical studies have implicated the entire cerebral cortex in the visual process.

A. TRANSMISSION FOR VISUAL REFLEXES

Some nerve fibers leave the optic tract and terminate in a midbrain structure, the superior colliculus, which consists of two bumps on the upper surface of the midbrain. In addition to receiving nerve impulses directly from the optic nerve, impulses are also relayed from the visual cortex, and the deeper layers of this structure receive input from the auditory and somatosensory systems.

The superior colliculus is believed to mediate purely reflex functions of the visual system because it projects fibers to various muscle groups of the eye. One example of a familiar type of visual reflex is blinking in response to an object that appears suddenly in the visual fields. Pupillary constriction in response to light and lens accommodation for proper focus on near or far objects are other types of visual reflexes.

The superior colliculus also projects fibers to the brainstem and spinal cord motor centers for control of head and eye movements. Thus, orienting movements of the eyes and head are probably mediated by this structure. It may be seen, then, that a great deal of the activity of the visual system is under the control of reflex mechanisms, and the superior colliculus is the center for mediating this activity.

DIRECTIONAL PROPERTIES OF VISION

The visible world consists of light sources and reflecting surfaces which emit or reflect light into the eye. The total panorama of visible sources available to the observer at a particular location is that observer's visible surroundings, or environment. For any particular position of the eye, head, and body, only part of the visible surroundings is in view; this part is called the field of view, or visual display.

The eyeball is suspended in its orbit by extraocular muscles and a series of ligaments and connective tissue. The extraocular, or extrinsic, eye muscles control the position of each eye in its socket. They may be grouped into three pairs: the medial and lateral recti, the superior and inferior recti, and the superior and inferior obliques. Each pair of muscles forms an

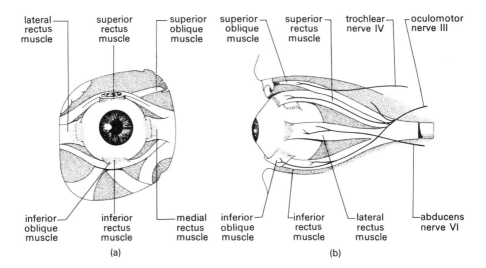

lateral rectus muscle | superior rectus muscle | superior oblique muscle | superior oblique muscle | superior rectus muscle | trochlear nerve IV | oculomotor nerve III

inferior oblique muscle | inferior rectus muscle | medial rectus muscle | inferior oblique muscle | inferior rectus muscle | lateral rectus muscle | abducens nerve VI

(a)   (b)

Fig. 6.9   The extraocular muscles. (a) An anterior view. (b) A lateral view. (Based on DeCoursey, 1968.)

antagonistic pair. The motor nerves to the extraocular muscles are the 3rd cranial nerve (oculomotor) running to the superior and medial rectus, inferior oblique, and inferior rectus; the 4th cranial nerve (trochlear) running to the superior oblique, and the 6th cranial nerve (abducens) running to the lateral rectus (Fig. 6.9).

The extraocular muscles are richly supplied with motorneurons; indeed, they have the smallest ratio of motor nerve fiber-to-muscle fiber of anyplace else in the body, and the movements which these muscles control are the fastest, most accurate, and most complex in the body. Most eye movements are designed to maintain the retinal image in the same position on the retina; this is the basic task of the eye muscles.

The tiny extraocular muscles cause rapid involuntary eye movements when we focus on a stationary object; these movements seem to be necessary to maintain form perception in vision. Experiments which have nullified the effects of these rapid eye movements have found that patterns fade and finally disappear entirely.

An important function in three-dimensional-space perception is also served by the extraocular muscles. Since these muscles control the convergence of the two eyes onto an object, as each eye converges onto an object, each eye views the object from a slightly different direction and sees parts of the object that the other eye cannot see. When two slightly different images are focused on the sensory receptors of each eye, perception of a single three-dimensional object occurs.

7

Motor Integration
and Control
of Movement

The observer of a smoothly coordinated motor performance usually does not realize that the performance represents a fantastically complex integration of many parts of the nervous system to produce the postures and movement patterns. In performing a basketball jump shot, a football forward pass, or an intricate dance routine, the complete movement patterns consist of reflexes, simple movements, and complex movements with precise spatial and temporal organization, meaning that the appropriate muscles are selected and employed at just the right time.*

How the nervous system produces a coordinated motor pattern has long been one of the major mysteries of the neurosciences. What accounts for the graceful performance of the skillful athlete or even the ordinary movements of daily life? For movement to be effective an appropriate group of muscles must be selected, each muscle fiber must be activated in the proper temporal sequence to the others and a precise amount of inhibition must be sent to each of the muscle fibers of muscle groups which oppose the intended movement. In addition to producing the contraction of a certain group of muscles the CNS must monitor the effects of its commands, it must coordinate the movements of the various segments of the body, and it must terminate a given phase in a movement pattern and proceed to the next phase.

In this chapter we will examine the motor mechanisms of the nervous system which are responsible for the integration and control of human movement patterns, but we shall have to emphasize that much is unknown about this aspect of human behavior.

---

*Spatial organization refers to the fact that the appropriate muscles must be selected. Temporal organization refers to the fact that muscle contraction or relaxation must occur at the appropriate time.

DEVELOPMENT OF MOTOR ORGANIZATION

At birth, the human infant possesses a number of built-in motor nerve circuits which produce synchronous movements. While most of these circuits are fairly simple, some are very complex. A few basic movement responses exist at birth, but others develop as extensions of the basic patterns as the nervous system matures. Basic human motor circuits and simple movement responses, then, are probably genetically established, while environmental conditions are responsible for the elaboration of the motor nerve network. That is, complex movement patterns are learned.

Learned movement patterns are controlled by the CNS, but practice has caused many of our movements to become complex automatic patterns. Walking is an example of a complex automatic pattern. Walking is learned very laboriously but once learned it is performed primarily by specific patterns of automatic nervous activity. Walking, running, hitting a baseball, shooting a basket are examples of remarkably skilled movements which we usually take for granted, forgetting their vast complexity, and the months or years of learning and practice required to master them.

MOTOR INTEGRATION AND TRANSMISSION NETWORK

A perennial goal in the study of the brain is to infer function from structure—to relate behavior to the organization of the nervous system. The traditional view of the brain in movement is that the highest level in its hierarchical organization is the cortex. Recent investigations seem to indicate that the structures participating in the integration and control of muscular movements include a complex of subcortical as well as cortical structures, each playing a highly specific role in the whole functional system which produces voluntary movement. That is why damage to different parts of the brain produces disturbances of different voluntary movements.

It is convenient to study the motor system by first identifying and describing the transmission network which carries motor impulses from their origins to the motor neurons which actually innervate muscle fibers, causing muscular contraction or relaxation. Having done that, the structures which are responsible for the motor impulses may then be identified and discussed. These structures may be treated as though the nervous system were composed of a series of levels and, starting from the top, the levels are the cerebral cortex, the basal ganglia, the cerebellum, the brainstem, and the spinal cord.

Each of the structures which contribute to motor integration and control plays a unique role. It must be emphasized, however, that the functional parts of the motor system are intimately interrelated and that in order to achieve almost any kind of complex motor behavior the entire system contributes to some extent. Thus, describing this system as a series of levels does not imply that the levels somehow function independently of one another. It is merely a convenient method for writing about them.

A. MOTOR PATHWAYS

Before we identify and discuss the functions of the various structures which control motor activity, it is necessary to describe the motor pathways over which impulses pass on their way to producing muscle contraction or relaxation. The sources of sensory information about the external world and our bodies are many and varied, but the means for control of voluntary movement in response to sensory information are few. There are at least 12 different kinds of sensory receptors, with their various pathways to the brain, but there are only two major motor pathways. These two motor pathways from the cortex to the spinal cord and the motor nuclei of the cranial nerves are (1) the pyramidal system, also called the corticospinal tract, and (2) the extrapyramidal system. These descending cortical and subcortical pathways represent the main instrument by which the brain controls movement.

1. The pyramidal system   This motor transmission network is made up of those neurons which originate in the cerebral cortex the axons of which descend to the spinal cord; thus, it is also called the corticospinal tract. The axons of this system are some of the longest found in the body. The name, pyramidal system, comes from the symmetrical wedge-shaped bulges its fibers form on the ventral surface of the medulla, just below the pons. The neurons of the cortex which send their axons down the pyramidal tract provide a direct channel from the cortex to the spinal neurons which in turn cause either muscle contraction or relaxation. This direct connection of the cortex with motor neurons ensures that the cortex very effectively and quickly brings about a desired movement (Fig.7.1).

About 40 percent of the axons of the pyramidal system come from cells of the motor cortex (a region just in front of the central fissure), about 20 percent come from cells of the somatosensory area in the parietal lobes, and the rest come from cells in other parts of the cortex. Pyramidal system neurons are of two types. One is the huge neurons in the motor cortex called "Betz cells," which are about 16 microns in size. These large Betz cells of each hemisphere of the motor cortex contribute about 34,000 large axons to the pyramidal system, which is only about three percent of the total axons of the system. The second type of pyramidal system neuron, and by far the most numerous, are small neurons which are distributed throughout the cortex

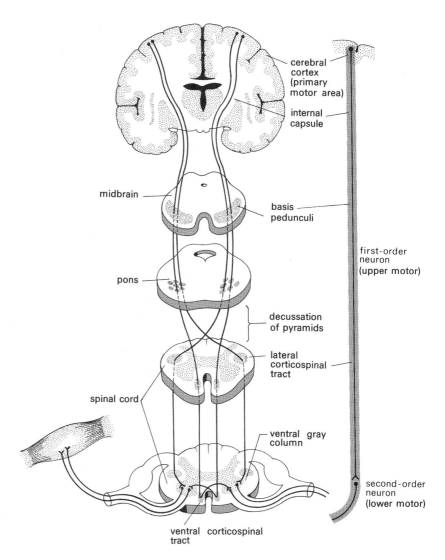

cerebral
cortex
(primary
motor area)

internal
capsule

midbrain

basis
pedunculi

pons

first-order
neuron
(upper motor)

decussation
of pyramids

lateral
corticospinal
tract

spinal cord

ventral gray
column

second-order
neuron
(lower motor)

ventral corticospinal
tract

Fig. 7.1   The pyramidal motor pathways. (Based on Langley *et al.*, 1969.)

and have myelinated or unmyelinated axons. These small unmyelinated and myelinated axons account for about 95 percent of the total corticospinal tract.

The pyramidal system axons leave the cortex, descend in the internal capsule, and pass through the pons, giving off collateral and direct axons to the motor nuclei of the cranial nerves for the control of facial, eye, and glandular activity. When they reach the medulla, collaterals and direct axons innervate cranial motor nuclei for the control of the pharynx, larynx, neck, upper back, and tongue muscles.

In the medulla, the pyramidal tract axons organize into bundles of axons, the pyramids, one pyramid on each side of the midline fissure. In the medullary pyramids, about 80 percent of the one million axons of each of the bilateral pyramidal tracts cross over the pyramidal decussation and terminate mainly on spinal cord interneurons, which in turn synapse on the motorneurons which control muscle action. About 50 percent of the crossed pyramidal axons end in the cervical region of the spinal cord while the other half end in lower parts of the cord. Uncrossed pyramidal axons continue through the pyramids and descend in the spinal cord. These axons then cross the midline of the cord a few at a time and synapse with motorneurons in the cord.

Most impulses descending over pyramidal tract axons do not go directly to the spinal motorneurons. Instead, they synapse on spinal interneurons, and these in turn relay the impulses to the spinal motorneurons, whose axons project out to muscle fibers.

It appears that the muscles especially controlled by the pyramidal system contain motor units with a relatively low ratio of muscle fibers. We noted in Chapter 3 that a low ratio of motor neuron innervation to muscle fibers permits smaller portions of the muscles to be independently controlled, which permits a pronounced precision and delicacy of movement. This aspect of pyramidal system control of delicate movement becomes evident when lesions are made in the pyramidal tract. Lesions produce a severe flaccid paralysis for a couple of weeks; then the proximal muscles of the arms or legs begin to recover and the shoulder or hip joint can be moved. Later, more distal muscles in the limbs may improve, but the fingers or toes rarely recover their former dexterity.

2. The extrapyramidal system   The second motor pathway is known as the extrapyramidal system. By definition, this tract includes all of the nonreflex motor axons not included in the pyramidal tract. The extrapyramidal pathway differs from the pyramidal pathway in two ways:

1. The chains of axons are interrupted synaptically in the basal ganglia, the pons, the medulla, or the reticular formation.
2. The axons do not pass through the medullary pyramids.

The extrapyramidal pathway originates in the motor area of the cortex, as well as in other cortical areas. The axons descend in the internal capsule and many terminate in various subcortical structures, especially the basal

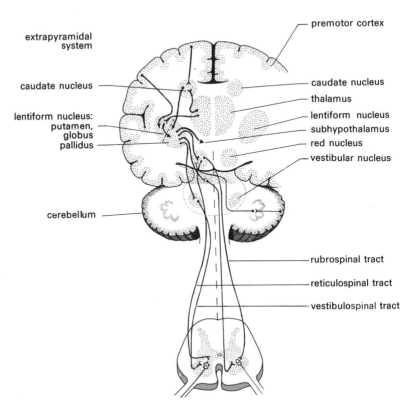

extrapyramidal
system

caudate nucleus

lentiform nucleus:
putamen,
globus
pallidus

cerebellum

premotor cortex

caudate nucleus

thalamus

lentiform nucleus

subhypothalamus

red nucleus

vestibular nucleus

rubrospinal tract

reticulospinal tract

vestibulospinal tract

Fig. 7.2 The extrapyramidal motor pathways. (Based on McNaught and Callander, 1963.)

ganglia, cerebellum, and thalamus, and in nuclei of the brainstem. Each of these structures and nuclei in turn has direct or indirect connections with each other (Fig. 7.2).

Extrapyramidal neurons have connections with many subcortical parts of the brain, and it is believed that these multiple connections serve to modify some of the operations of the pyramidal system—perhaps helping to refine and smooth out movements. Moreover, extrapyramidal neurons carry a large portion of the impulses for postural adjustment and reflexive gross movements.

3. Pathways to cranial nerves   Since motor activity of the head and neck is carried out by the muscles supplied by cranial nerves, the pathways which innervate the cranial nerves are not separated anatomically into pyramidal and extrapyramidal (Fig. 7.3). The reason for this is that most of these descending pathways terminate before reaching the medullary pyramids.

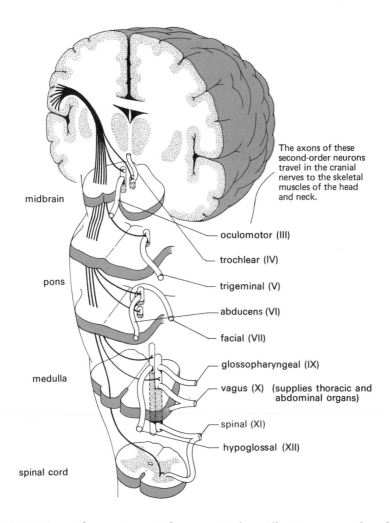

The axons of these second-order neurons travel in the cranial nerves to the skeletal muscles of the head and neck.

midbrain

oculomotor (III)

trochlear (IV)

pons

trigeminal (V)

abducens (VI)

facial (VII)

glossopharyngeal (IX)

medulla

vagus (X) (supplies thoracic and abdominal organs)

spinal (XI)

hypoglossal (XII)

spinal cord

Fig. 7.3 Motor pathways to cranial nerves. In the midbrain, pons, and medulla, motor fibers cross the midline and the upper motorneurons synapse with neurons in the nuclei of the cranial nerves. (Based on McNaught and Callander, 1963.)

B. THE MOTOR CORTEX

The region of cerebral cortex from which most neurons arise for motor integration and control is called the motor cortex area. This part of the cortex has a primary area which lies immediately anterior to the central fissure and a secondary area, known as the premotor area, which lies just anterior to the primary area, about 1 to 3 cm in width (Fig. 7.4).

The motor cortex area contains some 34,000 giant Betz cells and millions of smaller neurons. The motor cortex projects fibers to all association areas of the cerebral cortex and there are many descending fibers leading out of the motor area. Axons of these descending neurons pass from the cortex and descend through the internal capsule. Motor impulses reach the spinal cord motorneurons either by relaying in various subcortical levels or by projecting through the direct motor pathway to the brainstem and spinal cord. More of the axons arising from neurons in the premotor area terminate in the subcortical structures and nuclei of the brain instead of projecting directly to the spinal cord.

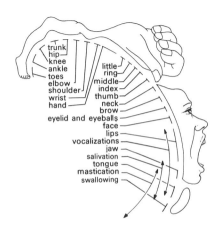

Fig. 7.4   The motor homunculus (little man) showing the extent of representation of the various body muscles in the motor cortex. (Based on Kimble, 1963.)

The motor cortex is topographically organized; that is, each part is responsible for specific muscles of the body. However, the different muscle groups of the body are not represented to the same degree in the motor area (Fig. 7.4). As a rule, the degree of representation is proportional to the discreteness of movement required of that part of the body. The hand and the mouth muscles have almost two-thirds of the total representation in the motor area. The large number of motor cortex neurons for innervation of the hand and face is one of the factors responsible for the fine degree of motor control humans have over these structures and reflects the importance of these parts to humans.

The "mapping out" of the human motor cortex was done by electrically stimulating the motor cortex during brain surgery on unanesthetized patients. Movements elicited by electrical stimulation of the motor cortex consist largely of flexion and extension of the arms and legs, opening and closing of the fists, and vocalizations; the limb movements are typically expressed on the side of the body opposite to the stimulation, but some ipsilateral activity may also occur. This technique gives an indication of what each portion of that part of the cortex may be used for; it does not use the motor cortex as it is employed by the stream of impulses which produce a voluntary movement. Therefore, movements elicited by electrical stimulation of the motor cortex will not by themselves necessarily tell us the complete story about the role of the motor cortex in the control of movement.

The motor area receives its main direct stimulation from other cortical areas and from subcortical areas via the thalamus. There is a close functional interrelationship between the motor area and the somatosensory areas of the cortex. Indeed, many of the cells of the motor area extend back into the somatic sensory areas, and likewise cells of the somatosensory areas extend forward into the motor area. The two areas may be said to fade into each other. Electrical stimulation of the anterior parts of the somatosensory cortex often evokes muscle contractions, while stimulation of certain parts of the motor area evokes sensory experience. In addition to the motor-somatosensory relationships, numerous association fibers from diverse areas throughout the cortex are major sources of input to the motor cortex.

Subcortical influences to the motor area come from feedback circuits involving the basal ganglia, cerebellum, brainstem, and even the spinal cord, as well as from peripheral afferent sources through subcortical nuclei. For example, the strongest sensory input to a particular portion of the motor cortex arises from the body part the movements of which it controls. Thus, the motor cortex hand area receives its strongest input from receptors in the hand.

The motor cortex serves to coordinate highly complex and skilled movements resulting from complex innervations on the motor area from other parts of the CNS. As Eccles (1973) says, "The motor cortex. . .is not the prime initiator of a movement. . . . It is only the final relay station of what has been going on in widely dispersed areas in your cerebral cortex."

Damage or destruction of the motor cortex evokes a loss of the fine voluntary movements, particularly of the fingers and feet. Effects are more prominent in the distal muscles than in the proximal muscles of a limb. Small lesions in the motor cortex do not always paralyze particular muscles but may prevent certain movements.

C. THE PREFRONTAL CORTEX

Also important in the control of movement is the prefrontal area of the cerebral cortex, which consists of both anterior poles of the frontal lobes of the brain. This area lies anterior to the primary and secondary motor areas, and is the most anterior part of the cerebral cortex (Fig. 7.5). The prefrontal cor-

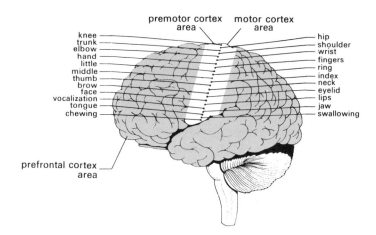

premotor cortex   motor cortex
area   area

knee
trunk
elbow
hand
little
middle
thumb
brow
face
vocalization
tongue
chewing

hip
shoulder
wrist
fingers
ring
index
neck
eyelid
lips
jaw
swallowing

prefrontal cortex
area

Fig. 7.5 Location of cortical areas which are responsible for certain types of motor activity. There is a representation of each of the different muscles of the body in the motor area. (Based on Guyton, 1964.)

tex has many complex reciprocal connections with other cortical regions. It also has rich reciprocal connections with the thalamus, hypothalamus, and other subcortical areas which appear to mediate emotion and motivation.

For many psychologists and neurologists, the prefrontal area is the most fascinating part of the brain, probably because it embodies the unique difference between the brains of other animals and of humans. Experimental and clinical evidence suggests that it must be included in the cortical areas responsible for motor behavior, and numerous studies on this part of the brain allow us to make several generalizations on its motor functions.

It seems that one role of the prefrontal area is related to regulatory activity in the form of correct evaluation of external impressions and the purposive direction and selection of movements in accordance with the evaluation obtained. Monkeys with prefrontal area lesions typically become less proficient with delayed response tasks (tasks where the subject is not allowed to make the appropriate response until after a lapse of time) and they find it more difficult to eliminate previous learning than normal monkeys. Luria (1966) reported that humans with a massive lesion of the prefrontal lobe cease to compare their performance with their original plan and they can no longer ascertain whether the action does in fact correspond to the plan. These individuals, therefore, do not notice their actions no longer correspond to the original plan. Thus "prefrontal" patients are perseverative; that is, they find it difficult to change from one solution of a problem or form of response to a different one. This behavioral syndrome is particularly evident in reversal learning problems and in other problems in which a previously correct response must be inhibited or a new response now becomes the appropriate one (Milner, 1964).

There is evidence that the prefrontal area also plays a prominent role in such things as judgment, planning for the future, ambition, conscience, and abstract thinking. Lesions in this part of the cortex reduce the ability to use good judgment; the individual responds rapidly, impulsively, and with no apparent evaluation of the consequences. In a way, then, the prefrontal area may have somewhat of an inhibitory effect on other brain areas, causing one to hesitate and plan one's response and its possible consequences before responding.

Damage or destruction to this part of the brain produces striking personality changes. There is a loss of drive and ambition, but the most dramatic changes are a lack of self-consciousness and freedom in social relationships, sometimes to an obnoxious or embarrassing degree.

Finally, extensive loss of abstract thinking or reasoning ability accompanies prefrontal area lesions. Simple problems requiring reasoning become extremely difficult to solve.

D. THE BASAL GANGLIA

We are now ready to examine the lower levels of the motor system—that is, below the level of the cerebral cortex—and one of the most important subcortical levels for coordinated movement is called the basal ganglia. The basal ganglia are the highest centers for motor control in birds and lower animals that have little cerebral cortex.

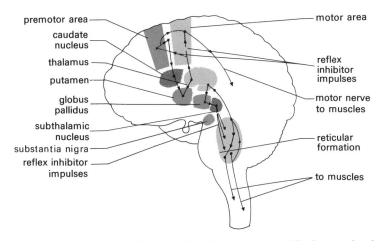

Fig. 7.6   The basal ganglia, showing their innervations with the cerebral cortex and various structures in the brainstem. (Based on Guyton, 1964.)

The term "basal ganglia" is nonspecific; it refers to masses of neurons clustered into large nuclei in the inner layers of the cerebral cortex and in the upper part of the mesencephalon. There is no agreement as to what cerebral ganglia constitute the basal ganglia, but the structures most frequently listed are the caudate nucleus; the putamen; the globus pallidus; the subthalamic nucleus; and the substantia nigra (Fig. 7.6).

There are two major fiber inputs to the basal ganglia; first, the ascending reticular formation; second, the motor areas of the cerebral cortex. The latter represents the highest and most important portion of the extrapyramidal system. The basal ganglia also have two primary output pathways: the first pathway descends through the thalamus and makes connections with various subcortical structures throughout the diencephalon, the midbrain, and the brainstem. The second output pathway ends in a part of the thalamus which projects fibers upward into the cerebral cortex. These output pathways allow the basal ganglia to influence spinal cord as well as cortical motor mechanisms. This massive network of input and output fibers of the basal ganglia apparently serves to facilitate and inhibit a wide variety of movements.

Actually, very little is known about the precise function of most of the various basal ganglia except that they function together in a loosely knit unit to perform controlling functions for coordinated movement behavior. Recent findings by Evarts (1973) indicate that the primary motor function is to generate slow movements. This is not to suggest that the basal ganglia function solely in the control of slow movements but at least a large portion of the basal ganglia is preferentially involved in the control of slow movements. The output of the basal ganglia, which presumably serves to modulate cortical output and control slow movements, goes to the motor cortex by way of the thalamus. Further discussion of the role of the basal ganglia appears later in this chapter.

E. THE CEREBELLUM

The cerebellar level is another brain level that is essential to well-coordinated, complex motor function. The cerebellum is a large, profusely fissured structure located posterior to the brainstem. It is an essential integrative center for postural adjustments, locomotion, and many other reflex activities. It also appears to play an important role in the preprogramming and control of rapid, ballistic movements.

The cerebellum is divisible into two hemispheres and a midline connecting portion, the vermis. Each of the two hemispheres is joined to the brainstem by three peduncles—the superior, middle, and inferior—composed of nerve fibers. The superior peduncle connects with the midbrain, the middle with the pons, and the inferior with the medulla. The cerebellum also has in-

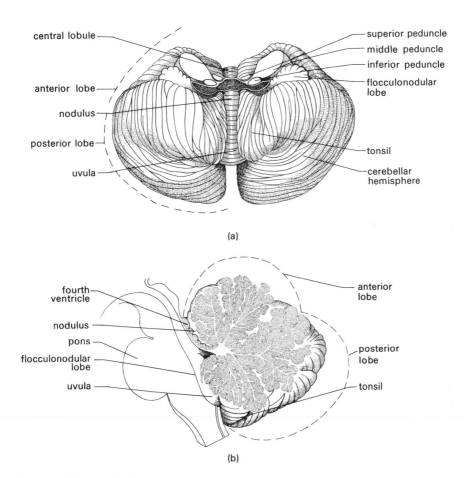

Fig. 7.7 The cerebellum. (a) A view of the anterior part of the cerebellum. This part is just behind the brainstem. (b) A sagittal view. (Based on Langley *et al.*, 1969.)

direct connections by way of the peduncles with the cerebral cortex and the spinal cord (Fig. 7.7).

The cerebellum has a cortex of gray matter which is similar to the cerebral cortex, and it has an interior of both white and gray matter. Its cortex is elaborately convoluted to increase its area; in fact, the fissures are much deeper and more closely spaced than those of the cerebral cortex. The interior gray matter consists of four cerebellar nuclei (dentate, emboliform, fastigial, and globose nuclei) which receive collateral axons from the afferent fibers projecting into the cerebellum and efferent connections from the Purkinje cells of the cerebellar cortex.

Anatomically, the cerebellum is served by two types of afferent fibers, the climbing fiber and the mossy fiber, a single type efferent neuron, the Purkinje cell, and several types of indigenous cerebellar neurons. The climbing fibers begin outside the cerebellum in other regions of the brain and project into the cerebellar nuclei and cortex, synapsing on a one-to-one basis with the Purkinje cells, and they exert a strong excitatory effect on the Purkinje cells. Whereas each climbing fiber connects with a single Purkinje cell, the mossy fibers do not synapse directly on Purkinje cells but on the interneurons of the cerebellum, and thus ultimately indirectly innervate many Purkinje cells. This form of input may inhibit or stimulate the Purkinje cell (Fig. 7.8).

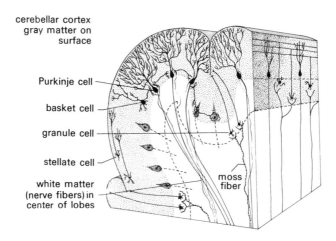

cerebellar cortex
gray matter on
surface

Purkinje cell

basket cell

granule cell

stellate cell

white matter
(nerve fibers) in
center of lobes

moss
fiber

Fig. 7.8 Cross section of interior of cerebellum, showing the network of cells which transmit nerve impulses through it. (Based on McNaught and Callander, 1963.)

Cerebellar output involves two stages. First, Purkinje cell axons project into the cerebellar nuclei and synapse there. Second, the cerebellar nuclei neurons project axons to brainstem nuclei and to the thalamus. Purkinje cells are inhibitory, but the cerebellar nuclei neurons are excitatory. The origins of excitatory input to the cerebellar nuclei neurons seem to be the collateral transmission from the climbing fibers and the mossy fibers (Fig. 7.9).

The cerebellum receives nerve impulses from a variety of sources—the somatosensory, visual, auditory, and motor areas of the cerebral cortex, various nuclei in the brainstem, the reticular formation, and sensory receptors. Cerebral cortex axons destined for the cerebellum follow a route

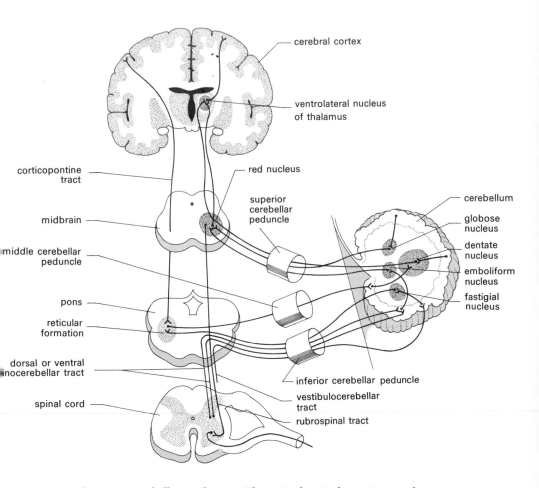

Fig. 7.9 The main cerebellar pathways. The reticulospinal tract is not shown. This tract extends from the reticular formation to the spinal cord and fibers in this tract terminate on anterior motorneurons. (Based on Langley *et al.*, 1969.)

through the internal capsule to the pons. There they synapse on neurons projecting into the cerebellum. The cerebellum also receives numerous inputs from brainstem nuclei. Sensory impulses from the proprioceptors, the receptors in the muscles, tendons, joints and vestibular apparatus project into brainstem nuclei, where they synapse on cerebellar afferent neurons whose axons ascend to the cerebellar cortex. Collectively, these signals transmit space-and-modality-specific data to the cerebellum which may be used in the control of fine movements of the limbs and in the monitoring of information pertaining to location or stages of movement involving an entire limb.

Also, sensory impulses from other sensory modalities give off collaterals to brainstem nuclei which in turn project axons to the cerebellum.

As noted above, efferent impulses from the cerebellar cortex pass into one of four nuclei which lie on the interior of the cerebellum (Fig. 7.9). Efferent pathways from the cerebellum then project to various brainstem nuclei where they join the extrapyramidal tract. Thus, there are cerebellar brainstem feedback loops. Ascending efferent cerebellar fibers enter the thalamic nucleus which projects to motor areas of the cerebral cortex. It may be seen that impulses which leave the cerebral cortex may ultimately return by way of the cerebellum; thus, the cerebellum is part of a dynamic cerebral-cerebellar feedback loop.

There have been many attempts to correlate cerebellar and body areas to ascertain whether one portion of the cerebellum is concerned with upper-limb function and another part with lower-limb function. Although investigations of this kind have been moderately successful in lower animals, the only localization known with any certainty for humans is that relating a hemisphere of the cerebellum to the same side of the body; thus, control is not contralateral as it is in the cerebral cortex. It has also been found that upper limbs have greater representation in the cerebellum than the lower limbs have. Investigators are in general agreement that the cerebellum does not contain a precise somatotopic map, such as those found in the somatosensory and motor cortex. There seems to be, instead, a large overlap of inputs and any small region in the cerebellum will receive inputs from a very large number of sources.

Several neuroscientists have proposed models of cerebellar function and with each model there is general agreement that cerebellar output plays a significant role in regulating movement although the manner or degree of control hypothesized by these scientists differs considerably (Eccles, 1973; Evarts, 1973; Llina, 1975).

It has long been known that the cerebellum is concerned primarily with the control of all complex movements. It has been commonly believed that the major role of the cerebellum is the control of movement in response to feedback from the proprioceptors after movement had begun; but recent investigations have shown that changes in cerebellar activity occur prior to the initiation of movement. Several neuroscientists have indicated that the cerebellum may actually have a key role in the initiation of fast, ballistic movements through its connections with the motor cortex via the thalamus. This is not to suggest that it does not have a feedback role in movement control, because it does indeed appear to have as one of its functions a kind of feedback loop circuit during motor activity. It receives data from various sensory modalities concerning the position of the body in space. It also receives information from cortical areas concerning the direction and amplitude of the intended movement. When the body parts deviate from the intended movement pattern, the cerebellum appears to initiate necessary adjustments via its connections with the cerebral cortex and brainstem motor pathways. This model, then, suggests that one of the cerebellar functions is to compare efferent and afferent signals, adjusting the movement so that the two sets of signals coincide.

Damage or destruction of the cerebellum results in various movement disabilities, depending on the damage, which supports the model of this structure as a regulator of motor activity. Disequilibrium, tremor, disturbances in timing and coordination, and overactive reflexes are some of the common effects of cerebellar damage. Cerebellar damage causing coordination deficiencies results in voluntary movements that are slow to start, have inaccurate direction of movement (so the moving part stops too soon or too late), and wild jerky movements, which are made in an effort to correct directional errors. Figure 7.10 illustrates the movement dysfunction of a patient with cerebellar damage in one hemisphere. Characteristic of cerebellar damage is muscular tremor that is most severe during voluntary movement and least severe when the muscles are at rest, a condition just opposite to basal ganglia damage. Since voluntary modification of the functions of the cerebellum seems to be impossible—we are never directly conscious of the functioning of the cerebellum—defects resulting from cerebellar damage or disorders cannot be voluntarily controlled or modified in any way.

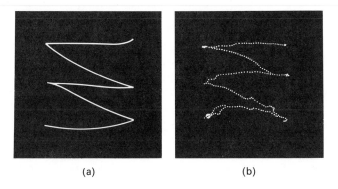

(a)   (b)

Fig. 7.10 A small electric bulb which flashed at 25 times per second was placed on the finger of a normal subject (a) and on the finger of a subject (b) with cerebellar damage. There were two columns of three red lights and the subjects' task was to point with their outstretched arm as quickly as possible to the succession of red lights from one and the other column. Meanwhile the movement, as revealed by the flashing light, was recorded by a fixed camera. (Based on Holmes, 1939.)

CONTROL OF MOVEMENT BY THE BRAIN

The traditional notion about voluntary movement has been that the motor cortex is at the highest level of motor control and subcortical structures are at a lower level, but recent research suggests that the situation is not that simple. Findings by Evarts and his colleagues (Evarts, Bizzi, Burke, DeLong, Thach, 1971; Evarts, 1973) show that the basal ganglia and cerebellum, as well as the motor cortex are activated prior to movement, and this has changed traditional ideas about the functional relations of these three structures. It now appears that the entire cerebral cortex sends signals to both the basal ganglia and the cerebellum, and these two structures recode this information and then send a new pattern of signals back to the motor cortex. The motor cortex, according to this view, is more directly connected with the spinal motorneurons than either the basal ganglia or the cerebellum.

This recent view of the interdependence of subcortical and cortical structures in the organization and control of movement also suggests that the signals from the basal ganglia and the cerebellum to the motor cortex play a specific role in certain kinds of movements. These two structures appear to have complementary roles, with the basal ganglia controlling slow movements and the cerebellum controlling quick movements; that is, the primary motor function of the basal ganglia is to generate slow movements, whereas one of the functions of the cerebellum is to preprogram and initiate rapid movements.

Evarts (1973) has reported that microelectrodes implanted in the brain show that motor cortex activity is involved with both slow and fast movements but the basal ganglia are preferentially active in slow movements while the cerebellum is preferentially active with fast, ballistic movements. Thus, damage to the motor cortex produces paralysis whereas damage to the basal ganglia or the cerebellum causes abnormality instead of abolition of movement.

The victim of a basal ganglia disease, such as Parkinson's disease, can frequently carry out high velocity movements quite normally but may have great difficulty starting a slow movement with the same muscle group. Conversely, damage to or disease of the cerebellum results in a movement abnormality that is almost the opposite of that caused by dysfunction of the basal ganglia. In the case of cerebellar dysfunction, muscular tremor is most severe during rapid voluntary movement and least noticeable while the muscles are at rest.

The present state of knowledge about the control of movement by the brain suggests that the cerebral cortex plays a supporting rather than a dominant role. Structures in the interior of the brain appear to be at a higher functional level of the system, judging by their position in the neural chain of command that triggers and controls movement. This implies that the primary function of the motor cortex may be the refinement of motor control rather than the actual initiating of movement.

Luria (1970) has suggested that voluntary movement control may be conceptualized into four components and that the components are mediated by different parts of the brain. The first component is the somatosensory system of sensory signals from the muscles, joints, and vestibular apparatus of the inner ear. Although simple ballistic movement patterns can be performed without feedback from the somatic system, several investigators have shown that humans find it difficult to regulate complex, coordinated movement patterns only by way of efferent impulses from the brain to the muscles. It seems important for the brain to receive feedback from the proprioceptors to correct the programs of impulses directed to the motor-neurons.* This somatosensory base is provided by the somatosensory primary cortex and its nearby association areas. If this part of the cortex is damaged or destroyed, the individual not only loses certain sensations but is unable to execute a well-organized voluntary movement.

A second component of voluntary movement is the spatial analysis component. A voluntary movement must be precisely oriented toward a certain point in space. This spatial analysis depends upon association areas of the parieto-occipital lobes. Malfunctions in these parts of the cortex result in a disturbance in which the sensory base of the movements is normal but the individual fails to exhibit precise spatial organization of the movement. Right and left spatial relations may be confused. Inability to make appropriate spatial movements even in a familiar place may result. Even the ability to distinguish east from west on a map or the position of the hands on a watch may be lost.

Although the sensory and spatial components are basic to the organization of voluntary movement, they are still inadequate to allow the execution of a movement pattern. A voluntary movement requires temporal organization, or sequential linking. In Luria's (1966) words, "a skilled movement is a kinetic melody of interchangeable links." As one part of a movement is completed, the motor impulses must be shifted to another link, and so on. Only in this way can an organized movement pattern be made. It appears that the premotor cortex (the secondary area of the motor cortex) is responsible for the sequential interchange of individual links of a movement pattern. When this part of the cortex is damaged, a skilled movement disintegrates. The individual loses the ability to block, or inhibit, one of the links of the movement and to make a transition from one link to another, even though the sensory feedback and spatial orientation aspects are present.

---

*It has been found, however, that motor performance, and even learning, can occur in the absence of proprioceptive information. This will be discussed more fully in Chapter 14.

Another component of voluntary movement involves purposive conduct or stable intention; that is, an effective movement must be carried on in a goal-directed manner, taking in all of the factors about the present stimuli, previous experiences, and the consequences of just-performed movements. If the prefrontal areas are damaged, the somatosensory component, spatial organization, and plasticity of the movement remain but goal-directed movements are replaced by inappropriate repetitions of already-completed movements or impulsive responses to the stimuli. Luria (1970) reported that a patient with damage to the prefrontal lobe wrote a letter to the noted Russian neurosurgeon, Burdenko, that went like this: "Dear Professor, want to tell you that I want to tell you that I want to tell you..." and this was repeated for page after page.

It should now be clear that the old notion that voluntary motor behavior is formed in the narrow areas of the motor and premotor cortex is inaccurate. The areas of the brain contributing to the creation of a voluntary movement include a complex of cortical and subcortical structures, each playing a very specific role in the entire functional system. Of course, there is much that is still unknown, and this whole area of study is still in its infancy. The next few years promise to be exciting ones for more precisely specifying the role of the various brain mechanisms in voluntary motor control.

8

Motor Integration and Control: The Brainstem and Spinal Cord

In this chapter we continue our examination of the various levels for motor integration and control of human movement. In the last chapter, we examined the cortical, basal ganglia, and the cerebellar levels as well as the motor pathways. The brainstem and spinal cord levels for motor function are the subjects of this chapter.

THE BRAINSTEM

The next level for motor integration and control is the brainstem. The two major structures of the brainstem are the pons and the medulla, and they contain numerous nuclei that are concerned with the control of motor activity. The reticular formation, extending throughout the brainstem, also projects ascending and descending signals to influence motor behavior when it is stimulated.

Input to the brainstem arrives from many sources. Axons from all of the sensory systems pass through the brainstem and they give off many collaterals which then synapse on brainstem nuclei neurons. In addition, the cerebellum, cerebral cortex, and the basal ganglia have projections into the brainstem. This area of the nervous system is, then, an integrative area for combining and coordinating all sensory information with motor information. Information from these various sources is then used to control many of our involuntary movements.

A. BRAINSTEM REFLEXES

The brainstem plays an essential part in the more automatic types of motor activity. Much of our postural, locomotor, cardiovascular, respiratory, and gastrointestinal activity is mediated by the brainstem, and a great deal of this activity is carried out in the form of reflexes.

A reflex is the simplest functioning unit of nervous activity, and many functions of the nervous system are performed by reflexes. In fact, much human behavior is reflexive. A reflex is a relatively constant pattern of response or behavior that is similar for a given stimulus. Reflex behavior might involve glands, i.e. sweating, as well as muscles.

The word reflex is from the Latin meaning bending back. This is very appropriate because to bring about a reflex nerve impulses travel from a sensory receptor along a sensory axon to the CNS; there the impulse "bends back" and moves away from the CNS, along a motorneuron axon, to activate a muscle or gland to bring about a response (Fig. 8.1).

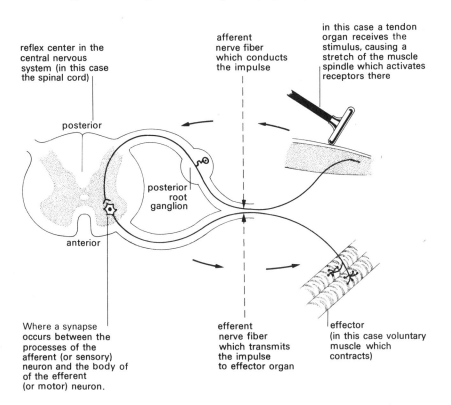

Fig. 8.1 Basic nervous unit for reflex behavior. (Based on McNaught and Callander, 1963.)

Four basic nervous units are necessary in reflexes:

1. A receptor—all of the sensory receptors in the body are potential receptor organs for reflexes.
2. An afferent neuron—a sensory neuron projecting to the CNS.
3. An efferent neuron—a motorneuron from the CNS to muscles or glands.
4. An effector—all of the muscles and glands are effector organs.

A fifth unit consisting of one or more interneurons is characteristic but not essential. The total pathway is called a "reflex arc" and it can function independently of higher brain centers. This independence, however, is not typical of nervous reflexes.

1. Respiration and cardiovascular reflexes

Two essential life-maintaining processes, respiration and cardiovascular regulation, have reflex control centers in the brainstem. Breathing depends entirely upon the cyclical inspiration and expiration of air from the lungs, and this activity is produced by the diaphragm and the intercostal muscles. Control of the neural activity of these respiratory muscles resides primarily in neurons the cell bodies of which lie in the medulla. Recording of electrical activity in the respiratory center of the medulla has demonstrated that certain neurons fire off in perfect synchrony with inspiration and others discharge synchronously with expiration. Although this vital center is continually subject to a variety of stimuli, its basic functions of automaticity and rhythmicity are a result of reflex connections, and the stimuli from the environment or from the body itself which have an accelerating or retarding action on either the inspiratory or expiratory neurons produce these changes in a reflex manner.

The cardiovascular control center is also located in the brainstem. Although cardiac muscle is capable of self-excitation and nerves to the heart merely alter the basic inherent rate and are not actually required for cardiac contraction, there are, nevertheless, important neural connections which modify cardiovascular activity. Indeed, this center is essential for blood-pressure regulation, and damage to it or destruction of it causes almost immediate death.

The cell bodies of the neurons of this control center are located in the medulla, and the axons of these neurons make complex connections with autonomic nervous system* neurons which influence blood-pressure regula-

---

*The autonomic nervous system (ANS) consists of neurons located in the central nervous system and peripheral nervous system which controls the response of smooth muscles and glands. It functions to control and regulate the internal environment of the body. A full examination of this part of the nervous system will be made in Chapter 23.

tion and cardiac activity. The neurons of the cardiovascular center are innervated by afferent neurons whose receptors are in the carotid artery and in the arch of the aorta. (The aorta is a large artery and its arch is located just above the heart.) As the carotid artery passes through the neck, the wall of the artery is thinner than usual and here there are nerve endings which are highly sensitive to stretching; there is a similar area for stretch receptors in the aorta. These stretch-sensitive receptors help to regulate arterial pressure and heart rate. Of course, other parts of the vascular network also contain stretch-sensitive receptors and they keep the medulla constantly informed about arterial and venous pressure.

The aortic and carotid arteries also contain receptors which are sensitive to the concentrations of arterial oxygen, carbon dioxide, and hydrogen ions. These receptors send information to the cardiovascular center for reflexive control to accommodate the oxygen demands of the cardiovascular system. Other information from sensory receptors of all kinds and from the higher brain centers impinges on this center. The heart rate and vascular system pressure at any moment reflect the various inputs to this center.

2. Righting reflexes

Postural reflexes for righting, walking, and other body positions have their centers in the brainstem. Sensory impulses originating in the vestibular apparatus are sent through the appropriate cranial nerve to the brainstem and synapse on neurons which are used to contract muscles for upright posture and to control muscles of the eyes. The vestibular apparatus, a part of the membranous labyrinth of the inner ear area, has sensitive hair cells which produce neural impulses when displaced. A more detailed description of this structure was given in Chapter 5.

Information from the vestibular apparatus is used for two basic purposes: First, to control the muscles which regulate the eyes so that in spite of movements of the head, the eyes remain fixed on the same point; second, for maintaining upright posture.

Extensive study of postural reflexes has identified four groups of righting reflexes—reflexes which function in righting responses. These righting reflexes are:

1. The labyrinthine-righting reflexes.
2. The neck-righting reflexes.
3. Body-righting reflexes from tactile stimulation.
4. Optic-righting reflexes.

Righting reflexes are concerned with maintaining the body in an orientation to gravity.

These reflexes have been studied by sectioning parts of an animal's brain in such a way that the midbrain and thalamus are left intact but higher brain levels cannot influence the behavior. The result is called a "thalamic preparation."

The labyrinthine-righting reflexes may be observed in a blindfolded animal with intact labyrinths. When the animal is held, head down, by the pelvis or hind legs, its head will remain in an upright posture, as far as possible, regardless of how the pelvis is rotated. Such reflex head movements are absent in labyrinthectomized (labyrinths removed) animals; thus, these reflexes must depend on the functioning of the vestibular apparatus. These reflexes hardly exist in a newborn human, but they develop in the first few months, and as they develop they help the growing child in the various postural tasks of lifting its head, sitting up, and finally standing.

The neck-righting reflexes concern the position of the neck with respect to the head. If the body is tilted, the labyrinthine reflexes restore the head to an upright position. As the head is brought upright, the neck becomes twisted in relation to the head which triggers the neck-righting reflexes causing the upper and then lower parts of the body to be brought back in line with the head.

The body-righting reflexes may be induced in a blindfolded labyrinthectomized animal by asymmetrical stimulation of the skin, such as lowering the animal in a lateral position onto a surface. In this case, even if the head of the animal is held firmly in the lateral position, its body will right itself. This is an example of the body-righting reflex.

The optic-righting reflexes play a major role in postural orientation in most higher animals, and the orientation of the head is controlled mostly by vision. A blindfolded thalamic preparation animal with labyrinths removed will display disorientation of its head until the blindfold is removed and the eyes are allowed to fixate on the environment. At that point, the optic-righting reflexes will cause the animal to attempt to attain an upright head and body position.

In the normal individual, all of these righting reflexes function together to maintain the upright posture. In the disoriented position, a sequence of events, called a chain reflex, occurs. For reorientation, the head leads the way through the mediation of the optic and labyrinthine reflexes, then the upper body is lined up with the head by the functioning of the neck-righting reflexes, and finally the lower body rotates into line with the upper positions.

It is clear that maintenance of upright posture depends on several sensory modalities, in addition to the vestibular receptors. Vision as well as tactile stimulation of the skin plays a critical role. Persons with defective labyrinths, even when blindfolded, are largely able to compensate for their disability in postural tests.

Much human movement behavior involves the assuming of certain postures, and reflexes play an important role in this behavior. In the adult, postural reflexes are integrated with complex learned movement patterns. The infant, however, does not possess a functional cerebral cortex, and thus exhibits postural reflexes in a primitive form.

3. Tonic reflexes

Another type of postural reflex which is mediated mainly, but not exclusively, by brainstem centers is called tonic reflexes. Tonic reflexes are concerned with the control of the position of one part of the body in relation to other parts, but not in relation to gravity. The tonic reflexes last as long as the head is held in a given position. The two tonic reflexes which are of particular interest in movement behavior are the tonic neck reflex (TNR) and the tonic labyrinthine reflex (TLR). The first results from stimulation of the neck-muscle receptors and the second from stimulation of the vestibular apparatus.

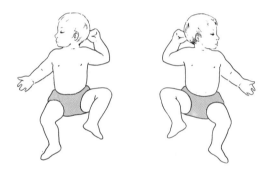

Fig. 8.2 Tonic neck reflex (fencing position) in an infant. (Based on Deutsch and Deutsch, 1966.)

Tonic neck reflexes may be noted in human infants during the first six months after birth. During this period, the cerebral cortex has not gained control over lower reflex centers. The tonic neck reflex manifests itself by a rotation of the head to one side causing stimulation of joint receptors in the neck which results in extension of both limbs on the side to which the face is rotated; at the same time, there is a relaxation of the limbs on the side toward the back of the head (Fig. 8.2). Lowering of the head (ventriflexion) causes a flexion of the arms and an extension of the legs. Elevation of the head (dorsiflexion) causes an opposite response. This reflex may be seen in the active behavior of a four-footed animal, such as a cat. As the cat lowers its head to eat food on the ground, the forelimbs relax. When the head is elevated, there is usually some relaxation in the hind limbs.

In humans, TNRs are obscured as motor development continues. They blend into the overall righting reflexes by helping to assure that the body follows the head in spatial orientation.

In tonic labyrinthine reflexes, isolated from tonic neck reflexes, when the individual is moved into different positions in relation to gravity the extensor tonus changes in the same way in all four limbs. The tonus is maximal in the supine position and minimal in the prone position. In human infants, the TLR produces stereotyped extension in all the limbs when the child is placed in a supine position; the prone position produces flexion in all the limbs. The TLR is masked by more complex reflexes as the infant matures (Fig. 8.3).

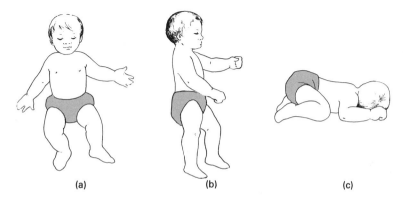

(a)   (b)   (c)

Fig. 8.3 Tonic labyrinthine reflexes. (a) All limbs in extension in the supine position. (b) Under limbs extended in side position. (c) All limbs in flexion in prone position. (Based on Gardner, 1969.)

The TNR and TLR are most easily seen in decerebrate (brain severed from the brainstem and spinal cord) animals. They are not easily detected in intact humans after the first few months of life, but they may be seen in some clinical conditions. This does not mean, however, that these reflexes are obliterated in the mature person. It means, instead, that they have become subservient to more useful motor control patterns. Hellebrandt and her associates (Hellebrandt and Waterland, 1962; Hellebrandt, Schade, and Carns, 1962) have demonstrated the presence of these reflexes in normal adults, and they have shown that these reflexes function especially during stressful motor activity to reinforce muscle contraction and extend endurance. More recently C. George (1970, 1972) has demonstrated facilitative and inhibitory effects of the tonic neck reflex upon grip strength of children five to seven years of age. Although the reflexes are not readily apparent, they probably play a vital role in the coordination of limb and body movements into an organized pattern.

THE RETICULAR FORMATION

One of the critically important brainstem mechanisms for the control of reflex movements and coordination of motor activity is the reticular formation.
Since the structural components and the overall functions of this mechanism
were discussed in an earlier chapter, they will not be repeated here.

Some reticular formation axons descend into the spinal cord, and it is
through these descending fibers, called reticulospinal fibers, that the reticular formation exerts many subtle influences in controlling basic patterns
of reflex connections to conform with postural needs or specific motor commands from the cortex or related extrapyramidal centers. Reticular formation excitation may cause enough spinal facilitation to cause movements—even complete postural adjustments. Usually, however, the reticular formation functions to facilitate or inhibit motor adjustments and
therefore modifies instead of elicits postural and phasic actions.

THE SPINAL CORD

The lowest level of organization for control of motor movements is the gray
matter of the spinal cord. In the anterior horn of the cord are two types of
spinal motorneurons. The first is called the alpha motorneuron; its cell body
is located in the spinal cord and its axons and collaterals pass through
spinal nerves to terminate on extrafusal muscle fibers, which are the main
skeletal muscles. It is through these neurons that impulses must pass on
their way to skeletal muscles. The gamma motorneuron is the second type of
spinal motorneuron; its cell body lies in the cord also and its axons and collaterals also pass through the spinal nerves, but the terminals end on the
specialized muscle fibers of the muscle spindle, the intrafusal muscle fibers.
Impulses from these motorneurons initiate the "gamma loop" servomechanism* which will be discussed below.

A. ALPHA MOTORNEURONS

Alpha motorneurons are the final common pathway for transmission of
motor impulses from the brain to the skeletal muscles. They have rather
large diameter axons averaging between 8 to 20 millimicrons, and they conduct impulses at velocities of around 100 meters per second. Their cell
bodies lie wholly within the CNS and their axons pass through cranial and
spinal nerves to end at neuromuscular junctions with skeletal muscle fibers.

---

*A servomechanism is any control system for maintaining an operation according to
a certain predetermined plan. A simple example is the thermostat.

It is only through the individual cranial and spinal motorneurons that the initiation, maintenance, or modulation of movement is possible.

Each alpha motorneuron cell body may have from 100 to over 15,000 synaptic endings on it which converge from many different sources. The activity or inactivity of the motorneuron depends upon the sum of the excitatory and inhibitory synaptic activity impinging upon it at any moment. If the sum of input is strongly excitatory, the motorneuron fires impulses at a rate reflecting the intensity of the stimulus; if the sum of synaptic input is predominately inhibitory, the neuron does not fire; finally, if the sum of input is excitatory but not enough to reach a threshold potential, the neuron is said to be facilitated.

On the average, each alpha motorneuron in the spinal cord innervates approximately 150 muscle fibers; thus, stimulation of one alpha motorneuron results in the contraction of 150 extrafusal muscle fibers, assuming the stimulation is strong enough to achieve the threshold potential of the muscle

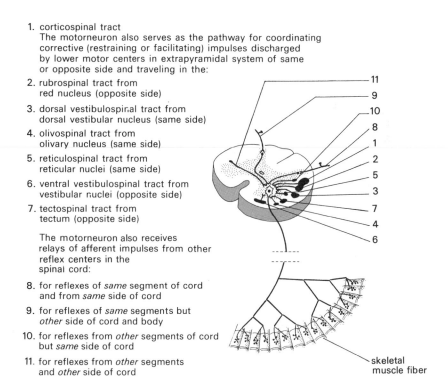

1. corticospinal tract
   The motorneuron also serves as the pathway for coordinating corrective (restraining or facilitating) impulses discharged by lower motor centers in extrapyramidal system of same or opposite side and traveling in the:

2. rubrospinal tract from
   red nucleus (opposite side)

3. dorsal vestibulospinal tract from
   dorsal vestibular nucleus (same side)

4. olivospinal tract from
   olivary nucleus (same side)

5. reticulospinal tract from
   reticular nuclei (same side)

6. ventral vestibulospinal tract from
   vestibular nuclei (opposite side)

7. tectospinal tract from
   tectum (opposite side)

   The motorneuron also receives relays of afferent impulses from other reflex centers in the spinal cord:

8. for reflexes of *same* segment of cord
   and from *same* side of cord

9. for reflexes of *same* segments but
   other side of cord and body

10. for reflexes from *other* segments of cord
    but *same* side of cord

11. for reflexes from *other* segments
    and *other* side of cord

skeletal
muscle fiber

Fig. 8.4   The final common pathway. Each anterior motorneuron serves as a pathway for impulses originating in other parts of the nervous system. (Based on McNaught and Callander, 1963.)

fibers. As you recall, a single alpha motorneuron and all the extrafusal muscle fibers innervated by it are called a motor unit (Fig. 8.4).

B. GAMMA MOTORNEURONS

Like the alpha motorneurons, the cell bodies of gamma motorneurons lie entirely in the CNS and their axons pass through cranial and spinal nerves, but their terminals end at junctions on the intrafusal muscles of the muscle spindle. There are at least two distinct types of intrafusal muscle fibers: nuclear chain fibers and nuclear bag fibers. The former are the smallest and are contained entirely within the spindle capsule and have only a single column of nuclei through their equatorial region. The larger fibers, the nuclear bag fibers, pass beyond the capsule and attach to the connective tissue of the extrafusal muscle fibers. The nuclei are centrally located and are swollen into a baglike structure. There are some functional differences in these intrafusal fibers, but these will not concern us here.

While alpha motorneuron fibers often divide to produce upwards to 100 terminal junctions, individual gamma neurons supply only a few different extrafusal fibers, although one gamma neuron may innervate several spindles within the same skeletal muscle. Gamma neuron axons are small (2 to 8 millimicrons) and conduct impulses at a lower velocity (10-50 m/sec) than the alpha neurons. About one-third of the total motorneurons of the spinal cord are the gamma type. The intrafusal muscle fibers which are innervated by the gamma fibers are too few and too small to contribute to contraction of skeletal muscles; their contraction, instead, results in stretching their central, noncontractile portions, where the spindle sensory receptors are located, causing these receptors to fire off.

As noted in Chapter 5, lying in parallel with the main muscles is a specialized structure, the muscle spindle, containing intrafusal muscle fibers with their own motor nerve supply and sense organs which are stimulated when the spindle is stretched or the intrafusal muscles contract. The spindle receptors may be activated in two basically different ways: (1) By contraction of intrafusal fibers; (2) By any event which lengthens the skeletal muscle and thus stretches the muscle spindle. Spindle afferents enter the CNS and synapse on alpha motorneurons which supply the same extrafusal muscle group of which the spindle is a part. The result is a contraction of the extrafusal muscles.

When gamma motor signals cause contraction of the intrafusal muscle fibers, this stretches their central regions and stimulates the spindle afferents. They synapse on the alpha motorneurons of the same muscle group causing contraction of the extrafusal fibers which shortens the intrafusal fibers, unloading the stretch on the spindle afferents. Thus, when the extrafusal muscle contraction reduces the length of the intrafusal muscle fibers, they cease firing because a steady state of the extrafusal muscles and intrafusal muscles has been achieved. It may be seen that the complete reflex mechanism constitutes a "follow-up servomechanism," the skeletal muscle length tending to follow changes in the spindle length. The spindle afferents themselves do in fact record not length but the difference in length between extrafusal muscle and spindle; they are misalignment detectors.

The actual activation of skeletal muscles can occur in two ways: (1) By direct signals from the alpha motorneurons; (2) Indirectly, via the gamma loop; that is, gamma signals cause intrafusal muscle contraction, stimulating spindle afferents, which stimulate alpha motorneurons, which in turn produce extrafusal muscle contraction. It appears that in normal body movements the motor systems play mutually cooperative roles. Thus, the CNS has two pathways through which neural commands may be transmitted to control skeletal muscle contraction, one by way of the alpha motorneurons and the other by way of the gamma motorneurons.

It is likely that in voluntary movements pyramidal and extrapyramidal tract impulses stimulate both alpha and gamma motorneurons in a synchronous manner. The alpha motorneurons are stimulated to fire impulses so as to bring about skeletal muscle contraction. Simultaneously the gamma motorneurons fire so as to contract intrafusal fibers and set up the gamma loop. Direct motor supply to the gamma neurons enables the spindle to adjust intrafusal fiber length during active contraction of extrafusal muscles, thus eliminating or minimizing unloading by resetting intrafusal length.

The net effect of intrafusal muscle shortening over the range of movement to coincide with the shortening of the extrafusal fibers is that if the extrafusal fibers are suddenly stretched, the muscle spindle will be stretched and spindle afferents will discharge, producing increased extrafusal muscle contraction and reflexively reducing the stretch.

It has been suggested that some voluntary movements are actually produced solely by the gamma loop system, especially slow movements and postural adjustments. The notion here is that the gamma loop system actually drives the contraction of skeletal muscles. That is, signals from the motor tracts supply the appropriate impulse code to the gamma neurons to bring about, through the gamma loop, the appropriate contraction of the extrafusal muscles to produce the intended movement. One advantage of driving the main muscles through the gamma loop is that the valuable self-regulating or servo properties of the stretch reflex are maintained at all lengths during the movement. On the other hand, movements initiated indirectly via the gamma loop would suffer delay from conduction time to and from the muscle, so for fast starting movements this system would not be very effective.

At the present there is a consensus that it is unlikely that any movements are initiated solely by the gamma loop. "Coactiviation" of the alpha and gamma motorneurons seems to be the more accepted notion with regard to motor control, though each system perhaps is preferential for some types of movements. For example, it has been speculated that for fast starting movements the descending motor tract signals probably converge primarily on the alpha motorneurons while gamma motor inputs are primarily employed for smooth, continuous control.

When performers wish to make a quick, forceful movement, they can increase the forcefulness of the movement by quickly stretching the muscle group that will then be used to bring about the movement. By stretching the muscle, they stimulate the spindle afferents which send impulses to the alpha motorneurons serving that muscle group. Simultaneously they can voluntarily send impulses to these same alpha motorneurons via the pyramidal and extrapyramidal tracts. The effect will be a summing of impulses upon these alpha motorneurons, and a maximal contraction of the appropriate skeletal muscles. For example, stamping the foot hard against the floor, thus stretching spindles in the gastrocnemius (calf) muscle, just before jumping, will result in a higher jump than if this is not done.

C. OTHER SPINAL MOTORNEURONS

In addition to the alpha and gamma spinal motorneurons, many other neurons in the gray matter of the cord are capable of assisting in certain kinds of organized motor activity. You will recall from the previous chapter that most pyramidal system (corticospinal tract) axons terminate on interneurons located in the spinal cord gray matter. Thus, the motor impulses are usually transmitted through interneurons before finally reaching the spinal motorneurons that control muscles. Other motor fiber pathways, besides those of the pyramidal tract, terminate on the interneurons, too.

In the anterior horns of the cord there is also an important interneuron, called the Renshaw cell which, when stimulated, serves to inhibit the antagonistic muscles of those which are contracting. This activity is called reciprocal innervation.

D. SPINAL REFLEXES

Like the brainstem, the spinal cord performs important motor functions in the form of reflexes. Spinal cord reflex arcs vary from simple two-neuron arcs to complex arcs which involve literally hundreds of neurons. Some of these reflexes serve to protect the body from injury while others initiate postural adjustments.

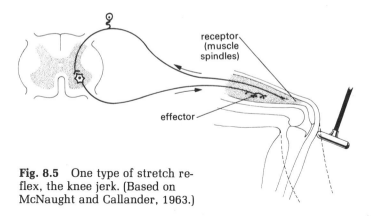

Fig. 8.5   One type of stretch reflex, the knee jerk. (Based on McNaught and Callander, 1963.)

1. Stretch reflexes

The stretch, or myotatic (muscle-stretching), reflex is the simplest of the spinal sensory-motor reflexes, since its basic structure consists of only a single sensory neuron and a single spinal motorneuron, and this type of reflex arc is referred to as monosynaptic because of this characteristic.

The knee jerk exemplifies a phasic type of stretch reflex (Fig. 8.5(a)). To produce the knee jerk, the subject is seated and one leg is crossed over the other at the knee. Then the patellar tendon (located just below the knee cap) of the hanging leg is hit. The tendon stretches the quadriceps muscles, which stretches muscle spindles embedded in the quadriceps. The spindle receptors are stimulated and send impulses to the spinal cord which synapse with alpha motorneurons and efferent signals are transmitted back to the quadriceps. The result is a quick muscular contraction causing the lower leg to jerk forward. While this movement may not have much functional value, it does have clinical significance. If a reflex can be elicited, it demonstrates that both sensory and motor nerve connections are functional.

In this type of reflex, the muscle is stretched quickly and all the muscle spindles within it are excited simultaneously. All the muscles are activated at once, resulting in a brief forceful movement. Additionally, there are static types of stretch reflexes. When a muscle is slowly stretched, only a few muscle spindle receptors are stimulated at one time. This causes varying muscle fibers to be activated. This type of neuronal activity produces a more sustained contraction—a contraction in which only a relatively few muscle fibers may be functioning at any one time.

The primary purpose of the stretch reflex is to oppose changes in muscle length, especially sudden changes. The functional significance of the stretch reflex during voluntary motor activity is not clearly understood, but it is believed that this reflex functions to "damp" movements to prevent jerkiness and "overshooting" (hypermetria) during movement, since jerkiness of movement and "overshooting" do result when the stretch reflex is lost from a body segment.

2. Flexion reflexes

The arrangement of three or more neurons is the most common reflex arc. In a three-neuron reflex arc, an interneuron mediates between the sensory neurons and motorneurons. Actually, this is an oversimplification, for seldom would we find just a single interneuron in a reflex arc. More often, a number of interneurons connect an afferent and an efferent neuron to form a reflex arc, and there may be a whole chain of them leading up and down the spinal cord from one segment to others. This would be considered a multisynaptic reflex (Fig. 8.6).

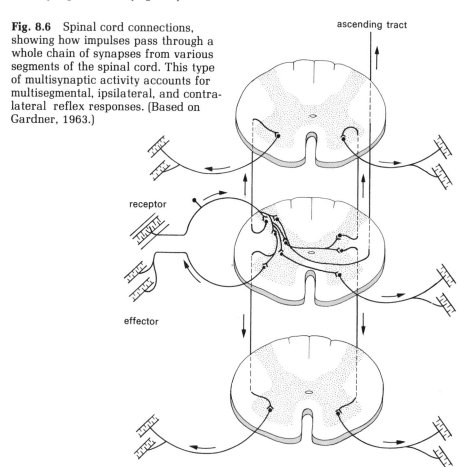

Fig. 8.6   Spinal cord connections, showing how impulses pass through a whole chain of synapses from various segments of the spinal cord. This type of multisynaptic activity accounts for multisegmental, ipsilateral, and contralateral reflex responses. (Based on Gardner, 1963.)

The flexion reflex is complex and is considered to be a classic example of a multisynaptic reflex connection. The flexion reflex consists of a contraction of the flexor muscles while reciprocal connections with the antagonistic extensor muscles cause reciprocal inhibition, resulting in relaxation of the extensors. This interaction of muscle groups permits movement of the stimulated limb away from the source of stimulation. In its classical form the flexor reflex is elicited most frequently by stimulation of pain receptors by application of a pinprick, heat, or some other painful stimulus. Pain causes withdrawal of any injured portion of the body from the object causing the injury.

One example of a flexion-reflex arc follows: If you touch a hot stove, the heat and pain receptors in your fingers will generate nerve impulses. These nerve impulses will be received by sensory neurons, transmitted to interneurons, and then along alpha motorneurons to effectors. When the nerve impulse leaves the motorneuron and finally arrives at the effectors in your fingers and arms, you withdraw your hand from the hot stove. This entire series of events can occur in less than 20 milliseconds. If some other part of the body besides one of the limbs is stimulated, this part also will be withdrawn from the stimulus; but the reflex may not be confined entirely to flexor muscles; therefore, this reflex is frequently called the withdrawal reflex.

The fiber pathways for eliciting the flexor reflex do not project directly from sensory neurons to the alpha motorneurons; instead they pass first into the CNS neuron network. Thus, a three-neuron arc is the shortest possible circuit for eliciting a flexor reflex. Actually, most of the impulses of the reflex travel over many more neurons than this and involve diverging circuits to spread the impulses to the necessary muscles for withdrawal and inhibitory circuits to inhibit antagonistic muscles.

A stimulus that causes contraction of a muscle usually inhibits the antagonistic muscle. So antagonistic muscles work as a pair and when one contracts, the other is reflexively inhibited, thus allowing the limb to move. This is called reciprocal inhibition. For example, when the flexor muscles contract there are opposing muscles which must simultaneously relax so as not to interfere with the withdrawing motion.

3. Crossed extensor reflex

Another type of reflex which often functions in conjunction with the flexor reflex is called the crossed extensor reflex. Usually, when a flexor reflex occurs in one limb, impulses pass to the opposite limb causing it to extend. Extension of the opposite limb, therefore, aids in pushing the entire body away from the object causing the painful stimulus (Fig. 8.7). A similar reflex plays an important role in all locomotor behavior; a flexion movement in one

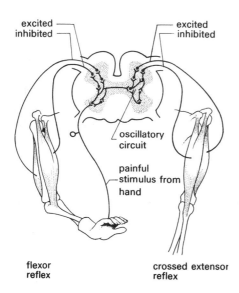

excited
inhibited

excited
inhibited

oscillatory
circuit

painful
stimulus from
hand

flexor
reflex

crossed extensor
reflex

Fig. 8.7 The flexor reflex and the crossed extensor reflex showing their neuronal mechanisms. This also illustrates reciprocal inhibition. (Based on Guyton, 1964.)

limb causes a reflex extension of the opposite limb. In the lower limbs, this action assists in supporting the weight of the body and maintaining the desired posture when the stimulated leg is lifted. Thus, it is at the spinal cord level that postural adjustments are initiated.

Of course, the total pattern of muscular adjustments required to complete gross coordinated movements is complex, but this complex sequence that constitutes locomotion is primarily reflexive. The basic reflexes that contribute to motion are simple. Reflex flexion of one leg initiates a reflex extension of the opposite leg. This oscillation back and forth between extensor and flexor muscles seems to result from reciprocal inhibition. Postural reflexes maintain or restore the equilibrium of the body during and after movement.

4. Extensor thrust reflex

One of the most complex reflexes in the body is the extensor thrust reflex, which is another reflex important to postural adjustment. This reflex helps to support the body against gravity. It is initiated by pressure on the footpads. The pressure excites the cutaneous skin receptors in the footpads and causes automatic contraction of the extensor muscles of the leg. This reaction involves a complex circuit in the interneurons similar to that responsible for the flexor and crossed-extensor reflexes.

Pressure on the footpad of a decerebrate animal (brain severed from the brainstem and spinal cord) will cause the foot to extend against the pressure that is being applied to it. Indeed, if the animal is placed on its feet, the footpads will reflexively stiffen and the limbs will support the weight of the body. This illustrates that standing posture does not depend upon higher-brain-level function but instead is a product of reflexes.

5. Muscle–tendon protection reflex

A reflex that protects the muscles and tendons is the so-called clasp-knife reflex. Skeletal muscles do not attach directly to bones; instead they are connected with tendons, which attach to bones. In the tendinous ends of skeletal muscles lie the Golgi tendon organs which are stimulated by tension on the tendons of a muscle group. Contraction of muscles produces tension and thus stretch on the tendon receptors and when their threshold potential is achieved, impuses are transmitted into the spinal cord. The Golgi tendon afferents synapse in the spinal cord upon interneurons which innervate alpha motorneurons which innervate the same muscle fibers from which the stimulated tendon afferents connect.

The interneurons on which the Golgi tendon organ axons terminate secrete an inhibitory transmitter substance, so the effect that tendon afferent transmission has is to inhibit the activity of the alpha motorneuron, causing a relaxation of the muscle fibers connected to the stimulated tendon organs. Golgi tendon organs respond with a greatly increased rate of discharge when the tension produced by muscle contraction is very high. It appears that one of the main functions of these receptors is to serve as a safety device, inhibiting the muscle group when the force it generates is great enough to damage the tendons or muscles. De Vries (1972) has suggested that the clasp-knife reflex may be employed by motor performers to prevent muscle soreness. When a muscle group has been stimulated through exercise, the muscle fails to relax completely. The incomplete relaxation brings about localized ischemia (lack of blood). The ischemia, in turn, brings about pain, which tends to trigger further muscular contraction, so a vicious cycle is begun which produces a spasm-type of response in the muscle and considerable soreness results. This spasm theory of muscle soreness suggests that to break the spasm, a reflex mechanism must be employed to relax the contracting muscles.

With muscle cramps a commonly used technique is to put the muscle into full stretch, hold it there. This usually brings about the clasp-knife reflex because the Golgi tendon organs are stimulated by the intense tension caused by the stretch. De Vries has found that if performers will engage in static stretching (not bouncing) immediately after a workout, muscle soreness is greatly diminished. Static stretching is done by slowly and fully extending the joint and then holding it there for a few seconds. Of course, when there is known rupture around a muscle, stretching should not be employed.

SOME GENERAL REFLEX CHARACTERISTICS

In this chapter several specific types of brainstem and spinal cord reflexes have been identified and discussed. It should be obvious that reflex activity plays an essential role in motor integration and control. Therefore, it is necessary to examine some general characteristics of reflex activity.

A. STRENGTH OF REFLEX RESPONSE

The strength of a reflex response increases as the intensity of the stimulation increases. So if there is an increase in the strength and duration of the stimuli, there will be an increase in the number of impulses arriving in the spinal cord or brainstem which will cause an increase in the intensity of the response. This phenomenon may be understood in the context of spatial and temporal summation. An increase of intensity of stimuli will increase the number of neurons firing and this will activate more motorneurons, causing more muscle fibers to contract, which will bring about a greater contraction of the whole muscle. Also, increasing intensity of the stimuli will increase the frequency of firing in each neuron, causing more frequent contraction of the muscle fibers and a more forceful contraction of the whole muscle.

B. REFLEX LATENCY PERIOD

Even in the simplest reflexes there is a time lapse between the time a stimulus impinges on the sensory receptor and a response occurs. Basically, there are three factors that determine the latency between stimulus and response; they are: speed of transmission over nerve fibers, time required to cross the synapses, including the neuromuscular junction synapse, and the time required for the muscle to contract. The speed of impulse transmission depends upon the diameter of the nerve fibers involved. As you recall, the larger the diameter of a nerve fiber, the faster the rate of transmission. It takes time for the impulse to cross synapses because it must go through an electrical-to-chemical-to-electrical process. The more synapses, the greater the reflex latency. Finally, time is required for muscle fibers to contract after they have received motorneuron impulses.

C. REFLEX AFTEREFFECT

Reflexes may display muscular or glandular activity even after the stimulus has stopped. This is called an aftereffect, or after-discharge. For example, a sensory receptor may be stimulated and a muscle caused to reflexively contract but when the stimulus is withdrawn the muscle may continue to contract for a brief period (normally less than a second). The reason for this is little understood, but one theory hypothesizes that the impulses from the sensory neuron are spread to many interneurons and thus the alpha motorneuron receives impulses at slightly different times, causing it to fire a successive series of impulses, thus prolonging the muscle contraction. This type of process is possible through a repetitive type of circuitry, which is known to exist in the nervous system. These repetitive circuits, along with reflexes, are one means by which reflex muscular contractions can occur rhythmically.

DAMAGE TO THE MOTOR SYSTEM

Much of what is known about the motor functions of the various levels is based on studies on lower animals and on human beings who have had destruction in certain parts of the brain. The motor pathways from the cerebral motor areas terminate on motorneurons whose axons innervate skeletal muscle fibers. Destruction of any of these motorneurons or their fibers at any level is followed by a characteristic clinical picture. When nerve impulses cannot reach the muscle fibers supplied by the destroyed nerve fibers, there is a loss of motor control. Thus, damage to any part of the motor system causes incoordination of movement in certain muscles. Destruction of the cortical motor area results in a general flaccid paralysis, but substantial recovery takes place. Apparently, other cortical areas take over the functions of this area to some extent. Cortical destruction of areas outside the motor area often leaves the victim with the ability to move the limbs normally in simple tasks, but unable to plan and perform complex motor tasks. This condition is known as apraxia. Destruction of motorneurons of the final common pathway results in an irreversible and complete paralysis of muscles innervated by these neurons; the muscles gradually atrophy. When there is no regeneration of nerve fibers, the muscles eventually disappear and are replaced by connective tissue and fat.

9

Learning and Memory

Humans learn from their experiences; that is, they modify their behaviors on the basis of their experiences—they are said to be capable of adaptive behavior. Adaptive behavior is guided by our sensory systems and is, of course, concerned with the selective control of motor mechanisms, so the sensory and motor information which we have already examined will be useful in understanding adaptive behavior.

Complex motor behavior consists of a variety of movements, and these movement patterns must be learned. Although the individual muscle contractions which allow skilled movement are functional in early infancy, the repertoire of complex motor patterns is very small. The movement patterns which require the selection of certain muscle groups (spatial organization) and the contraction of these muscles in a precise sequential order (temporal organization) for skillful movement must be learned. Since all behavior is under the control of the nervous system, learned behavior must result in some modification in this system. Therefore, in this chapter we shall examine the present state of knowledge about what occurs in the nervous system when we learn.

UNDERSTANDING LEARNING AND MEMORY

The subject of learning and how learning and memory occur has been a central topic in psychology since its birth as a scientific discipline, and several elaborate theories of learning have been formulated. Indeed, there are entire college courses devoted to these theories of learning.

Unfortunately, many of the "learning theorists" have not been concerned with what actually occurs in individuals when they learn; rather they have primarily studied behavioral changes which result from various experimenter manipulations. They have manipulated stimuli, observed responses, and then described the responses as learning, or described the behavioral changes that result from practice, reward, or other conditions as learning. In other words, a vast amount of the psychological study dealing with learning has merely described the modifications in behavior which resulted from varying environmental conditions rather than actually identifying and describing the physiological mechanisms which are involved in behavioral modifications.

Perhaps the famous Harvard psychologist, B.F. Skinner, best exemplifies this tradition in learning theory. He believes that since we cannot observe what goes on inside the brain during learning we should stop worrying about how information is transmitted and stored and concentrate instead on creating the behavior which indicates that one possesses that information. According to Skinner, behavior should be broken down into small pieces, reinforced systematically, and in due course shaped in a way that adds up to learning.

Learning theories which focus upon the modification of overt behavior are certainly valuable and they have led to some significant educational and psychotherapeutic developments, but they have not advanced our understanding of how learning actually occurs. For example, describing the response characteristics and performance of an automobile does not help us understand how an automobile engine works—what causes the response characteristics. You have to open up the engine, look inside, and learn how the combustion of gas pushes the pistons, which cause the crankshaft to rotate, which causes the axle to turn, which causes the wheels to turn, to really "understand" how an automobile works.

A. LEARNING AND THE NERVOUS SYSTEM

Learning anything new must involve changes among the billions of neurons in the brain. What we must do to understand how learning occurs is to examine the mechanism that is most involved in behavior—the nervous system. It is a fundamental fact that the changes in behavior called learning are in the last analysis a result of changes in the nervous system. It seems unwise to study about learning without studying about the nervous system, for all of the remarkable functions of learning are mediated by this system.

Learning may be viewed as a neural change which occurs as a result of experiences with stimuli in the environment. That is, it is the internal process assumed to occur whenever a change in performance, not due to maturation or fatigue, exhibits itself. The entire set of conditions responsible for learning is partly internal and partly external to the individual.

B. MEMORY

Closely related to learning is, of course, memory. The ability to learn obviously requires memory. The word memory is really no more than a label used to indicate that people do retain information. Memory is the learned capability for reproducing something, and it is commonly measured by a recognition or recall test (J.A. Adams, 1967). Thus, if I practice a tennis stroke today and can perform it tomorrow, it follows that I have retained something that enables me to recall the movement pattern.

Memory, then, is the retention of the effects of learning of any kind. Specifically, it is the process as well as the product by which the individual stores information. As such, it is assumed to involve some modification in neuronal structures. The postulated neural correlate of memory is called the memory trace.

In any discussion of learning it is difficult to put memory into one category and learning into another. Learning and memory are inextricably related; it is artificial to speak of the learning process as isolated from memory. We, therefore, use the term "learning–memory" frequently in this chapter.

C. PRESENT KNOWLEDGE ABOUT LEARNING–MEMORY

The physical process that underlies the functional changes we call learning has provided a fascinating challenge to many scientists, and the study of the neural basis of learning–memory has been interdisciplinary. Such biological sciences as neuroanatomy, neurophysiology, biochemistry, in addition to psychology, have made important contributions to the work on learning–memory. The basic question that these investigators have been pursuing is exactly what happens when an organism is in the process of learning. The past 50 years of intense research have produced much information about neural mechanisms in learning–memory, but much of the research has raised more questions than it has answered. So our most difficult problem in discussing learning–memory in this context is that we do not yet know the exact neural processes by which it occurs. But, although present knowledge concerning the nervous system's function in learning–memory is far from complete, students of human motor behavior cannot ignore the anatomical and physiological functioning of the nervous system if they are to acquire some understanding of the learning process.

D. LEARNING–MEMORY MECHANISM FUNCTIONS

There are at least four fundamental interrelated functions which a learning–memory mechanism must perform. First, external and internal stimuli impinging on the individual, which constitute experience, must be detected, selected, and registered, or coded, into neural impulses; this might be called a registration function. Second, the coded data about that set of stimuli must be stored; this would constitute a storage function. Third, access to that coded information must be available to retrieve the specific experiences from storage; this would be a retrieval function. Fourth, the retrieved information must again be decoded into neural activity which in some manner recreates the sensations and qualities of the original experience or initiates responses; this might be considered a readout function (Fig. 9.1).

Previous chapters which dealt with sensory integration, and motor integration and control are related to the first and fourth of the functions above. This chapter focuses on the second and third functions of learning–memory. However, since research has been overwhelmingly concerned with memory storage rather than retrieval, we shall have to limit our attention more to this function in examining the neural basis for learning–memory.

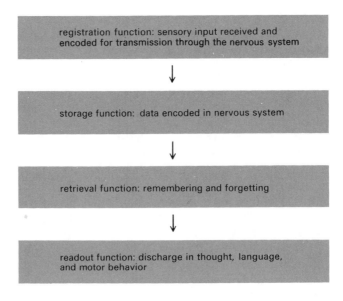

Fig. 9.1 Functions of a memory-learning mechanism.

THEORIES OF LEARNING–MEMORY

The physiological events which must occur when we observe changes in response on the behavioral level have interested scholars for many centuries. Theories about learning–memory prior to the 20th century were mostly based upon myth, superstition, religious teaching, and primitive physiology. The Greek philosopher, Aristotle, taught that the heart was the seat of memory and the brain was a radiator which cooled the blood. A group of pseudoscientists of the 18th and 19th centuries, called phrenologists, thought that the brain was a compartmentalized structure which had separate compartments for intelligence, judgment, speech, humor, etc. (Fig. 9.2).

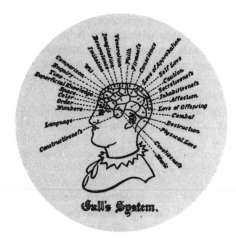

Fig. 9.2   The phrenologists' view of the brain.

A. LOCALIZATION OF MEMORY

In the early years of the 20th century, one of the popular theories was that memories were localized into a single region of the brain. This notion was probably a carryover from phrenological theory, but more significant were the findings from electrical stimulation experiments during the latter decades of the 19th century. These "brain stimulation" experiments had mapped out the somatosensory and motor areas of the cerebral cortex and had shown that sensations and movements could be evoked in certain regions of the brain, depending on where the stimulation was made. This

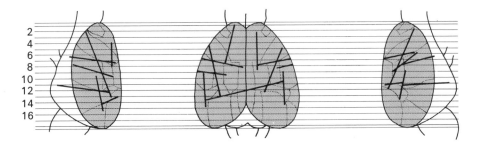

Fig. 9.3   Rats' brains were incised by Karl S. Lashley of Harvard to determine the role of cortical connections in memory. This diagram shows the brain of the rat from the top (center) and both sides. Each heavy line represents an incision made in a single rat. None of the cuts impaired maze-running performance. (Based on Lashley, 1950.)

line of work suggested that a similar localization of function might be present in the brain for memories.

The idea that memories are localized in the brain leads to the conclusion that if the site of memories is removed the memories will be obliterated. Thus, numerous lesion (meaning to destroy tissue) and ablation (meaning to remove tissue) experiments in which various parts of the brain were destroyed or removed were performed in an effort to find the seat of memory. These studies have failed to locate the site or the connection of any pathways responsible for memory. Of course, certain behaviors, especially those based upon complex sensorimotor integration, can be severely disturbed by localized brain destruction, but it is difficult to show unequivocally that memory for some specific event is localized in a particular restricted point in the brain.

Karl S. Lashley, an eminent neurophysiologist, studied the question of brain localization in great detail. Working with laboratory animals of various species (rats, monkeys), he trained the animals to perform some task. He then made deep incisions through different regions of the brain (Fig. 9.3). He reported that these structurally catastrophic conditions caused little memory loss to the animals. Lashley's work, in short, offered no support for the notion that specific areas of the brain act as repositories for memory, into which information to be remembered is stored and from which it is retrieved on demand.

Experiments of this kind on animals and clinical studies of humans led Lashley to formulate his "laws of mass action" and "equipotentiality," which assert that the loss in learned response following ablation is a function of the volume of brain tissue removed or destroyed rather than its location (Lashley, 1950).

Neural mechanisms which mediate learning–memory of language in humans apparently possess some anatomical specificity because there is a permanence of certain memory defects in humans, such as agnosia (inability to recognize familiar objects) and apraxia (inability to carry out purposeful movements in the absence of paralysis), due to temporal lobe impairment. Thus, particular brain regions may play a critical part in the consolidation of memories about certain specific classes of events in humans.

Although there is evidence that certain brain areas may have memory functions, investigators have been moving away from viewing the brain as having centers and regions with specific memory functions. This is primarily because of the discouraging results of experiments designed to localize memory functions since, when primary sensory projection areas are left intact, there is little evidence that localized brain impairment interferes differentially with specific memories.

B. DYNAMIC REVERBERATING MEMORY

Another theory that garnered some popularity around the turn of the century proposed that an experience establishes a continuing electrical activity in a certain set of nerve circuits which then continue to reverberate, and the persistence of these active circuits corresponds to our memory of the experience. According to this theory, when this dynamic trace, or reverberating activity, stops, we lose that memory (Fig. 9.4).

Several rather simple studies have been conducted to test whether memory is purely a dynamic mechanism, with closed loops or reverberating circuits, as the storage process, and the results indicate rather conclusively that this theory is incomplete. If, as this theory suggests, memory consists of active electrical circuits, anything that shuts off the electrical activity, or dramatically disrupts it, should destroy memories. The brain's electrical activity has been stopped or disrupted in several ways. Using lower animals,

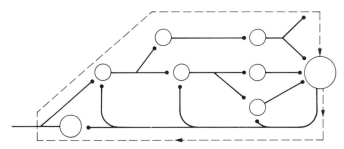

Fig. 9.4   Reverberating neural circuit. Dashed arrow indicates directions of conduction of impulses. (Based on Vander *et al.*, 1970.)

body temperature has been reduced until all brain activity has ceased; normal temperature was allowed to return. After this procedure, it was found that the animals suffered no impairment of performance on a previously learned task—memory was not lost. In another technique, vigorous electric shocks have been delivered to the brain, which momentarily disrupts normal electrical activity. After recovery, the animals' retention of learned tasks was found to be unaffected.

Thus, it appears that memory does not depend entirely upon an active mechanism, or purely dynamic process. This, of course, does not preclude the possibility that the initial dependence of memory necessitates reverberating circuits, for the initial experience does trigger the passage of impulses in the nervous system. Indeed, experimental evidence from studies in which electrical activity in the brain is disrupted shortly after the learning experience has shown an impairment of memory. This will be discussed more fully below.

C. CONSOLIDATION MEMORY THEORY

One of the central questions which contemporary learning–memory investigators have debated is whether the primary physical modification in the nervous system is an active, dynamic, mechanism whereby a series of circulating neural impulses fire continuously with specific spatiotemporal patterning in a reverberating, or closed loop, manner or whether there is a permanent structural change in the physical or chemical properties of neurons in the brain. The former notion, as we discussed above, postulates that as long as impulses are circulating, they give rise to specific behavior responses, which could be classed as memory. Clearly, this theory is incomplete because investigations to test its validity showed that memory does not depend entirely on an active trace of some kind. However, numerous studies have shown that a reverberating electrical trace appears to exist, and even be necessary for memory to develop, for a short time after an experience but then ceases, presumably consolidating memory in the process by producing some structural modification in the brain.

The picture that is beginning to appear from recent research is that there are at least three stages in the learning–memory process. First, as information is received it is transduced at the receptors into a physiological representation which is very briefly stored in what is called a sensory storage system. There is considerable evidence that information persists in a sensory store for two to three seconds for vision and perhaps up to 15 seconds in other sensory modalities (Averback and Sperling, 1961; Eriksen and Collins, 1968; Bliss, Crane, Mansfield, and Townsend, 1966; Wickelgren, 1966; Posner and Konick, 1966). It seems that this representation is transformed into a new code and retained temporarily in another storage system which is of relatively short duration. This second system is called short-term memory (STM). In this stage, there is a fairly brief period during which the relatively fragile and labile trace of an experience is maintained by a transient reverberative process. This phase decays within a few seconds or minutes, but before doing so the short-term electrochemical process causes a series of events in the brain which leads to a subsequent long-lasting phase, representing long-term memory (LTM), during which the memory trace is consolidated in the form of a structural modification of the nervous system, presumably by means of specific biochemical or structural alteration in the neurons. The three processes are viewed as being interrelated in that the activity mechanisms presumably assist in the development of the structural change.

Although there is no universal agreement about the details of this three-stage memory theory by neuroscientists, this theory is dominant in the current literature and commonly goes under the name of "Consolidation Memory Theory." That is the name we shall refer to it in this book.

The original consolidation memory theory was advanced by Müller and Pilzecker (1900). They hypothesized that information is initially stored in some form of dynamic electrical activity and is gradually converted into structural changes at the synapses. More recently Hebb (1949), Konorski (1967), and Eccles (1973), to name only three of the more influential scientists in this field, have supported and extended the consolidation theory. Although the details of their writings vary, common basic concepts and hypotheses are easily discernible and they are sufficiently similar to provide a composite model of memory. Briefly, it is suggested that following a learning experience a continuing process of neural activity occurs in the form of reverberating electrical activity until a memory trace is firmly consolidated, or stored, in the form of some structural and/or chemical change.

According to memory consolidation theory, the first stage in consolidating a memory occurs immediately after the experience, and may be viewed as an image of a stimulus which is maintained for from 1 to 15 seconds after the physical stimulus ends. Another brief period follows which consists of dynamic electrical events; this stage is referred to as short-term memory (STM).

One thing that is clearly implied from consolidation theory is that if the electrical events in the short-term stage of memory are interrupted, the final stage, or LTM, will not be triggered, and memory of the experience will be lost. This prediction has been supported by numerous studies which have shown that if the brain is disturbed soon after a learning event, memory storage is disrupted.

Whereas STM has limited capacity, in general it seems that LTM has virtually unlimited capacity. Moreover, although information in STM may be lost completely and leave no permanent record, it is possible that no complete loss of memory occurs among materials which have reached LTM. Whether one can retrieve, or remember, certain information may be dependent upon such factors as the precise way the information is stored, the available cues to the subject for locating the information, and so on. Loss of information from LTM may involve it becoming misplaced in the complex associative structure of memory, rather than actually being eliminated. The loss is like losing a golf ball; the ball still exists (probably out there in the rough), but the owner cannot locate it. On the other hand, there may actually be a loss of information over time or the information may be interfered with by previously learned or subsequently learned information. The theories of forgetting information presumed to be in LTM will be more fully discussed in Chapter 16 under the section entitled "Retention."

1. Evidence for short-term memory

There is a considerable body of clinical and experimental evidence which supports the consolidation memory theory. If, as the consolidation theory suggests, there is a period of continuing electrical activity after an experience which gradually triggers the consolidation of a memory trace, or LTM, then anything that interferes with, or disrupts, STM, will prohibit the LTM stage from forming.

Perhaps the most compelling clinical support for consolidation theory comes from head injury in humans. After a severe head injury, there is usually a period of unconsciousness. When consciousness is regained, there is frequently a loss of memory of events just before the accident; common exclamations are: "What happened?" "Where am I?" "How did I get here?" This condition is known as Retrograde Amnesia (RA). With RA, memory loss occurs from the second before the accident and becomes less pronounced for events occurring some time before. In other words, there is typically no impairment of memory other than for very recent events. Russell (1959) reported that of over 1000 cases of head injury which he studied in only about 13 percent was there no report of RA. Amnesia was reported for events occurring from a few seconds to 30 minutes before the injury in about 67 percent of the cases; in the other cases there was RA for periods longer than 30 minutes. It appears, then, that the injury to the head causes electrical disruption of events which are in STM and thus prevent the STM from triggering the LTM stage. There is no memory deficit for events occurring some time before the accident, presumably because they were already in LTM and therefore not affected by momentary electrical disruption caused by the accident.

Experimental work with electroconvulsive shock (ECS) is more convincing with regard to consolidation theory. In ECS a rather substantial electric charge is passed through the brain. It has been shown, both with humans and with animals, that shock, if given shortly after a learning experience, produces a retention deficit. It has further been shown that as the interval between the learning and the application of the ECS increases, the learning deficit decreases.

It would not be feasible to review all of the pertinent research in which ECS has been used, but a few examples should help to elucidate the findings in which this technique was employed. Halstead and Rucker (1968) used ECS to interfere with STM in mice. A mouse was placed on a platform under an intensely bright light. To escape the light, the mouse quickly stepped into a nearby hole. Once in the hole, it received a foot shock. The next day under the same conditions, the mouse would not step into the hole, presumably because it remembered being shocked when it stepped in the hole. However, if a mild electrical current was passed through its brain immediately after the foot shock, the next day the mouse would not hesitate to run into the hole to escape the light. Apparently, the electrical current disrupted the STM process. But if the electric current was not passed through the mouse's brain for some time after it received the foot shock, the effect on the mouse's memory was much less, suggesting the information had reached LTM, and therefore was not bothered by electric shock, before the electric current was applied.

Similar experiments have been conducted using a step-down procedure with rats. Rats placed on a platform will step off of it consistently. If the rat is shocked when it steps off the platform, it "learns" to stay on the platform. However, if a rat is shocked when it steps off the platform and its STM is interfered with by a mild electrical current being passed across its brain, thus disturbing the STM process, when tested the next day the animal acts as if there were no memory of the foot shock and it steps down off the platform. When a long time interval is allowed between the foot shock and the electrical current through the brain, the rat "remembers" the foot shock, and will not step off the platform again. It appears that the STM process has now had time to establish the long-term processes before it was disrupted.

Clinical work in which ECS therapy has been used with human patients in an effort to correct certain "mental" dysfunctions has shown that the patients are not only disoriented immediately after the ECS treatment, but they are also confused about events immediately before the ECS. In other words, the ECS treatment frequently produces a genuine Retrograde Amnesia.

Experiments in whch anesthetic and convulsant drugs, such as ether, sodium pentobarbital, and pentylenetetrazol, were administered to animals soon after learning trials to interfere with STM have generally yielded results comparable with ECS experiments. On the other hand, stimulant drugs have been injected into animals shortly after completion of learning periods, and the animals were tested for learning retention after the drugs had worn off. Comparisons with control animals (those who learned the same task but did not receive an injection of stimulant drugs) demonstrated the superiority of the drug-treated animals. Investigators have concluded that the results with the stimulant drugs could best be interpreted as showing that these drugs improve memory consolidation by facilitating the short-term memory process.

It may be seen that the evidence for some sort of short-term memory process which gradually produces a long-term memory trace is rather convincing. However, the exact way in which this short-term mechanism functions has not been ascertained. The most generally accepted hypothesis at this time is that the neurons in the brain record a sensory input by means of a pattern of neural activity and that a reverberating circuit is established in a set of neurons and the nerve impulse circulates many times in a closed, self-exciting, circuit until some type of permanent process develops to "stamp-in" or consolidate the data and cause LTM. This process—a reverberating circuit for STM and a permanent storage mechanism—seems to be confirmed in the experiments mentioned above.

2. Motor short-term memory

The STM concept of consolidation memory theory was formulated from observations of verbal, visual, and auditory memory and most of its support has come from work involving these tasks, but within the past decade there has been a growing interest in whether verbal, visual, auditory, and motor memory follow the same laws. In most experiments on motor STM, blindfolded subjects have pushed a slide or turned a lever through an arc (from 5° to 160°) which was preset by the experimenter. Either immediately or after rest intervals from 5 to as much as 120 seconds, the subjects attempted to reproduce the extent of movement originally performed. There have been a number of variations on this procedure, of course.

The investigations so far provide for only a few tentative conclusions. One rather consistent finding is that there is spontaneously forgetting in STM regardless of whether the retention interval (the time between a practice trial and a retest) is filled with an interpolated task.* Adams and Dijkstra (1966) were the first to report that errors on a test of kinestetic recall was an increasing function of the retention interval and others have reported similar findings (Posner and Konick, 1966; Posner, 1967).

Although the findings are contradictory with regard to the effects on motor STM of an interpolated task, it seems that task-related interference is

---

*An interpolated task is a task of some kind that is inserted between trials in an experiment. The subject must perform the interpolated task during a retention interval.

a powerful source of forgetting. Conversely, verbal tasks and certain other "unrelated" tasks that subjects have had to perform as interpolated tasks have not produced consistent interfering effects. Several investigators found that, just as with STM for verbal responses, the pattern of retention of voluntary blindfolded movements declined significantly when subjects had to perform interpolated kinesthetic tasks; in other words, kinesthetic recall is subject to interference when the interpolated task involves certain types of movement of attention-demanding tasks (Jones, 1974; Patrick, 1971; Stelmach and Wilson, 1970; Williams, Beaver, Spence, and Rundell, 1969). Other investigators have reported that STM, for blind positioning movements is not much affected by verbal-type and certain other "unrelated" interpolated tasks (Adams and Dijkstra, 1966; Posner and Rossman, 1965).

The evidence is still conflicting about whether memory for movements over short periods is similar to that for verbal, auditory, and visual materials, but in a recent review of this topic, one of the most active of the researchers on motor STM, George Stelmach of the University of Wisconsin, concludes that:

...motor memory does not deserve its own memory compartment fragmented from verbal, auditory, and visual memory, but...motor memory is somewhat unique only in that it involves the recall of motor responses. The decision as to whether this memory needs to be fractioned into a separate memory system must await further research.

3. Evidence for long-term memory

How memories are consolidated and stored for LTM has challenged the efforts of numerous scientists. Although there is no general consensus on the neural basis of LTM, the current theories may be grouped into two major categories: chemical theories and morphological theories. These theories are certainly not mutually exclusive, because a change in structural relationships (morphological change) is possible through a modification in molecules (chemical change). Indeed, this is exactly what Sir John Eccles, the Nobel laureate in neurophysiology, has recently proposed (1973). We will discuss this theory later.

There is a growing body of research on the subject of LTM which points very strongly to chemical processes. Indeed, the biochemical bases of memory are the subject of widespread current investigations, and general developments in biology and in biochemistry itself are responsible for this trend. One of the most important factors stimulating biochemical studies on memory has been the remarkable advances in the field of molecular biology in the past two decades.

The most current chemical work on memory has been focusing on the possibility that the neural change is in a modification of the chemical structure of the neurons of the brain. Basically, it has been proposed that slight changes occur in the molecular structure of brain cells as a result of learning, and these molecular changes "store" the information in coded form.

Scientists who have been interested in the chemical correlates of memory have performed experiments in which they taught various things to animals and then analyzed the chemical composition of the animals' brains. They have theorized that the brain from an untrained animal should be chemically different from that of a trained animal, and their research has tended to support this belief. These experiments have generally confirmed the view that an organism's brain chemistry is subtly altered by experiences the organism has.

The nucleic acids and nucleoproteins have been studied extensively over the past 15 years. At the present time, the most promising substance appears to be the nucleic acids. Ribonucleic acid (RNA), an essential intracellular chemical found in every neuron in the nervous system, is believed by a number of scientists to be the substance which is modified in LTM, and therefore, to be responsible for storing information. An RNA molecule is a large complex unit, consisting of thousands of subunits. The potential number of different arrangements of subunits within the RNA molecule is enormous, and each different arrangement creates a distinct RNA molecule capable of causing the synthesis of distinct protein molecules.

Most functions of living cells are controlled either directly or indirectly by proteins, so control of protein synthesis in the cell indirectly controls the function of the entire cell. Cells must manufacture proteins from simple components, and RNA acts as an enzymatic template (mold) for the synthesis of protein in cells. The major role of RNA, then, is to determine and control the specific form of proteins that are synthesized within a cell.

For various reasons, RNA has been identified as the logical candidate for the role of the "memory molecule." Since the amount and structure of RNA seems to be altered by neural activity, and since this altered state could result in modified protein synthesis, and therefore modified functions of the cell, RNA has been proposed by some theorists as the structural component for the memory process.

Considerable evidence has accumulated in the past 15 years that suggests that RNA must play a vital role in memory consolidation. Studies have demonstrated that:

1. RNA synthesis is increased in nerve stimulation.
2. There is an increase of RNA synthesis in learning situations.
3. Base ratios of RNA change during learning.
4. A decrease in RNA adversely affects learning and performance.

5. Chemical stimulators of RNA synthesis, such as tricyanoaminopropene (TCAP), accelerate the rate at which consolidation is achieved.

6. An increase in RNA facilitates the storage of information and its retrieval.

7. RNA can be tnsferred from one animal to a second animal and the conditioned responses of the first animal will be transferred to the second.

Hyden (1965) and others have established the fact that a chemical concomitant of neural stimulation is a stimulation of RNA production. In addition to studies which suggest that RNA synthesis is increased in nerve stimulation, studies by Morrell (1961) and others have demonstrated that there is an increase in RNA synthesis in learning situations. Hyden (1965) has also found that there is a qualitative change in RNA base ratios, in addition to the quantitative increases; that is, RNA changes its basic character following learning.

Several investigations (John, 1967; Dingman and Sporn, 1964) have explored the effects of interference with RNA synthesis or destruction of RNA on the memory process. Using different experimental techniques, investigators have found that impairing RNA synthesis disrupts normal storage and retrieval of information. For example, ribonuclease, an enzyme that destroys or breaks up RNA, will destroy memory as well. Conversely, facilitating RNA synthesis by chemical means or increasing RNA by massive doses results in an enhanced ease of acquisition of new responses and storage of information. Essman (1965, 1966) reported facilitative effects of TCAP in learning situations, but conflicting reports have also appeared, and thus the status of TCAP as a "learning facilitator" is in doubt.

The strongest yet most controversial support for the chemical theory of LTM comes from the so-called memory-transfer experiments. In the early 1960s James McConnell (1962, 1964) and his Planarian Research Group at the University of Michigan reported that if planarians (a simple flatworm) were conditioned to respond to a light stimulus, then cut in half and the lower half allowed to grow a head and become a complete organism (planarians can do this), what was once the tail end of the planarian will respond to the light stimulus. More startling, though, was their report that if conditioned planarians were ground up and fed to unconditioned cannibalistic planarians, the cannibalistic flatworms appeared to acquire part of the training by ingestion. Similar findings have been obtained when the RNA of a "trained" animal has been injected into another animal.

Several hundred successful "memory-transfer" experiments have been reported in the scientific literature in the past 15 years. Various species of invertebrates and vertebrates have been used as subjects. It appears that the transfer of learning that is found in these studies is due to the incorporation by the "naive" organism of stable chemicals from the trained donor which has been altered in a specific way by learning, and RNA is the most commonly implicated transfer chemical in these experiments.

A few studies of chemical transfer of RNA have been attempted on humans by Cameron and Solyom (1961). RNA was given intravenously or orally to subjects suffering from arteriosclerotic or senile memory defects with some positive effects and evidence of improved memory function. There has, however, been very little follow-up on Cameron's work in recent years.

It has been suggested by some investigators that perhaps RNA is not the primary agent for data storage, but instead is an agent for the transfer of information to protein. These investigators, on the basis of their research, suggest that the synthesis of new brain proteins is crucial for the establishment of the LTM process. They have shown that, if new proteins are prevented from forming in the brain, the LTM process never becomes established, even though the STM process is not interfered with.

A number of studies on the effects of blockage of protein synthesis on memory have been conducted in the past few years (Flexner et al., 1963; Agranoff, 1967). Using chemicals, such as puromycin, which are known to block protein synthesis, the investigators have injected the substances into experimental animals and observed the effects. These substances have been found to have disruptive effects on the consolidation of memory. Additionally one investigator discovered that puromycin blocked retention of learned responses if injected shortly after the training session, but had diminishing effects on LTM as the time of injection after the training period increased. Experiments of this type suggest that the memory process which mediates long-term storage is dependent upon protein synthesis (Agranoff, 1967).

Morphological theories of memory have been popular among some neuroscientists for over 70 years. These theories suggest that changes in the relationship between neurons occur during the formation of a memory trace. Since it is known that nerve impulses pass from one neuron to another via the synapses, the synapse has long fascinated learning theorists, for this juncture has seemed to be a likely candidate for involvement in learning–memory because of its key role in the transmission of impulses.

It has been suggested that new synaptic relationships are established or that existing synapses become more efficient when new information is transmitted to the brain. These modifications of synaptic relationships might take the form of enlarging or shrinking of synapses or increasing or decreasing the actual number of synapses as the result of use or disuse. It might also take the form of increasing or decreasing secretion of transmitter substance.

One of the earliest morphological theories of learning–memory is that neuronal activity causes neurons to proliferate new presynaptic terminals and enlarge the existing ones, thus increasing contact with neighboring neurons. The first theory of this type was proposed by Tenzi about 80 years ago. He suggested that the passage of nerve impulses may produce metabolic changes which increase the volume of the conducting cell and cause its processes to approach neighboring cells more closely, thereby establishing an "associative bond."

Several investigators over the past 30 years have reported that nerve fibers swell as they transmit nerve impulses, and the swelling lasts for minutes, hours, even years. It has recently been reported that dentritic branching is considerably greater in the cortex of animals reared in groups in a complex environment than in littermates reared individually in laboratory cages (Volkmar and Greenough, 1972). An interdisciplinary group of scientists at the University of California have also reported more dentrite spines* in animals exposed to an "enriched" environment than in littermates from an "impoverished" environment. In addition, they found that the synaptic junctions of the animals from the enriched environment averaged about 50 percent larger in cross section than similar junctions in littermates from impoverished environments. More will be said about the research of this group later in the chapter (Rosenzweig, Bennett, and Diamond, 1972).

The neurons from brains of older persons do have a more extensive branching than those of young persons, and this fact has been cited as evidence that learning alters the structure of neurons. It has been suggested that the poor memory of older persons for recent experiences is a result of the inability of their neurons to further proliferate and bring about learning. This view has little research support at the present time.

The increased branching in neurons that has been reported presumably provides increased surface for synaptic contacts, and when combined with the reported alterations in the size of individual synapses this might conceivably underlie some forms of information storage in the brain.

Deutsch (1971) has provided evidence that synaptic conductance is altered as a result of learning and that it is probably the postsynaptic membrane that becomes increasingly more sensitive to acetylcholine with time after learning. Increasing the amount of learning leads to an increase in conductance in each set of synapses without, according to Deutsch, an increase in their number.

The eminent neuroscientist, Sir John Eccles, has proposed that both chemical and morphological changes occur in the consolidation of memory.

---

*Dendrite spines are tiny "thorns" or projections from the dendrites of a nerve cell which serve as receivers in many of the synaptic contacts between neurons.

He suggests that in the process of learning, the experience leads first to specific RNA modification and this in turn to specific protein synthesis, and "finally to synaptic growth and the coding of the memory" (Eccles, 1973).

There is a substantial body of literature about long-term memory of motor skills, but this literature is framed almost exclusively in "behavioral" terms, and is not concerned with morphological or biochemical changes that occur in the nervous system. The topic of LTM typically goes under the title of "retention" in the motor behavior literature. Since there is so little research on LTM for motor skills (although many of the LTM studies with lower animals have used motor responses), and in keeping with custom, LTM for motor skills will be examined in this book in Chapter 16 in a section called "Retention."

Whether motor STM and motor LTM are separate processes, as has been fairly clearly confirmed for other forms of memory, is still an unanswered question. Some differences in memory characteristics have been demonstrated for motor memory, but at the present, there is no definitive reason to propose entirely different processes; thus, the consolidation memory theory appears generally applicable to motor memory.

PRESENT STATUS OF CONSOLIDATION MEMORY THEORY

It should be evident from the discussion above that there is no definitive answer as to exactly what changes in the nervous system correlate with the behavioral modifications which we call learning. Although some changes must occur in the nervous system as a result of learning, our present state of knowledge is not much more than speculation about what the changes are, and where they occur. Moreover, although there has been speculation that memory processes for motor memory are different from those underlying other forms of memory, there is no compelling evidence at this time for this position. The consolidation memory theory seems to provide the best approximation of the learning–memory process, and it admittedly is very general and imprecise.

To review, this theory suggests the following sequence of events. First, stimuli which impinge upon the sensory organs are transduced and coded in the form of nerve impulses and transmitted to the brain. This process probably initiates neural activity which momentarily outlasts the stimulus; this activity then becomes recoded, possibly in the form of reverberating circuits. This phase, so-called short-term memory, has a capacity of about seven to eight items or stimuli. The "hold time" for items in STM seems to vary from a few seconds up to perhaps an hour or more. Gradually, the neural representation of the stimulus event is transformed into a structural change in the brain. This transformation from a dynamic activity to a consolidated memory is the so-called long-term memory. If the STM process is disrupted, the long-term process cannot take place and the stimulus event cannot be recalled. Present knowledge does not permit a definitive exploration of LTM, but recent studies of the biochemical correlates of learning–memory suggest that molecular changes occur in the neurons whenever an individual learns something. The molecules most frequently identified as being involved in LTM are RNA and protein. There is also evidence that morphological changes in the form of changes in the relationship of synapses may also be involved in LTM.

IMPLICATIONS OF CONSOLIDATION MEMORY THEORY

Although the mysteries of learning–memory are as yet unraveled, the information that has emerged permits experimentation with various conditions, and these experiments, while they have been done primarily with laboratory animals, provide implications for human learning–memory. In future years these implications will surely be explored. Two examples of studies in which conditions were manipulated will illustrate the kinds of studies that relate learning–memory to experimental control.

A. THE USE OF DRUGS TO IMPROVE LEARNING–MEMORY

James McGaugh (1965), building on the consolidation memory theory, hypothesized that he could improve learning by increasing the robustness or the survival time of STM by administering a drug to increase the vigor of the reverberating process or the ease with which the long-term process develops. Using chemical compounds like strychnine and metrazol, which are CNS stimulants, McGaugh improved the intellectual level of animals.

McGaugh first tested the maze-learning ability of two different strains of mice—one hereditarily a maze-bright group, the other hereditarily a maze-dull group. Some animals from each strain were injected with different doses of the stimulant drugs shortly after each learning trial to ascertain whether they would improve their ability to retain what they had learned on that trial. Some mice received no drug treatment. With the optimal dosage of the drugs, the chemically treated mice were 40 percent better at remembering their learned tasks than were the untreated mice, provided the drugs were given within 30 minutes or so of the training. Indeed, under metrazol treatment, the hereditarily maze-dull mice were able to perform better than their hereditarily superior but untreated mice. This treatment might be called a "chemical memory pill."

Several other investigators have studied the effects of various chemicals on learning–memory in recent years. The results of these studies can be generalized in this way: barbiturates, anticholinergic chemicals, or substances which produce depressant effects tend to impair learning–memory. On the other hand, stimulants, anticholinesterase substances, and convulsant drugs in subconvulsive quantities, even when supplied after the learning experience, tend to facilitate learning–memory. Here again, studies of this type have been done primarily on laboratory animals, but they raise the question of whether learning–memory may be affected by similar manipulations with humans.

A curious phenomenon related to drugs and learning is so-called state-dependent learning. It has been known for some time that if animals drugged with alcohol, sedatives, or antianxiety drugs learn to perform a task while under the influence of one of these drugs, they frequently cannot perform the task when they are not under the influence of the drug, but when the drug is again administered the task is performed well. On the other hand, tasks that are learned while not under the influence of drugs may not be able to be performed while drugged and only able to be performed well in an undrugged state. State-dependent learning in humans has been reported by Overton (1969). He reports on one study that suggests that students who take stimulants while studying may forget what they learned when the effects of the drug wear off. This type of information has many implications for motor learning, since drugs are becoming increasingly used.

Much interest and concern has arisen in recent years about the administration of drugs to quiet disruptive children in school. Several years ago it was discovered that learning and overall school achievement could be enhanced by the administration of certain drugs to children who normally had difficulties in school because they were overactive, distractible, or impulsive. This practice has come under increasing criticism by parents and physicians and it will probably not gain widespread support in the near future.

B. ENRICHED ENVIRONMENT AND LEARNING–MEMORY

Another approach to understanding the physiological correlates of learning–memory has been undertaken by an interdisciplinary group of scientists at the University of California, Berkeley, (Rosenzweig et al., 1972). They took the position that if learning–memory involved anatomical and chemical changes in the brain, then one should find that an animal which has lived a life replete with opportunities for learning and memorizing would develop a brain morphologically and chemically different from that of an animal which had lived an intellectually impoverished life.

At weaning time they divided rats into two groups. Half of the rats were placed in an intellectually enriched environment (ECT) and the other half in a deprived environment (IC). All conditions were held the same except the ECT group lived together in one large cage, were provided with many rat toys, and they were given lots of handling and care. They were taught to run mazes, and in general were given an "enriched" environment. In the meantime, the deprived group lived in barren cages, devoid of stimulation of any kind. After about 30 days of this treatment all the animals were sacrificed, their brains dissected, and various chemical and histological analyses were performed. The brains from the rats from the enriched environment—and presumably, therefore, with many more stored memories—were found to have heavier and thicker cortexes, a better blood supply, larger brain cells, more glia cells, and increased activity of two brain enzymes, acetylcholinesterase, than did the brains from the animals which had led lives less "enriched."

In one of the studies by these investigators, after a 30-day period of either environmental complexity (EC), which is an environment similar to ECT, but with no training or isolated control (IC) conditions, rats were given a 30-day period where both groups were pretrained and tested on reversal discrimination problems. The EC group was significantly superior to the IC group. Within the EC group high and significant correlations were found between the behavioral scores and the cortical–subcortical ratios of cholinesterase and between the behavioral scores and the cortical–subcortical ratio of brain weight.

These studies point to the importance of providing an environment that is rich in stimuli, an environment that provides a great many opportunities for the learner to interact with persons and objects. Since the human brain develops rapidly in the first three years, the infant's environment should be replete with opportunities to move and to handle objects. Indeed, if these opportunities are denied the child in the first few years of life, no amount of education may compensate for this early deprivation.

10

A Neuropsychological Model of Motor Behavior

This chapter serves as a bridge between the preceding chapters on the structure and function of the nervous system and the following chapters which are directly concerned with human motor behavior. With the exception of content dealing with the structure and functions of the autonomic nervous system, our specific examination of the nervous system is complete. In the remainder of the text, content from previous chapters will be foundational as we examine human motor behavior.

The study of motor behavior is concerned with an analysis of the processes involved in the performance and acquisition of motor skills and with an identification of the factors which enhance, deter, and limit human motor behavior. Those who study motor learning and performance seek to discover principles and (it is hoped) laws regarding human motor behavior, which, if accomplished, will make possible predictions and control over complex motor activity. In attempting to understand the complexities of motor learning and performance, it is helpful to have reference to a conceptual framework for studying this subject. In this chapter a framework is presented which identifies the basic functional and neurological components of motor learning and performance. The framework is in the form of a model. A model is a unifying structure which facilitates the conceptualization of some phenomenon and it functions to provide a pattern or guide to how a system works. It may also be viewed as an analogy which advances understanding and leads to new inferences.

The basic notion behind model development is that first it identifies the components of a functional system and second it gives one an overview of how the system functions. Once one is familiar with the components of a system and how they work, one can begin to control the system, modify it, and predict how the system will respond if certain variables, or forces, are applied to it.

BASIC COMPONENTS OF A MOVEMENT MODEL

Any approach to model building abstracts the common characteristics from the multitude of activities and categorizes them into components of function which are more easily understood. Reference to the model is then made to determine the relative functioning of each component with respect to the entire system. The model proposed here is based on a review and synthesis of other models which have been discussed for motor learning and performance (Adams, 1971; Bernstein, 1967; Craik, 1948; R. Davis, 1957; Gentile, 1972; Laszlo and Bairstow, 1971; Welford, 1968b); however, several of the other models only partially describe the components in motor learning and performance, and most of them do not give any attention to the neural mechanisms involved.

The general assumption which will be made with the model described in this chapter is that complex motor behavior may be viewed as an information-processing activity guided by feedback control mechanisms which enable adaptive processes to occur. The view of human behavior is an adaptive information processing system is a view which has come to have increasing influence in psychology.

From this perspective, information in the form of physical energy (light, sound, mechanical, chemical) impinges on the individual and serves as a stimulus to the sense organs. This information is coded into electrical energy at the sensory receptors where it then takes the form of electrical impulses which are sent over sensory nerve cells to the central nervous system. In the brain and spinal cord, present information is integrated with stored information (memories) and this process results in information (in the form of electrical impulses) being sent to the muscles and glands to produce a response of some kind. The response produces feedback information (in the form of nerve impulses) to control and direct the immediate response and/or may produce adaptive behavior for future responses to a similar stimulus situation.

Since the information from the environment is "picked up" by structures of the nervous system, transmitted over nerve fibers, integrated and interpreted by nerve cells, and muscles and glands activated by the mediation of nerve cells, it is obvious that recognition of the critical role of this system must be an integral feature of any model of motor behavior. Indeed, a successful model of motor learning and performance is unlikely to emerge without consideration of the functions of neural mechanisms. Therefore, the composite of the model to be described in this chapter is called a neuro-psychological model.

A. FUNCTIONAL COMPONENTS

Before presenting the complete neuropsychological model, it may be well to review two simple models which illustrate the basic functional and neurological components of motor behavior. The first model relates to the functional components of motor performance and is shown in Fig. 10.1.

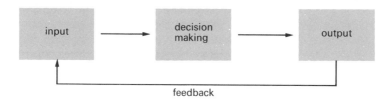

Fig. 10.1   The basic functional components of motor behavior.

1. Input

Input is made up of all the stimuli which are impinging on a person at any given time. The total amount of input is sometimes referred to as the "display." There are relevant and irrelevant stimuli in a display; relevant stimuli are those which are important for the present moment and irrelevant stimuli are those which are not needed nor used for the immediate situation.

2. Decision making

Decision making refers to the process of integrating and interpreting input and determining, or deciding upon, the appropriate response which should be made to relate the stimuli to a response.

3. Output

Output is the response (or behavior) in the form of muscular action or glandular activity.

4. Feedback

Feedback refers to the information, or restimulation, which is produced by the output. Feedback may be intrinsic to the task; that is, the movement execution itself may also produce feedback information, or the feedback may be augmented as it is when an instructor gives information about the consequences of the movement.

B. NEUROLOGICAL COMPONENTS

From the simple functional model, we may consider the neurological mechanisms which are related to the components above. A simple model of this kind is shown in Fig. 10.2

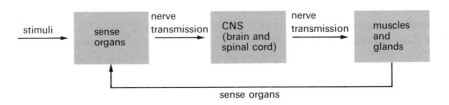

Fig. 10.2   The basic neurological mechanisms for motor behavior.

In relating this model to the first one, we see that *input* is received via the sense organs. The brain and spinal cord serve the *decision-making* function, and *output* is mediated by the muscular and glandular system. *Feedback* is mediated by the various sensory organs. The information is transmitted from one part of the model to other parts via neural transmission.

A NEUROPSYCHOLOGICAL MODEL

We are now ready to examine an elaboration of these simple models, with an emphasis on motor learning. This detailed model, shown in Fig. 10.3, more precisely illustrates the functions and neural mechanisms for motor learning.

The components of this more elaborate model are described below.

A. STIMULI

Holding (1965) suggests that motor learning involves the integration of three kinds of information: first, information about what is to be achieved; second, information from the task itself; and third, information about the results of the performance itself. This information impinges upon the various sensory systems and serves as stimuli to the individual.

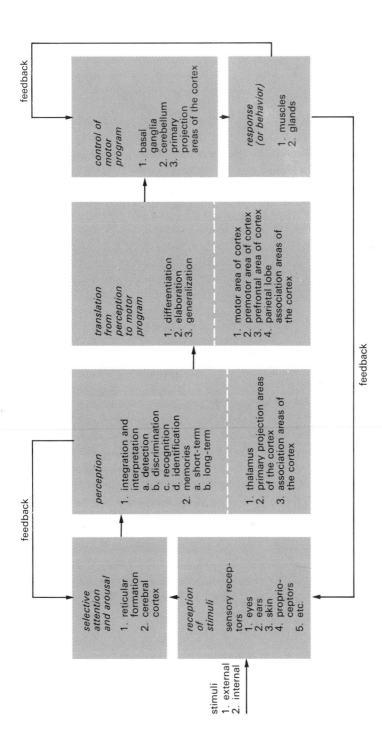

Fig. 10.3   A model of the functional and neural mechanisms for motor behaviors.

Successful motor learning and performance depend on an individual's ability to pick up stimuli within the environment and to transmit this information to various parts of the body for a response. Various stimuli impose upon the motor performer in sports: visual stimuli in the form of equipment teammates, coaches, opponents; auditory stimuli such as the sounds of balls being hit, voices of teammates, coaches, opponents, and starting signals; mechanical stimuli imposed by the pressures of opponents in boxing and wrestling and the pressure of water in swimming. There are, of course, many other stimuli which could be mentioned.

Stimuli which impinge upon the individual are of two basic varieties, external and internal. External stimuli are in the form of light energy, sound energy, mechanical energy, thermal energy, and so on, originating outside the organism. One form of internal stimuli arises from mechanical or chemical energy operating from within the individual. For example, pressures on internal organs by movement stimulate receptors in the muscles and joints of the body, and hormones serve as chemical stimulators for certain target cells of the nervous system. Another form of internal stimuli arises from the cognition, or thinking, mechanisms in the brain. One extraordinary feature of the human nervous system is this self-generation of information—what we call thinking and imagination. Stimuli (external and internal) are transmitted as electrical impulses throughout the nervous system over nerve fibers via an electrochemical process.

Motor learning normally relies heavily upon the functioning of various sensory systems, especially the visual, auditory, and proprioceptive systems. Fitts and his colleagues (1964; Bahrick et al., 1954) have suggested that during the initial stages of motor learning the individual relies heavily upon visual information. According to Fitts (1951), "visual control is important while an individual is learning a new perceptual-motor task. As performance becomes habitual, however, it is likely that proprioceptive feedback, or 'feel,' becomes more important."

Visual information has been postulated as the major error-correcting mechanism used by the learner. Fleishman and Rich (1963) concluded that individuals with greater capacity for utilizing visual information make more rapid progress in the early phases of skill learning. Rock and Harris (1967) have shown rather decisively that in the early phases of motor skill acquisition, vision is completely dominant over touch (they include proprioception in their use of the word touch). Pew (1966) showed that after a period of practice learners shift from visual control of individual movements to the use of visual feedback for periodic monitoring for correction or modulation of the pattern of movements.

The importance of proprioception to motor performance cannot be overlooked, however. The proprioceptors keep one apprised of the position of all segments of the body and the rate of movement at all times, and they provide the only constant source of sensory information. Complex human movement is virtually impossible without functional proprioceptors.

1. Neural mechanisms for the reception of stimuli

The neural mechanisms for reception of external and one form of internal stimuli are the sensory receptors throughout the body. It is through the sensory systems that we are in contact with our environment. They are sensitive to a wide variety of stimuli which impinge upon the organism. (Stimuli which are formed in the cognitive mechanisms will be discussed later in this chapter in relation to motor program formation and control.)

For external stimuli, the first task of the sensory receptors is to transduce (change from one form of energy to another) the stimulus energy into electrical energy. This process is accomplished in different ways by the various sensory systems. The next task is to transmit the electrical current which has been produced by the stimulus into the central nervous system. Basically, this transmission network is as follows: Impulses travel over spinal nerves and enter the spinal cord where they travel up one of the spinal cord tracks, and synapse in the thalamus before traveling up to the cerebral cortex. For sensory transmission via the cranial nerves, the process is essentially the same only the impulses do not enter the brain from the spinal cord.

B. SELECTIVE ATTENTION

The individual cannot and does not process all the stimuli in the immediate environment. One of the most critical factors in motor behavior is the ability to select and attend to only the relevant stimuli in the environment and to ignore the irrelevant stimuli. It is possible for one to direct one's attention to any stimulus in the display by choice, but normally the multitude of stimuli from the various senses that impinges upon an individual is largely ignored and only a very limited range of stimuli is selected for attention out of the multitudes bombarding the sensory systems.

This division of stimuli into relevant and irrelevant information occurs very rapidly, so that certain stimuli are inhibited or augmented. Evidence of various kinds strongly indicates that the sensory systems and the CNS have limited capacity for handling data and many of the sensory data are irrelevant to appropriate behavior, so only a part of the incoming information can be selected for processing, and attention is focused on only a part of the stimulus display. But how can stimuli be divided into relevant and irrelevant categories? It appears that there is a wide variety of factors which govern the distribution of attention. Such properties of the stimuli as intensity and novelty (or change) are important, while other factors such as set, motivation, and expectancy are certainly important too. Experience within the environment leads to an appreciation of which aspects of the environment convey little relevant information and which will be useful for appropriate responses, and indeed which will and which will not require a response. Thus, in many cases attention is probably determined by the past experiences of the person—or the person's memories of stimuli.

Attention is certainly determined to a large extent by the ongoing sensory information—especially the information that just proceeded it. In other words, as one "chunk" of information is perceptually processed, feedback is sent to the selective attention mechanisms to regulate them to screen out information which the perceptual mechanisms have deemed irrelevant.

Finally, attentiveness is affected by the nature of the task demands. Many studies in which the task required vigilance (monitoring an instrument, such as a radar screen, in which a significant event rarely and irregularly occurs) or repetitive performance have found a substantial decrement in performance over time periods of one-half hour or hour, with the most marked decrement occuring in the first 15 minutes.

The entire body frequently takes part when a particular stimulus has been selected for attention. These bodily activities include changes in position (turning the head for visual focus or for better hearing), orienting toward the source of the stimulus, changes in sensitivity of the sensory system (widening of the pupils), modification in the ongoing electrical activity of the brain, and widespread changes in autonomic nervous system activity. These activities are accompanied by modification in arousal which produces a maximum receptivity and readiness to respond to the stimulus.

Information and cybernetic theories seem to provide the clearest concepts for describing how selective attention functions. In the past 25 years, concepts and theories which have been developed in the area of cybernetics and information theory for use with highly sophisticated electronic instruments, such as computers, have come into use by those who are attempting to discover how the nervous system handles information. Although the nervous system is vastly more complex than any computer, in many respects it has functions which are analogous to those of the computer. It follows, then, that concepts and theories developed for designing and perfecting computers may have some relevance to explaining neural function.

Information theory in the service of electronic instrumentation suggests that the chain of processes from input to output involves the channeling of information from one point in the system to another point. It follows that with any information system there is a finite capacity to channel the information in any X time period. When the channel capacity is overloaded, several mechanisms may be brought into play to accommodate the situation (omission, queuing, filtering, approximating).

That the human nervous system possesses a limited channel capacity is confirmed by everyday observation as well as by experimental research. For example, when we attend to one set of stimuli, we have to ignore others. Anyone who has tried to attend selectively to one person's speech in the presence of competing conversations has experienced what is called the "cocktail party phenomenon." Cherry's (1953) research of presenting different information to the two ears and having subjects shadow one (repeat back) showed that subjects could not report about information coming to the opposite ear (except for their name or changes from verbal to music). A phenomenon called the "psychological refractory period" provides additional experimental support for the notion of a single channel capacity in human neural function. When an individual must react to a second stimulus very shortly (less than 250 milliseconds) after reacting to a first stimulus, the reaction time to the second stimulus is slower than the reaction time to the first stimulus. This is called the "psychological refractory phenomenon" and the explanation for it is that while the channel processing capabilities of the nervous system are being used in processing the first stimulus, information about the second must wait, thus delaying reaction to it.

Vogel-Sprott (1963) found that stimuli which are irrelevant to the visual focus necessary for correct performance can alter motor efficiency markedly. The presentation of irrelevant stimuli beyond the center of attention or visual focus was found to retard response to irregular signals for action. Schlesinger (1954), on the basis of considerable research, indicated that individuals vary in their abilities to distinguish the relevant from the irrelevant stimuli and maintain asn attentive set.

Although the use of the word attention implies that when persons are attending to one thing they cannot simultaneously perform something else, this is, of course, not true. Tasks can be performed simultaneously if one of them does not require too great attention. Walking, for example, requires very little attention, once learned, and other tasks can be performed simultaneously, such as talking, or thinking.

Through early practice experiences learners develop an ability to selectively attend to certain aspects of the display, and it is only after they can do this that they are able to develop an effective movement pattern. As motor skill learning proceeds to advanced levels, performing the task demands less and less active attention. Thus, a person highly skilled in a sport can perform while devoting attention to other matters, such as tactics and surveying the playing conditions. Various types of motor tasks demand quite different intensities of attention; less complicated tasks require less attention, since presumably fewer control mechanisms are needed for their execution.

People are most likely to remember information to which they have given their fullest attention, and anything which assists learners to attend to the information they are to retain may improve their subsequent performance. The educator can presumably influence skill learning and performance by instructions to the learner on how to allocate attentional capacities. The important role of the teacher-coach with regard to selective attention is described by Whiting (1972):

> ...one of the criteria on which a teacher...or coach might be judged successful is his ability to make his trainee's attention selective by pointing out toward what part of the display his perceptual systems need to be oriented and the information he is to try to abstract. Unsophisticated teachers may fail to appreciate that the beginner in a skill may not be utilizing the same information as the expert....

Thus, to the extent which instructors are aware of this aspect of developing skill, they may be able to find more effective means of directing the attention of the learner.

1. Neural Mechanisms for Selective Attention

There is considerable controversy in the neuropsychological literature as to what the neural mechanisms of attention may be and, in particular, whether attention involves a peripheral "filtering," or "gating," of sensory inputs or CNS mechanisms. (See Moray, 1970, for an excellent review.) It is well known that impulses transmitted through the ascending afferent pathways do not maintain constant strength from reception at the sense organ to arrival in the cortex; indeed, there is evidence for regulation of afferent input at several levels in the nervous system. Thus, interference with afferent impulses from the sensory receptors, other than those pertaining to the subject of attention, is an obvious possibility. This afferent blockage could occur any place along the sensory pathways, from receptors to the primary cortex areas; it might also occur in the collateral paths that are found in the reticular formation.

Research on this topic suggests that the selective attention mechanisms may have two parts—one part which may not utilize the cerebral cortex of the brain and a second part which does involve the cortex. Perhaps the most interesting aspect of selective attention is that it does not seem to depend completely upon cortical mechanisms. For example, experimental evidence suggests that the reticular formation may play an important role in regulating sensory transmission. Hernandez-Peon et al. (1956) have shown that the inhibitory effects of stimuli may be mediated by the reticular formation. They say:

The blocking of afferent impulses in the lower positions of a sensory path may be a mechanism whereby sensory stimuli out of the scope of attention can be markedly reduced while they are still in their trajectory toward higher levels of the central nervous system. This central inhibitory mechanism may, therefore, play an important role in selective exclusion of sensory messages along their passage toward mechanisms of perception and consciousness.

Both facilitatory and inhibitory effects as a result of reticular stimulation have been reported for the retinal ganglion cells and optic tract (Dodt, 1956; Granit, 1955), transmission of kinesthetic and cutaneous pressure (Hagbarth and Kerr, 1954), olfactory and auditory stimuli (Adey et al., 1957; Galambos, 1956; Kerr and Hagbarth, 1955).

Lesion studies by Sprague et al. (1961) support the idea that an important component of the attention mechanism is found in subcortical structures in the midbrain. Jabbur et al. (1971) demonstrated that the cuneate nucleus (the first synaptic relay receiving ipsilateral afferent input from upper thoracic and cervical body segments) modified transmission of somatic sensory impulses. In a recent study of human auditory attention, Picton et al. (1971) concluded that "attention is mediated not by selective gating of inputs at the periphery but by specialized processing of relevant stimuli at higher levels of the sensory system." With regard to subcortical attention filter mechanisms acting on the input from various sense organs, Welford (1968) says, "How such a filter works and how many stages it entails are matters for future research to decide."

Cortical mechanisms for attention are no better understood, but there is good evidence that the cortex has an important attentional role. Hugelin and Bonvallet (quoted in Berlyne, 1960) have shown that the cortex is capable of powerful and selective inhibition of the reticular formation. Sokolov (1960) has suggested that models for familiar stimulus patterns are formed in the cortex and any stimulus which is not in accord with the models will open these pathways for this stimulus, thus producing attention to it, but if non-novel or repetitive stimuli match the models, cortical mechanisms inhibit subcortical mechanisms, especially the reticular formation. Although this notion is rather speculative, Sokolov has produced some research which supports the plausibility of the theory.

C. AROUSAL

Arousal refers to the state of wakefulness or alertness of the individual. A certain amount of arousal is necessary for optimal motor learning and performance. Arousal facilitates the cortex and enhances transmission throughout the brain, making it more effective in processing incoming sensory information. It also activates various mechanisms throughout the body for preparing the body for action.

Arousal may be viewed as having two dimensions: a background level and a stimulus-specific arousal level. First, the background level of arousal refers to the general state of the individual which varies with the time of day, spontaneous neural activity, and many other factors. The stimulus-specific arousal response is triggered by novel and changing stimuli as well as by cortical activity, i.e., thinking about a certain thing.

The stimulus-specific arousal response brings about an alert, even emotional, state of the individual. The basic cause of this response is a novel or unexpected stimulus, but the perception of stimuli as threatening also produces arousal. If a stimulus is constantly repeated, this response decreases, thus representing habituation of the response. There is growing evidence that some aspects of stimulus-specific type arousal are important for optimal performance, memory storage, and enhanced rates of learning. Mahut (1964) reported that learning was facilitated with cats learning a two-choice task when a reticular formation was stimulated during the learning trials. Reticular stimulation just before the task trials had no effect on learning while stimulation during the ten seconds immediately after each trial disrupted learning. Sage and Bennett (1973), using college students, found that shock treatment which enhanced arousal produced increased learning rates on a pursuit motor task. Other investigators have reported that high states of arousal may inhibit immediate performance but may actually enhance learning.

Arousal may facilitate performance as well as learning. Fuster and his associates (Fuster, 1958; Fuster and Uyeda, 1962) studied the effect of electrically stimulating the reticular formation of monkeys on performance of a previously learned tachistoscopic discrimination task. Number of errors and reaction time were reduced under reticular stimulation. Numerous other investigators have found that increasing arousal increases performance output.

Of course, there is a good deal of evidence which indicates that very high states of arousal cause a disorganization of behavior and a reduction in quality of performance. The notion of an optimum level of arousal for performance was first formulated over 60 years ago by two comparative psychologists; it carries their names as the "Yerkes-Dodson Law" (1908). In the intervening years the validity of this notion has been supported many times, and a number of variables have been identified which influence optimum arousal (Duffy, 1962).

1. Neural mechanisms of arousal

It was Moruzzi and Magoun (1949) who first identified the neuroanatomical basis for arousal. Their ideas have been extended in recent years by many other scholars, especially Hebb (1966). The primary location of arousal structures is in the brainstem and midbrain, and the reticular formation has probably received the most attention with respect to the arousal function. As described in an earlier chapter, this structure extends from the medulla up to the lower thalamus with branches into the posterior hypothalamus.

Thus deep within the brain is a kind of inner brain which monitors all incoming sensory data and is richly interconnected with other brain structures, including the cortex. It is capable of controlling the general activation of the cortex as well as the excitability of localized cortical areas. The integrated reticular formation, therefore, provides the energizing aspects of motivation and general behavior.

D. PERCEPTION

The beginner in motor skill learning situations typically tries to first "understand" the task demands and formulate an image of the movement or "general plan" (G.A. Miller et al., 1960). Thus, an "overall" plan of the performer becomes the guiding influence which directs and monitors the output. The motor organization initially used is usually based upon prior learned patterns. The process by which sensory information is obtained about the task, organized, integrated, and interpreted to produce meaning of the incoming data and a movement plan involves perception.

Perception is essentially an organizing process and past experiences play a leading role in this process. The process of perception involves detection, discrimination, recognition, and identification of incoming information for an interpretation; then the oncoming information takes on meaning. Perception is an important component in motor behavior because all complex motor learning and performance require perceptual function.

The simplest perceptual task is detection. Detection requires the individual to merely indicate when a predefined stimulus event has occurred. The lowest stimulus intensity which can be detected is called the threshold; rather the threshold varies with the type of stimulus, level of the subject's motivation, quality of instruction, and other variables. As perception develops, the individual comes to detect properties of stimulation not previously detected, even though they may have been present. Through growth and experience with the world of stimulation, detection becomes more sensitive and precise. One of the most important variables related to detection is the background "noise" stimulation already present in the nervous system. A complete signal-detection theory has emerged which involves differences in both theory and method from the old classical threshold notion but it is beyond the scope of this book to examine this particular theory.

Another perceptual task is discrimination. Discrimination occurs when a "stimulus event" is defined as a difference between two separate stimuli on some attribute (e.g., Do these two stimuli seem different: yes or no? Are these two pitches different? Are these offensive maneuvers different?). Improvement in perceptual skill through discrimination seems to be closely related to selective use of stimulus cues; with experience, there is a greater noticing of the critical differences with less noticing of irrelevancies. For example, experienced athletes are not as easily fooled by fakes and deception used by opponents during a contest.

Recognition is a higher order perceptual task. Recognition is an awareness that an object, person, or event is familiar and the individual can choose that item previously learned from among several items. Finally, identification is an even higher order perception which is exhibited when an individual is given minimal information about the stimuli under investigation and can provide a personal response (e.g., What is this word? What defense is the opponent using? What kind of serve did the tennis opponent just make?). As these abilities become precise for each task, the individual improves in ability to deal with environmental stimulation.

Perception implies the relating of present information to stored information in the form of memories. As noted in the previous chapter, the theory that memory depends upon at least a two-stage process is dominant in neuropsychological theories of learning–memory today and is commonly referred to as the "Consolidation Memory Theory." This theory, as you recall, proposes an early, and relatively brief, period (less than five minutes) during which the relatively fragile and labile trace of an experience is maintained by a transient reverberative process in the nervous system. This phase decays within a few seconds or minutes but before doing so the short-term electrochemical process produces a second series of events in the brain which leads to a subsequent long-lasting phase during which the memory trace is consolidated in the form of a structural modification of the nervous system, presumably by means of specific biochemical and/or morphological alterations in the neurons. The two processes are viewed as being interrelated in that the dynamic activity mechanism (first stage) presumably assists in the development of the structural change (second stage).

Perceptual abilities vary between individuals and within a single individual over time. Wober (1966) noted that there is a variety of individual differences in the use of sensory information; that is, individuals have different primary modes of perceptual processing. Some persons give preference to visual information while others give preference to kinesthetic or auditory data. Wober found cultural differences in perceptual preference as well as differences based upon educational backgrounds. There is a wealth of data showing individual differences in perceptual style with regard to visual figure-ground ability. Finally, differences in perceptual speed are well documented in the "reaction time" research literature.

This information about the development of preferred forms of perceptual modes suggests that environmental influences, such as sports experiences, may affect hierarchical modes of perception. Thus, the athlete may become more perceptually adaptive with experience. Of course, some athletes may have innately superior perceptual modes for sports.

In sports performances the perceptual aspects of the tasks are sometimes quite important and other times they are not too important. In basketball, football, and baseball, performers must not only execute certain movement patterns but they must perceptually organize a great deal of information about their own locations, the positions of their teammates and opponents, the score, and time period of the game so that the most effective movements can be selected for that situation. In other sports, such as shot putting, gymnastics, and diving there is a minimum of perceptual data necessary for carrying out the task. In these latter sports, perceptual data are used in learning the task, but not so much in performance; that is, current information does not greatly affect the performance, since the movement pattern tends to be basically preprogrammed.

1. Neural mechanisms of perception

The various stimuli that impinge upon the individual are processed by a complex system at various levels of the nervous system, from the sense organs to the highest centers in the brain. All of the sensory systems are important in perception for they provide the "raw material" out of which perception arises. Other mechanisms which are responsible for perceptual activities are located in the thalamus, in various subcortical structures of the brain, and in various regions of the cortex. These all play decisive roles in the analysis, coding, and storing of information.

Sensory receptors are sensitive to a variety of stimuli and it is from these structures that the elementary processes of perception begin. At these organs energy impinging upon the individual is transduced to neural impulses and transmitted into the brain.

Each sensory modality has a primary projection (or cortex) area that sorts and records the sensory information and a secondary area which organizes and codes the information. Then there are cortical association areas where the information from different sensory systems overlaps and is integrated for interpretation to lay the foundation for the organization of perception. Among these areas in the cortex are the primary visual, auditory, and somatosensory areas. A description of these neural structures and functions was presented in Chapter 4 and will not be repeated here.

E. TRANSLATION FROM PERCEPTION TO MOTOR PROGRAM

A response to perception which serves as stimulus to effector function may be viewed as a translation process; that is, there is a translation from perception to a series of detailed muscular units. Perceptual information must be converted to a muscle command, or what several investigators call "a motor program." Newell *et al.* (1958) noted that the concept of motor organization becomes more operational and succinct when defined as programs. They say, "The vaguenesses that have plagued the theory of mental processes and other parts of psychology disappear when the phenomena are described as programs."

A motor program may be viewed as a set of neural units which is structured before a movement sequence begins, and that makes it possible for the entire sequence to be "run off" uninfluenced by peripheral feedback. Of course, the actual motor program selected on any occasion is adapted to the demands of that occasion. Presumably the precise motor program selected varies from one occasion to another, since performance requirements vary from one occasion to the next, even when a movement seems to be repeated exactly.

Basic to any model of motor learning is the notion of an existence of hierarchical organization whereby motor programs may be modified on the basis of new and accumulated information. Thus, the motor program mechanism is viewed as changing or maintaining its program with experience to achieve enhanced adaptive behavior (or improved performance levels).

Laszlo and Bairstow (1971) propose what they call a standard (STD) which "is the global memory trace of a given task, incorporating all available information relevant to the task." The STD, then, "forms the central comprehensive precept about the task." This information is transmitted to the motor programming mechanism the function of which is the structuring of motor programs; that is, it selects the appropriate motor units and the proper timing of these units. The most effective motor programs will be selected when the STD provides explicit and detailed information to the motor program unit.

For humans no motor programs for coordinated motor activity exist at birth—only mass activity and reflexes. Recent research with lower animals indicates, however, that whole programs for the control of movement patterns can be stored within the CNS (Camhi, 1971; Kennedy, 1967; Wilson, 1964, 1968).

The development of human motor programs progresses through several stages, beginning with differentiation. Differentiation means to sort out, to recognize the difference. It is the process by means of which a mass of homogeneous nerve cells develops into a specialized unit. Through differentiation, a motor program (or movement pattern) takes place in certain order. Movements are divided into coordinated parts rather than disembodied movement; only the necessary movements to carry out a task are used. From differentiation, learners elaborate—they find many ways to make a variety of movements to carry out a task. Thus, several motor programs are developed to produce the same or similar result. From differentiation and elaboration, generalization of motor programs develops. This is a process whereby motor programs may be applied to new and different tasks; that is, motor programs developed to perform a certain task may be utilized to perform other tasks.

The discussion above is related most directly to movement activities which require enactment of different movements as environmental conditions change (such as fielding a thrown ball) but there are movement activities in which environmental conditions remain fairly constant from response to response: The latter type of activities have been called "closed skills" and the former "open skills" by Poulton (1957) and the idea of a continuum of skills was proposed by Knapp (1961). For closed skills the objective of the learner is to ascertain an effective motor program and duplicate this program with each response. Sports such as shot putting, diving, and gymnastics would be classified as sports in which closed skills dominate. It may be seen that closed skills depend upon strength, endurance, power, and technique for performance. Since environmental conditions remain relatively static for the task, the learner attempts to develop consistency of execution for optimum goal attainment. Open skills demand an entirely different learning strategy. Open skills are employed in a changing environment, and the selection of the appropriate response is variable as is the environment. Sports such as basketball, soccer, and baseball would be classified as sports in which open skills dominate. Since environmental conditions may vary from one response to another, the performer must have a variety of motor programs to accomplish the task. In addition to developing a variety of responses for differing environmental demands, the learner must develop a contingency strategy whereby the likelihood of using certain programs instead of others is developed. Thus the performer is able to anticipate which programs will be called for, and can therefore react faster when the time for movement arrives.

Motor tasks in which open skills must be executed place enormous demands upon the individual. Why is it that a skilled musician is able to maintain excellence well into old age while middle-aged athletes can no longer compete with the younger athletes? First, a musician follows a precise detailed program; each note, each bar can be anticipated. In most sports the opponent attempts to confound prediction, to foster suddenly the unexpected. With age one seems to need more time to respond to the unexpected and it is this coping with uncertainty that becomes harder with age. Abrupt reversal or modification of movement, the coding and transmission of the signals to the effector apparatus, the development and maintenance of states of optimal readiness, all of which are executed over a microscopic time scale, may take longer with increasing age.

1. Neural mechanisms of motor programs

The neural mechanisms for the formation of voluntary movements are quite complicated and are certainly not formed in the narrow area of the cerebral cortex called the motor area, as once believed. The entire frontal lobes are involved in the formations of intentions and programs for motor behavior. Furthermore, other cortical and subcortical mechanisms participate in the creation of a voluntary movement, with each mechanism performing a highly specific part in the whole functional system (Evarts, 1973; Hutton, 1972).

Traditionally, the focus in motor integration has been on the role of the cerebral cortex, but recent research has shown quite convincingly that the basal ganglia and the cerebellum receive information from the somatosensory, visual, and auditory regions of the cortex and recode this information, returning it to the cerebral cortex, via the thalamus, for use in formulating motor programs (Evarts, 1973).

Spatial organization is essential to the execution of a coordinated movement pattern, and it appears that association areas in the parieto-occipital region of the cortex are essential for the spatial analysis of input. Lesions in this part of the cortex cause losses in the ability to evaluate spatial relations and the individual confuses left with right and experiences confusion in evaluating body position while making a series of movements (Semmes, 1965; Semmes et al. 1955).

F. CONTROL OF MOTOR PROGRAMS

One of the central questions in motor behavior study is how a movement pattern is actually executed and controlled. In the execution of movements, two basic types of movement-control mechanisms have been proposed.

The first type of movement-control hypothesis proposes that the movement pattern is performed via a stimulus–response (S–R) process. This traditional notion of motor control postulates that movement control is based on a "serial chaining"–each component of the movement pattern is assumed to be triggered by feedback from various sensory receptors. This notion, called the "peripheral-hypothesis," is basically a simple S-R approach to movement. It suggests that once a movement pattern is initiated the response of one component of the pattern produces a stimulus (via proprioceptors) which serves as the stimulus for triggering the next response component, etc.

There are various kinds of behaviors in which this notion seems to hold. There are cases when the individuals' latency will likely suggest that they are providing themselves with the stimuli of n-1 in order to perform. A person asked to name the letter in the alphabet that comes after "H" typically has to cognitively recite the alphabet beginning with "A" before saying the correct letter. Or a person who is asked to recite nth line of a well learned poem typically has to begin at the beginning of the poem. Although the alphabet is well learned, few persons can recite it backwards. Findings of disruption of speech performance with elimination or brief delays of the sounds strongly suggest involvement of response-produced stimuli.

While the examples above suggest support for the "peripheral hypothesis," there is overwhelming evidence against it as a complete explanation of movement control. Many movements are executed too fast for response-produced stimuli to be useful. Lashley (1951) makes this point very succinctly:

The finger strokes of a musician may reach sixteen per second in passages which call for a definite and changing order of successive finger movements. The succession of movements is too quick even for visual reaction time. In rapid sight reading it is impossible to read the individual notes of an arpeggio. The notes must be seen in groups, and it is actually easier to read chords simultaneously and to translate them into temporal sequence than to read successive notes in the arpeggio as usually written.

Movement patterns, especially in some sports, are never executed exactly alike. Bartlett (1932) has offered a classic statement on the skilled movement pattern in sports:

We may fancy that we are repeating a series of movements learned a long time before from a textbook or from a teacher. But motion study shows that in fact we build the stroke afresh on a basis of the immediately preceding balance of postures and the momentary needs of the game. Every time we make it, it has its own characteristics.

One can write an "A" with both hands and both feet, even with one's teeth, if asked to do so, therefore learned S–R bonds could not account for this ability, other than with the normal writing arm (Black, 1949; Williams, 1960). There is also a mass of experimental data in which sensory feedback mechanisms have been blocked and the movement pattern could still be executed (Wilson, 1964, 1968; Kennedy, 1967; Camhi, 1971). Animals have learned movements when spinal deafferentation has completely abolished all sensation from the moving limb (Taub and Berman, 1968). Finally, relevant evidence from research raises interpretative problems due to the difficulty of specifying the stimuli that control learning prior to the development of serial chaining. Notwithstanding these problems with serial chaining, it may very well be that this type of mechanism is involved in performances characterized by invariant sequential movements, but it seems likely that the serial chaining mechanism is superseded for highly practiced tasks by some form of neural motor program that operates without sensory feedback (Greenwald, 1970).

If sensory feedback is not needed for the execution of a movement pattern, then it must be assumed that the movement patterns are represented centrally in the brain. Such a representation has been called a motor program. As noted above, the notion of a motor program is that when it is activated neural impulses are sent to the appropriate muscles in the specific sequence, timing, and force and impulses are largely uninfluenced by sensory feedback. Motor skill acquisition, according to this notion, is the construction of a motor program, not the building of an S–R chain.

This idea suggests a preprogrammed set of circuits in the central nervous system which is "set-off" and the programmed output is carried out without any ongoing control until it is completed. There is considerable evidence that entire movement sequences may depend solely upon the initial stimulation and not on subsequent feedback. It was Woodworth (1899) who over 70 years ago suggested that the pattern for simple motor responses is set up in advance of their beginning and is uninfluenced during the execution by any feedback, while complex responses may be preformed and initiated as a unit. More recently, Wilson (1964, 1968), Kennedy (1967), and Fentress (1973) among others have provided evidence for motor programs which function without sensory feedback.

Perhaps Camhi (1971) best summarizes the status of the "peripheral hypothesis" and the alternative notion that control is from a central control mechanism. He says, "My work shows that central-nervous-system networks, independent of the senses, can function in a wide variety of ways and give rise to kinds of behavior difficult to explain on the hypothesis that the nervous system is largely a reflexive mechanism." Thus, it appears that there are centrally controlled and governed motor program mechanisms for movement patterns.

Performance in the absence of feedback, or in any open-loop manner, could easily occur, but it could not account readily for modifications in movement execution during performance nor for improvement in performance. To account for movement modification and skill acquisition, a CNS closed-loop mechanism has been proposed by several investigators. Many movements require monitoring and modification until they are completed if they are to be executed effectively and if learning of correct movements is to occur. Thus, motor control is needed while the movement is in progress—adjustments frequently have to be made between one component of the movement and the next. Indeed, a fundamental assumption of closed-loop theories of motor behavior is that ongoing, response-produced feedback stimuli from a movement are fed back to a reference mechanism so that when a movement error occurs it can be detected and corrected. It has been suggested that the motor program signals the general patterning of a movement pattern and then sensory feedback causes adjustments for minor corrections that must be made. The specific mechanism presumably depends upon some kind of comparison process. Chase (1965a, 1965b) suggests a closed-loop system whereby feedback is processed by an "error detection unit" in the brain and if a mismatch occurs with the motor program, new directions are sent to the effector system. Von Holst (1954) has proposed a theory based upon the notion of neural comparison in the nervous system of afferent and efferent impulses. He says, "We shall propose that the efference leaves an 'image' of itself somewhere in the CNS, to which the re-afference of this movement compares as the negative of a photograph compares to its print." In essence, he suggests that a motor program (or brain command) which initiates a movement also produces an "efferent copy." The movements triggered by the motor program produce reafference, and if the reafference "matches" the efferent copy, no corrective action is called for. But if there is some difference between the two, the difference can either influence the movement itself or ascend to another center and produce a perception. In other words, if the motor program output at any second results in a reafference input that does not match the efferent copy, the mismatch results in a changed output pattern until the mismatch disappears. The efferent copy serves only as a template against which feedback is matched. In reference to this notion, Greenwald (1970) says:

A recently accelerating trend in the analysis of skilled performance is to regard the performer as an information processor who compares incoming sensory feedback from responses (reafference) with a stored representation of what feedback from correct performance would be (imaged reafference). Performance control is achieved by the information processor's detecting discrepancies between imaged and actual reafference, then generating responses that serve to reduce or eliminate disparities.

It has been suggested that there are actually two feedback loops operating to control motor programs: a short loop, which controls the immediate
timing and direction of each individual movement component; a long loop
which takes a longer time to operate. This long-term loop is primarily a product of visual, auditory, and proprioceptive feedback, while the short-term
loop is presumably a central loop and this loop feeds back to directly modify
the motor program component, since corrections made by it do not require
any new decision but are rather mere adjustments made to correct the accuracy and speed of the particular program in use. The existence of a "short
feedback loop" is supported by research on animals with deafferented
limbs. Animals with a deafferented limb that they cannot see have learned
to repeat movements, when by all normal considerations they should not
know where the limb is, whether it has moved, and if moved, in what way.
Since information about the topology of movements could not have been conveyed over peripheral pathways, it must have been provided by some central mechanism. Such a mechanism requires the existence of a purely
central feedback system that could return information about future movements to the CNS before the impulses that will produce these movements
have reached the periphery (Taub and Berman, 1968). Electrophysiological
evidence for such a mechanism has been demonstrated by Chang (1955), and
Li (1958), and Kuypers (1960) has identified anatomical evidence. It appears
to involve afferent collaterals from the medullary pyramidal tracts to the nuclei gracilis and cuneatus, then back to the cerebral cortex. Taub and
Berman (1968) have hypothesized that there may be several central loops.
They say, "if one were to set out a priori to construct a servo-mechanism
that was maximally effective and sensitive to control, one would certainly
establish a feedback loop at each level of the system from command center
to output."

It seems, then, that the motor program mechanism is essentially an
"order" to the effector mechanism and is carried out by means of two feedback loops—a short loop, taking about 30 milliseconds to make modification
when called for, and a long loop which takes about 200 milliseconds to be
effective in modifying movements. It appears that when a motor program
has been decided upon there is a comparison of feedback from the moving
body parts with the "motor program" and, when needed, corrections are
made without the issuance of new "orders" via the short loop and/or via
issuing new orders via the long loop (Welford, 1968, Wilson, 1964, 1968)
providing, of course, that the speed of movement is not too fast to prevent the
feedback transmission from being processed.

Sensory control and monitoring appear to play an important role in normal complex movements because disrupting or delaying the feedback disturbs the temporal execution of the task. Speech is blurred and stuttering

occurs, hand movements become irregular and misdirected. This has been well documented by Smith (1962, 1966) for vision, Chase *et al.* (1961a, b, and c) for sound, and Laszlo (1966) for proprioception.

Our discussion of a central mechanism for motor control has focused on control during the execution of a movement up to this point, but this closed-loop mechanism is believed to function also in the acquisition of motor skills. In outline, the view that a motor program is developed in motor skill acquisition under closed-loop control is as follows: First, a template, or image, is established which corresponds to the task. This is based upon the instructions and demonstrations which have been given about the task. Once a template has been established, the learner attempts to select from previously learned motor programs one that produces a movement pattern that most closely resembles the task demands of the current task. The learner then performs the task. The feedback from the execution is then compared with the template stored in memory. If there are discrepancies, the motor program is altered and feedback is again compared with the template and so on until the "intended" movement and the actual movement correspond and the correct movements are established.

It may be noted that according to this notion, feedback is not conditioned to subsequent movement, in an S–R chaining fashion, but instead feedback is used for making modifications in the motor program. Once the motor program is established, feedback can be eliminated and the task still performed correctly. Of course feedback does perform other functions, such as monitoring during a movement.

It may be seen that this closed-loop model of skilled acquisition regards the learner as an information processor who compares response-produced sensory feedback with a stored representation (template) of what feedback from correct performance should be. Improvement in skill is achieved by the individual detecting discrepancies between the template and the actual re-afference of feedback, then modifying the motor program to reduce or eliminate these discrepancies.

Perhaps the most popular of the closed-loop theories of motor learning is that proposed by Adams (1971). The Adams motor learning model postulates two memory states: A "memory trace" and a "perceptual trace." The first is a modest motor program that merely selects and fires a response rather than controlling a movement pattern. It must be cued to action, and the strength of it develops as a function of practice; that is, its strength is seen as increasing through stimulus–response pairing over practice trials. The perceptual trace is a mechanism which develops as the learner receives error information in the form of sensory feedback from task performance. It is assumed that visual, kinesthetic, and auditory feedback contribute sensory information to the building of the perceptual trace. It is the perceptual trace that the learner uses as a reference against which to compare and modify subsequent performance on the basis of feedback. In learning a skill, then, the learner uses feedback to make the next response different from previous ones—the learner uses the perceptual trace in relation to feedback and makes necessary adjustments on the next trial. The perceptual trace develops as a result of experiencing the feedback stimuli with each performance. The memory trace applies only to the choosing and initiation of a movement while the perceptual trace is also the reference mechanism used to evaluate the ongoing feedback from movement leading to error detection and correction processes. Empirical support for the theory has been demonstrated in learning self-paced positioning tasks and short, fast-timing movements (Adams, Goetz, and Marshall, 1972; Newell, 1974).

There are several characteristics of movement behavior under closed-loop control. First, with practice, and as motor programs become firmly established, dependence upon feedback may change from one sense modality to another. Fitts (1951, 1964) and Fleishman and Rich (1955) indicate that vision gives way to kinesthesis for movement cues and monitoring as proficiency is attained. Fitts (1951) states: "Visual control is important while an individual is learning a new perceptual-motor task. As performance becomes habitual, however, it is likely that proprioceptive feedback, or 'feel,' becomes more important." Thus, the unskilled musician, typist, gymnast, etc. uses vision for controlling movements while the skilled person in these tasks uses other cues. A second characteristic is that with practice the extent of a motor program becomes more complex, or larger. The typist advances from typing a letter at a time to complete words, and finally to full phrases; the musician progresses from single notes to melodies; and the athlete advances from phasic discrete movements to integrated movement patterns. A third characteristic is that the skilled performer uses feedback only occasionally to "check" on the progress of a pattern; thus, for the highly skilled performer sensory feedback may become largely unnecessary for successful performance.

The notion of a template, or "image," suggests that an important first task is to install in memory a perfect template. This may be done most advantageously by having the learner observe skilled performers before actually physically practicing. Observational learning studies have demonstrated marked facilitation of a variety of skilled performances directly following visual observation of another's performance. This matter will be taken up again in Chapter 21.

1. Neural mechanisms for motor program control

Various neural mechanisms are undoubtedly responsible for the movement control function. It is clear that three interconnected parts of the brain—the motor areas of the cortex, the cerebellum, and the basal ganglia—act together to control movement. As was noted in an earlier chapter, within the brain are masses of neurons collectively called the basal ganglia. These structures seem to exert important modulating influences on cortical output and are thus concerned with the regulation of motor programs. Recent findings indicate that the basal ganglia are preferentially active in slow movements; thus, they appear to regulate cortical influences so as to bring about smoothly coordinated movements. The second structure, the cerebellum, seems to serve as an important mediating structure for motor programs because of its profuse connections with the motor tracts leading from the cortex to the spinal cord. Ruch (1951) suggested that the cerebellum may function like a "comparator" of a servomechanism in that it receives a response image or efferent copy of the motor command and then it receives signals from the sensory systems about the resulting movement. These two inputs are compared by the cerebellum and, if there is a discrepancy, signals are transmitted to the cortex to alter commands to the muscles to correct the discrepancy. It has recently been suggested that the cerebellum may have a special role in actually preprogramming and initiating quick, ballistic movements. Evarts (1973) notes that "with a cerebellar disorder, muscular tremor is most severe during voluntary movement (fast movements) and least marked when the muscles are at rest." Thus, it appears that the basal ganglia and the cerebellum are complementary structures for motor control, with the basal ganglia controlling slow movements.

The motor area of the cerebral cortex is, of course, an important structure in the evocation and control of movement. Neurons from the cerebral motor cortex provide the most direct connections with spinal motorneurons, and damage to an area of the motor cortex usually results in paralysis of the muscles controlled by that area. Presumably, the motor area mediates the various feedback sources which operate during a movement and is the primary center for modification of signals to the muscles.

Since control of motor programs may follow a feedback pattern in which movements are monitored and modified if they are slow enough, one major source of feedback is from the visual, proprioceptive, and auditory systems. This may be considered the "long" feedback loop which was discussed in the previous section of this chapter.

Although very little is known about the exact neurological structures which might be functioning to effect the short-loop feedback which was discussed in the previous section of this chapter, it appears that the cerebellum is largely responsible for coordinating the timing activity in various groups of muscles. In order to modify muscular activity, the cerebellum receives information about position and movement from all sensory modalities. It sends signals directly to the motorneurons descending to the spinal cord and it also sends signals to the cerebral cortex, via the thalamus, to facilitate and time discharges over motor tracts. One of the main roles, then, of the cerebellum seems to be to take care of adjustments to movements by feedback. Eccles (1973) claims that all motor transmission over the motor pathway from the motor cortex is provisional and is subject to revision by the feedback operation of the cerebellar feedback loop. The existence of a purely central feedback system has been electrophysiologically and anatomically demonstrated and involves collaterals of the pyramidal tract. Pyramidal tract collaterals have been traced at different levels of their course and have been shown to play a role in the control of somatosensory afferents (Chang, 1955; Kuypers, 1960; Towe and Jabbur, 1961).

Neuroscientists have traditionally thought that comparison processes of a motor program and its "image" or "copy" occurred primarily in the brain, but Gibbs (1970) has suggested that some of the comparison between the motor program and feedback may occur at the muscle and spinal cord level. He has suggested that it may be possible that the "efference copy" of a motor program is represented in signals that go to the muscle spindles at the same time that signals go to the extrafusal motor fibers. The "copy" may cause the gamma efferent muscle fibers to contract to a certain extent at the same time that the extrafusal fibers are contracting. If the main muscle contracts to the same extent as the spindle muscle fibers, this mutual action means that spindle afferents will not be stimulated. However, if there is a discrepancy, the spindle afferents may be stimulated and thus, through their firing, bring the main muscle in line. This process may bypass the brain completely, or it may occur simultaneously with feedback to the brain. In any case it could result in a compensatory change in the movement to adjust the movement to correspond to the efference copy.

G. OUTPUT

The activity of muscles and glands constitutes the behavior (or response) which has been brought about by all the preceding neural activity. In the case of muscles, movement activity occurs.

H. FEEDBACK

The notion that feedback is a critical feature of complex motor behavior should be obvious to the reader by now. Powers (1973) notes: "All behavior involves strong feedback effects, whether one is considering spinal reflexes or self-actualization." The model presented here posits feedback in motor learning and performance as essential to some extent in various components of the system. Indeed organized closed-loop controls have been found to exist at all levels of the nervous system. As Miller et al. (1960) state, "The fundamental building block of the nervous system is the feedback loop," The importance of feedback to motor learning and performances is summarized by Held (1965):

In sum, the experiments I have described have led us to conclude that the correlation entailed in sensory feedback accompanying movement-reaffer-ence plays a vital role in perceptual adaption. It helps the newborn to devel-op motor coordination; it figures in the adjustment to the changed relation between afferent and efferent signals resulting from growth; it operates in the maintenance of normal coordination; and it is of major importance in coping with altered visual and auditory inputs.

Response-produced feedback is used not only to make certain that the motor program is carried out as intended but, more importantly, to correct errors if the movement is unsuccessful. Thus, stimuli produced by the learn-er's own behavior appears to play a critical role in the acquisition of skilled motor behavior. The movement-produced feedback enables the learner to systematically correct errors from practice trial to practice trial in order to develop a motor program which coincides with the learner's intentions (Howard and Templeton, 1966). Feedback, then, is not only a feature of the ongoing movement but various types of feedback which occur at the comple-tion of movements are important in enhancing motor learning.

The form of feedback that has been emphasized so far in this chapter is what is called "concurrent" feedback; that is, it is the type of feedback that the individual receives while actually performing the movements of a motor task. There is another form of feedback that is essential for skill acquisition. This second type of feedback is called "terminal" feedback, and we shall briefly discuss it now, since concurrent feedback has already been des-cribed in some detail.

Upon completion of a motor task, terminal feedback is needed by learn-ers to evaluate the "goodness" of their movements. They must decide whether their movements should be repeated or whether one or more com-ponents of the task need different motor programming. Learners receive terminal feedback of two kinds: knowledge of results (KR), which provides them with information about the outcome produced by their movements, and knowledge of performance (KP), which provides information about the move-ments themselves (Del Rey, 1971).

With regard to knowledge of results, Bilodeau and Bilodeau (1961) say, "Studies of . . . knowledge of results (KR) show it to be the strongest, most im-portant variable controlling performance and learning. It has been shown repeatedly . . . that there is no improvement without KR, progressive im-provement with it, and deterioration after its withdrawal." Fortunately, in many motor tasks KR is an intrinsic feature of the task. (The basketball shooter sees whether the ball goes in the basket; the tennis player sees whether the serve is in or out.) Since KR occurs after a performance, it may easily be provided in a variety of ways, such as films, videotape, and/or teacher instructions.

Information about the movement itself is called knowledge of performance, and it is concerned with such things as the temporal, spatial, sequential, and force aspects of the movement. KP may be supplied by teacher demonstration, verbalization about the movement pattern, or videotaped and filmed replays.

Several investigators have suggested that terminal feedback is primarily a source of information which a learner uses to formulate various hypotheses and strategies for selecting appropriate motor responses for subsequent performances. Presumably some sort of comparison process such as that suggested by Adams (1971) or Miller *et al.* (1960) mediates response enactment and thus provides a basis for adaptive behavior. The process may function in this way: The learner begins a movement with a template, image, or an "idea" of what movement pattern is to be executed, and then selects a motor program for task accomplishment. This program may be executed or for some reason the learner may not produce the intended motor program. In either case, the learner may accomplish or may not accomplish the task objective. If the intended program was executed and did accomplish the intended movement goal, presumably this will have reinforcing properties and will tend to produce the execution of the same motor program for subsequent responses. However, if the intended motor program was actually executed and the task objective was not accomplished, the learner becomes cognizant that the motor program is not right for the movement task. Selection of another motor program will probably be the outcome of this experience. Continued revision of the motor program after experiences of this kind usually produces a motor program–motor task match. A third situation occurs when the intended motor program is not executed and the task objective is not attained. In this case, the first strategy adopted by the learner would probably be to attempt the task using the intended program rather than repeating the incorrect program. This situation probably occurs most frequently during early learning trials, and cognitive efforts by the learner and/or guidance by an instructor would seem to be important for overcoming the problem. A final situation occurs when the learner does not execute the intended motor program but goal accomplishment is attained. From introspective evidence, it seems that the learner is surprised by this result. The learner obviously is reinforced by the result but may have difficulty duplicating the motor program, since it was not the one which had been intended. Learners in this situation frequently exclaim,"Now let's see, how did I do that?" as they undertake the task again.

1. Neural mechanisms for feedback

Feedback mechanisms for concurrent feedback have been discussed in earlier sections of this chapter and will therefore not be repeated here. Terminal feedback for human movement typically is mediated by the visual and auditory sensory systems. Seeing and hearing the consequences of movements constitute two of the most powerful sources of terminal feedback.

PROBLEMS OF MODELS

One of the problems in presenting schematic models of human behavior is that they convey the notion of a static system. Nothing could be further from the truth in actuality. The human neuromuscular systems are constantly active. All of the components in the model are in a continuous state of activity and change. Another problem with models of human behavior is that they are much too simplified for what actually is occurring. The human nervous system is a fantastically complex system and our understanding of its intricate functions is still quite incomplete.

11

Perception: Introductory Concepts

It is necessary to begin this chapter with a disclaimer. No attempt will be made in this chapter and the ones that follow in this section of the book to examine the subject of perception comprehensively. This topic has a vast and complex literature in the field of psychology; entire texts are devoted to such topics as theories of perception, perceptual learning, perceptual development, and even to the specialized topic of "perceptual-motor" behavior. In this text, only selected aspects of perception are examined, and in this chapter some of the general considerations of perceptual learning and development are dealt with while visual, kinesthetic, pain and speed of perception are examined in subsequent chapters. In each chapter only those aspects of the subject which seemed most appropriate for this text are discussed.

GENERAL FEATURES OF PERCEPTION

The only means that we have for getting information about our environment is by specialized sensory receptors, and that is why our senses are sometimes referred to as our "avenues to the world." They are the source of our knowledge of the world about us, and most behavior is a response to physical stimuli which have activated sense organs. Our sensory systems, then, provide us with the "raw" information which is necessary to make effective and efficient movements; indeed, motor learning and performance are largely dependent upon sensory data.

While there is a tendency to think of the "external" world as the major source of stimulation for an individual, this overlooks other important sources. Internal organs provide stimulation, and so do the movements of one's extremities as one moves through space. Action-produced stimulation is obtained by individuals, not imposed upon them. A stimulus, then, may arise from an empty stomach, a bending of the joints, or from the pull of gravity on the receptors of the inner ear.

Physical energy impinging upon an individual's sensory receptors provides the data out of which "meanings" arise. Activation of the senses may be viewed as the first stage in a multistage process for bringing order and organization out of the kaleidoscopic environment. The process by which sensory input is organized and formulated into "meaningful" experiences is called perception.

As you sit reading this book, if you should hear a sudden squealing sound followed by crashing noises on the street outside, you might guess that an automobile accident had occurred. But why would you surmise this? There is nothing about the sounds that enter your ear that requires such an interpretation. No, instead the sounds provide only the sound waves that are translated into spatiotemporal nerve impulses which are then combined with memories about streets, automobiles, and tires for an interpretation, or perception, of what has happened.

We are continually striving to make sense out of our world, to find out what the sensory information means. Perception is the process of organizing and giving meaning to sensory input, and therefore serves a useful function as a guide to behavior. Indeed, our behavior depends largely on how we perceive the world about us. Perception, then, helps to determine what responses we will make; thus effective and efficient motor behavior is highly dependent upon it. For this reason, many psychologists believe that the study of human perceptual development and learning is foundational to understanding behavior.

It should be obvious from what has just been said that the human nervous system does not restrict itself to a simple reaction to isolated stimuli; instead it responds to the spatial and temporal relationships between complex stimuli. These complex sensations are not simply and directly related to the physical properties of the component stimuli, and we do not understand the integrative action of the nervous system well enough to definitively discuss the physical or physiological bases for them at the present time. These "higher order" processes are therefore conceptualized as perceptions; this concept implying the operation of complex integrative processes which somehow transfer simple sensations into meaningful experiences that are not adequately described by reference to their physical properties.

DIFFERENCES BETWEEN SENSATION AND PERCEPTION

Historically, there has been considerable confusion over the words "sensation" and "perception." At one time perception was considered merely to be input to the brain, hardly different from sensation except more complex. Also, sensation was once thought to be a simple element in awareness, while perception was a combination of such elements. Extensive research in perception has made these notions obsolete.

Sensation is concerned with the ways in which the various sensory systems function. Sensation, therefore, may be defined as the activity of sensory receptors and the resulting afferent transmission. Perception, on the other hand, is the activity of mediating processes which integrate present input with past input. It is one of the intervening variables between a stimulus and a response.

Sensation may be viewed as a one-stage process that is not affected by learning; the same stimulus must have the same sensory effects on each repetition, except when fatigue develops. Perception usually demands a sequence of stimulations, and it is influenced by many factors, including learning, and its relation to stimulating events is variable. The same stimuli can produce different perceptions and different stimuli can produce the same perception. Evidence that perception is more than sensation is clearly demonstrated in viewing ambiguous, or reversible, figures; the same stimulus results in variability of perception. The significance of these figures is that two different perceptions can occur with the same sensory stimulation; that is, stimulus objects and their relationships to one another may be perceived—seen, heard, etc.—differently by different persons. There are, for example, notoriously wide variations in eyewitness accounts of accidents or crimes. Teachers are frequently appalled at the various perceptions which students have obtained from hearing exactly the same lecture.

One rather bizarre form of perceptual experience which illustrates quite dramatically the individual differences in perception is synesthesia, a word used to describe perceptions which intermingle different sensory modalities. For example, some people see each of the days of the week as a color, a smell, or as being spatially arranged in a complex order. Others experience letters and numbers in terms of colors and sounds, and there are people to whom music brings vivid perceptions of color.

SEQUENCE OF PERCEPTUAL ORGANIZATION

Stimuli impinging upon the organism in the form of physical energy provide the input for perception. These stimuli impinge upon specialized sensory mechanisms, each of which is particularly sensitive to a certain form of physical energy, which changes, or transduces, the physical dimensions of the stimulus into nerve impulses which are then carried over afferent neurons to the CNS. When the stimulus has been transduced into nerve impulses, the process of perception begins. While perception starts at the level of the sense organ, its organization continues to form as the impulses enter the CNS and ascend to the brain. In the subcortical areas of the brain, the nerve impulses become mixed with other signals from other senses and signals from other parts of the brain which inhibit, enhance, and thus recode the impulses as they continue their ascent to the cerebral cortex. In the cortex the signals are reorganized, modified, and integrated with other sense modality signals and with stored memories to produce a perception of the present experience. Verbal or motor behavior is the outcome, or output, of the total perceptual process.

In addition to making present information meaningful, perception is a core process in the acquisition of knowledge, or learning. Stimuli possess information which is extracted by the individual as learning; that is, information is acquired through experience and becomes part of the individual's storage of memories. This learning modifies the individual so that subsequent perception of the same stimuli will be different. Different people perceive the same stimuli in different ways because the stimulus activates different contents in their memory. Learning may also lead to thinking, which may be viewed as a manipulation of previous learning; the consequences of thinking modify the individual because new learning occurs; thus, the perception of stimuli is modified.

DEVELOPMENT OF PERCEPTION

An old argument is psychology is whether the organization of our perceptual experience is the result of learning or whether it is an innate function of the nervous system. The two classical positions on this question are represented by "nativism" and "empiricism." The first takes the position that perceptual organization is an innate function of the various sensory modalities; the second holds that perceptual organization is the result of learning. The nativism–empiricism controversy reached a peak of prominence during the 18th and 19th centuries. Beginning in the latter 19th century, this dichotomy began to be reinterpreted to some extent as a nature–nuture problem; that is, what has nature conferred that nuture further shapes? A brief review of the literature will serve to show the importance of both nature and experience in the development of perception.

A. EVIDENCE FOR THE INFLUENCE OF NATURE

Experiments on animals and human infants by Fantz (1966) and Gibson and Walk (1960) imply that animals possess a great deal of innate perceptual organization, and that certain basic perceptions such as visual figure–ground relations, depth perception, and auditory direction may be largely innate in humans. Fantz developed a simple method of studying the perceptual development of infants called a "looking chamber" (Fig. 11.1). He found that he could determine the direction the infants were looking by observing the position of their eyes. Assuming that the direction of vision indicated some awareness on the part of the infant, Fantz presented them with choices of patterns to view. The patterns consisted of plain and colored circles and outline drawings of a human face. He reported that infants even under five days of age prefer to view facelike objects. These findings indicate that some pattern vision is available within five days of birth and there appears to be innate preference for patterns which resemble a human face. Fantz concluded, "Clearly some degree of form perception is innate."

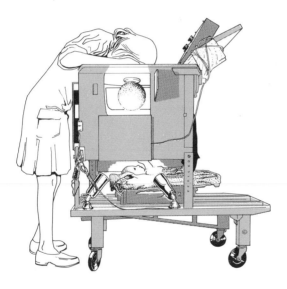

Fig. 11.1   This "looking chamber" was used to test the visual interests of human infants. The infant lies on a crib in the chamber, looking at objects hung from the ceiling. The observer watches through a peephole and records the attention given each object. (Based on Fantz, 1961.)

Gibson and Walk constructed a "visual cliff" (Fig. 11.2) which consisted of a transparent surface of glass under which was a solid center support surrounded on both sides by what looked like cliffs. The cliffs were covered with glass but they provided the viewer with an illusion of nonsupport. The cliffs on either side of the support were of different depths, one shallow and the other deep. The object of the experiment was to place a subject (animal

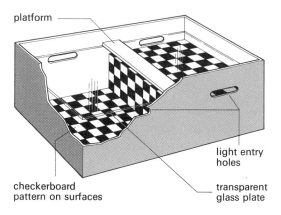

platform

light entry holes

checkerboard pattern on surfaces

transparent glass plate

Fig. 11.2 The visual cliff. (Based on Gibson and Walk, 1960.)

or human infant) on the center support and then induce the subject to move onto one of the nonsupport sides (Fig. 11.2). Most animals, when first learning to locomote, cannot be induced to move onto the glass above the deep "cliff" and very few human infants in the early stages of crawling will move onto the deep "cliff." Some animals with poor vision do not display these behaviors. It appears, therefore, that animals that depend upon vision for movement are able to discriminate depth when their locomotion is adequate, even when locomotion begins at birth; thus depth perception does not depend on experience.

B. EVIDENCE FOR THE INFLUENCE OF EXPERIENCE

There is, on the other hand, considerable empirical evidence which rather conclusively supports the notion that some perceptual organization requires experience. For example, Riesen (1960) found that when translucent covers were placed over the eyes of newborn animals and allowed to remain for long periods of time before removal, these animals, when the covers were removed, did not recognize forms in their environment, and they had a great deal of difficulty in learning to distinguish between simple forms. In subsequent research Riesen *et al.* (1964) and others have reared several species of animals in complete darkness and then studied the effects of the visual deprivation on visual perception. The findings of these "visual-deprivation" studies show conclusively that there is an initial deficiency in visual performance and the need for a period of visual experience seems to give clear evidence for the necessary role of learning, especially in the development of form and depth perception. But vision is not the only sensory modality in which sensory experience is important. Nissen, Chow, and Semmes (1951) obtained results similar to those reported by Riesen by restricting somato-sensory activity.

Numerous other studies have been carried out with a view to investigating the effects of different environments during infancy, especially the effects of some form of deprivation of early experience upon later behavior. By and large, the findings have indicated that animals deprived of early experiences are markedly poorer at various perceptual and motor tasks. For example, animals reared in a restricted environment are less active and poorer at problem solving than normal animals (Hymovitch, 1952). Thompson and Melzack (1956) raised dogs in a restricted and unstimulating environment and reported that these dogs proved to be poor learners. Sackett (1965) reported that monkeys reared in isolation were characterized later by grossly abnormal sexual and parental behavior.

Experimenters studying the role of experience in human perception cannot intentionally interfere with the development of perception in the human infant and for this reason animals have had to be used. But animals cannot report their perceptual experiences and, therefore, their usefulness is limited. Clinical opportunities have provided some chances to study human perceptual development. Human babies born with congenital visual defects are occasionally able to have the defects corrected. Hebb (1949) reported on a number of patients who had congenital visual defects which were subsequently corrected. He noted that these individuals could not identify patterns, objects, or faces when first exposed to them. Some of these individuals never attained normal visual recognition of complex forms, and long periods of learning were necessary to produce visual recognition. These conditions existed even when visual acuity was normal. Dennis (1960) reported that lack of varied experience in early childhood, insufficiency of cuddling, verbal communication and so on result in a general retardation of perceptual-motor development, and Davis (1940, 1947) described the pitiful cases of two girls who were extremely socially deprived in their first six years of life. The consequences of this deprivation were disastrous.

One type of human perceptual learning research involves experiments in which transformations have been imposed on the stimulus array; that is, it has been displaced in some manner. This is done by using an instrument which biases the stimulus information that reaches the sense organ. The basic issue is whether and how a subject adjusts to this distortion of stimulus information. Adjustment to the transformed array is usually referred to as "adaptation."

Over 70 years ago experiments were performed by Stratton (1897) with special glasses which inverted the retinal image that is normally projected onto the retina. He found that after a period of confusion the subject learned to adapt to the new image and the world was actually perceived rightside up. When the inverting glasses were removed, the subject momentarily per-ceived the world as upside down, but adaptation was accomplished rapidly. Recently, Kohler (1962) has repeated and extended some of these early experiments and has confirmed the findings of the earlier studies. These visual-inversion experiments suggest that visual direction is learned and that the orientation of the retinal image is unimportant to our perception of upness or downness.

Held and Freedman's (1963) experiments with prisms that displace the apparent position of objects in space provide additional support for the "perception-is-learned" position. They discovered an interesting dimension to this problem. They found that one of the important conditions for adjust-ing to displacement of the prism was the requirement of self-activated move-ment of the subject. The subjects who moved around with the prisms on soon adapted to them, but these who sat passively made very little adaptation to the prisms. They concluded that perceptual organization was learned and that perceptual learning was dependent upon self-initiated activity of the individual.

As indicated above, the intentional deprivation of experiences of human infants is not possible, but it is possible to do the opposite, that is, to increase sensory and motor experiences. In a recent study, using the techni-que of enhancement White and his colleagues (1964) advanced the occur-rence of accurate visually guided prehension in human infants from an average of five months to approximately three months. By increasing the mobility of infants and increasing sight of both the hands and near objects, development of sensorimotor coordination was enhanced.

The roles played by heredity, maturation, and experience in the development of perception are neither simple nor easy to resolve. It seems that our perceptual world is developed from certain innate abilities, but per-ceptual ability is continuously being modified as a result of maturation and experience. It also seems clear that sensory stimulation during infancy is necessary for normal perceptual development, and this sensory stimulation includes movement to produce stimulation.

C. SEQUENCE OF PERCEPTUAL DEVELOPMENT

Perceptual abilities of lower animal forms tend to be prewired, or pre-programmed, with little modification occurring due to experience. This is not true for humans. One of the unique characteristics of human behavior is the change in the manner in which maturing humans perceive the world These modifications are a combination of the normal maturational process and the experiences which the individual encounters.

Although there is an enormous amount of individual difference in normal human perceptual development, there are reliable consistencies in the stages of perceptual development. Of course, the normal developmental sequence depends upon the experiences of the maturing individual. Research has demonstrated that restricted, bland environments with little novelty and challenge inhibit full development of perceptual potential while environments which are rich in sensory stimulation, variety, social interaction, and opportunities to see and do produce adequate and often superior development of perceptual abilities.

At birth the human infant is basically a reflex organism, reacting in a diffuse manner to a variety of stimuli. But almost at once the sensory perceptual mechanisms begin to evidence selectivity to stimuli and begin to make discriminations in all of the sensory modalities. The neural mechanisms mature in conjunction with a variety of learning experiences, and the result is a typical pattern of perceptual development. It is beyond the scope of this book to make an extensive examination of the details of the perceptual developmental sequence of human life; other books are devoted entirely to this subject. (See, for example, Bartley, 1969.) We shall, however, briefly note some of the rather general characteristics of perceptual development, especially those of the first few years of life, when the foundations for perceptual abilities are being formed.

In its most general form, perceptual development tends to follow this sequence: (1) A shift in the hierarchy of the dominant sensory systems; (2) An increase in intersensory integration; and (3) Improvement in intrasensory discrimination (Williams, 1973b). One of the first perceptual modifications that occurs is the shift from the dominance of somatosensory receptors to greater utilization of visual and auditory information for modification and control of behavior. The visual system, especially, comes to dominate experiences with the environment, making possible the use of a much more refined, rich, and precise modality for extracting information than is possible with the somatic system. This use of visual cues, of course, allows children to make more rapid and precise judgments about their environment and in turn facilitates their behavioral responses to immediate stimuli.

The second general perceptual developmental stage is that of improved intersensory integration. Stimuli in the real world are multivariate, and the ways in which they may be perceived vary. For example, a dog may be seen, touched, or heard; a single cue may be enough for it to be perceived as a dog, but the use of multicues makes the task easier, and in some cases a richer perceptual experience. The well-known legend about the blind men who tried to identify an elephant demonstrates nicely the limitations of restricted sensory information. With improved intersensory integration, maturing children become more proficient at integrating what they see with what they hear, what they see with what they touch, and so on. Williams (1973b) summarizes this developing ability in this way: "[The child] can use visual cues and sound cues as well as tactile-kinesthetic [somatosensory] cues to help him adapt his behavioral responses to the precise environmental conditions in which he finds himself."

The third perceptual change is an improvement in intrasensory discrimination—each sensory system develops a more precise ability for detecting, discriminating, recognizing, and identifying stimuli. Improved intrasensory functioning manifests itself in the child's ability to detect and discriminate more details and differences in visual, auditory, somatosensory information, make precise judgments about speed, direction, and patterns of visual and auditory stimuli.

The consequences of these three basic perceptual developments are that children more readily adapt to the environmental demands of human life. This increase in perceptual ability enables children to gain greater control over their cognitive and motor behavior. Indeed, an inability to accomplish any one of these perceptual developmental changes restricts the individual's potential in certain spheres of life.

PERCEPTUAL LEARNING

The clear implication of the preceding section is that there is compelling evidence that perceptual abilities are modifiable by experience; that is, that a great deal of perceptual learning is an important aspect of behavior. Learning has been a major preoccupation of American psychologists over the past 80 years. The dominant orientation, the so-called Behavioral Psychology, has focused on the behavioral responses which are modified as a consequence of experiences or practice with a certain set of stimuli. This approach has been concerned with how one learns a list of nonsense syllables, chooses a correct response, acquires fear, etc. The emphasis has been on the actual behavior rather than on the processes which actually produced the change in behavior, for example, the perceptual learning that had occurred. Much behavior which is typically thought of in terms of the acquisition of competence in making specific responses depends for its successful execution on the growth of specific discriminations—a perceptual ability.

Gibson (1969) defined perceptual learning as "an increase in the ability to extract information from the environment, as a result of experience and practice with stimulation coming from it." The consequences of perceptual learning are "a better correlation with the events and objects that are the sources of stimulation as well as an increase in the capacity to utilize potential stimulation."

The main idea behind the notion of perceptual learning is that there are potential variables of stimuli which are not initially differentiated within an array of impinging stimulation, but given the proper conditions of practice and experience, they may become differentiated. As they do, perceptions become more specific with respect to the stimulation and have a greater correspondence with it. Thus, there is a modification in what the individual can respond to. The change, according to Gibson (1969) "is not the acquisition or substitution of a new response to stimulation previously responded to in some other way, but rather responding in any discriminating way to a variable of stimulation not responded to previously." In other words, perceptual learning is an increased ability to detect properties, patterns, and distinctive features of the stimulation—an increase in specificity with respect to a set of stimuli.

Studies of the acquisition of various skills show rather convincingly the consequences of perceptual learning. In industry, grading of products such as cheese, wool, cloth, and vegetables indicates quite clearly that trained personnel grade more accurately than untrained personnel do. Chick sexing—separating pullets from the cockerels shortly after they have hatched—and wine tasting are two commercially important perceptual skills which are learned after much experience of observing variations in the genitals of newborn chicks or tasting many kinds of wine. Other commonly acquired occupational perceptual skills are aerial photograph reading, oscilloscope reading, and X-ray plate interpretation.

There are numerous examples of perceptual skill learning in sports. Differentiating among a fastball, a curveball, and a knuckleball in baseball, differentiating between a fake and a real intent to move is important to performers in basketball, wrestling, boxing, football, and many other sports.

While instructional procedures in physical education have commonly concentrated on the control of response change, it is probable that it would be equally useful in many cases to train perception explicitly. Even in cases in which this has been done, the methods used were often haphazard. The use of systematic procedures for producing changes in discrimination ability may well shorten learning time and increase efficiency of final proficiency.

A. HIERARCHICAL ORDERING OF PERCEPTION

In an earlier section of this chapter, the sequential stages of perception were described, but perception itself is a complex task which has several subtasks. These subtasks have been extensively studied over the past half century and a body of literature has emerged which strongly suggests that these subtasks can be ordered into a hierarchy from the simplest to the most complex, with each successive step up in the hierarchy involving the extraction of progressively more information from the stimulus energy. This hierarchical ordering of perceptual segregations from the simplest to the most complex is: detection, discrimination, recognition, and identification. These were described in the previous chapter but will be reviewed here briefly.

A detection task is one in which the perception of the presence or absence of some aspect of stimulation is indicated by the subject. A tone, flash of light, a pressure on the skin, or some feature of patterned stimulation might be selected for detection. The subject typically makes some verbal remark such as "yes" or "no" or a brief simple movement, such as pressing a button as the indicator response. That learning can occur in even this simplest perceptual task has been shown using a variety of tasks. Improvements of acuity judgment have been found for the visual resolution of a pair of parallel lines (visual acuity) and two-point limen of the skin. In the latter, the task requires that the subject detect that the stimulation of two adjacent points on the skin is two stimuli instead of one. Absolute thresholds, in which the upper or lower limits of sensitivity are tested, have shown improvements in thresholds for all of the sensory modalities. Finally, detection of complex targets, such as a certain design (a so-called embedded figure) in a background which has been constructed to mask or camouflage it, is learned with practice with the task.

Discrimination refers to any noticing of differences between two or more stimuli presented simultaneously or in quick succession. Judgments of "same" or "different" or "more" or "less" are examples of a discrimination response. The smallest difference that can be consistently discriminated along a dimension such as weight or pitch is called differential threshold. Numerous experiments have demonstrated that differential threshold may be lowered (improved) by practice. Same or different discrimination of multidimensional stimulus arrays shows improvement with practice. For example one investigator had subjects practice making same–different discriminations of fingerprints and found considerable improvement. Another gave children practice in making discriminations among artificial graphic forms and found that the children improved their ability to discriminate among them (Pick, 1965; Robinson, 1955).

Recognition refers to noticing differences and similarities among objects when they are not presented simultaneously or nearly simultaneously in a stimulus array. Recognition demands judgments about whether or not an object is the same as the one perceived before—there is, thus, a requirement to distinquish an object from other objects. If subjects are shown a set of stimulus items and are later asked to pick out these items from a larger set of objects, they are being asked to display their recognition ability. The typical indicator response is "old" or "new," instead of "same" or "different" as it is in a discrimination task. As with other perceptual tasks, perceptual learning for recognition judgment has been demonstrated by several investigators.

At the highest order of perception is identification. Identification requires a unique response for each item presented. Making absolute judgments of tonal pitch, estimating a weight in pounds, estimating distances in feet in which the subject must respond with a specific response are examples of identification. Identification experiments in which the subject is asked to make absolute judgments on a single dimension such as estimating the distance from the subject to targets scattered over different distances, or absolute judgments of multivariate stimuli such as multidimensional color or sound stimuli, or identification of complex multivariate stimuli such as a human face or human voice, clearly demonstrate that perceptional learning occurs and indeed is essential for numerous human activities if the individual is to function in human society.

PERCEPTUAL TYPES

No two persons perceive an object or an event in exactly the same way. Differences in sensory system proficiency and stored memories will produce differences in perception. Furthermore, such factors as set (a temporary condition of individuals which makes them ready to respond in a certain manner), motivation, and even personality influence perception. The famous linguist, Benjamin Whorf (1961) after careful study of the Hopi and Shawnee languages concluded that people in different cultures categorize the world of sensations in different ways, and these categories are reflected in the language of the culture. The categorizations, then, determine what is perceived.

There appear to be characteristic ways in which individuals structure their world and thus perceive objects and events; thus, it is possible to speak of perceptual "types" of persons. One perceptual dimension of individual perceptual difference classifies persons as analytic, flexible, or synthetic, depending on how they perceive stimuli. Another perceptual classification is visual versus haptic,* and refers to the prominence given to vision or somatosensory stimulation. Persons vary in their perception of objects within a stimulus array, and those that are adept at distinguishing the figure

---

*The word haptic comes from a Greek term meaning "to lay hold of." It operates when a human or animal feels things with its body or its extremities.

from the background are said to be field-independent while those who are poor are said to be field-dependent. Levelers and sharpeners are classifications for individual differences in accentuating or minimizing differences between stimuli. A related classification uses the concepts reducers and augmenters to refer to persons who are relatively insensitive to sensory input and those who are acutely aware of sensory stimuli.

George (1952) differentiated among the analytic, flexible, and the synthetic. The first type of individual tends to perceive discrete parts of objects and fragments complex stimuli, seeming to "pull apart" and isolate for perceptual purposes. At the other extreme, the synthesizer tends to see the whole rather than minute parts, tends to generalize and synthesize objects and events; the synthesizer attempts to combine and relate stimuli. The flexible perceiver employs a changing perceptual style, depending on the nature of the stimuli and the particular situation. The perceptually flexible person has the ability to switch attitudes about a stimulus situation. Tasks which test the resistance to one form in order to visualize a second or third, or tests requiring the location of pictures of geometric design in more complex pictures evaluate perceptual flexibility.

Although both visual and somatosensory systems are used in perception of the environment, some individuals characteristically appear to give preference to visual impressions while others are more perceptually adept for somatosensory input. For the latter, tactual, manipulative, or movement experience richly supplements perception. For example, teaching letter and word shapes by providing manual inspection of the configurations, such as running the hand and fingers over the words, has been found to be effective with some children, but not for others.

Witkin (1950; Witkin et al., 1954) placed subjects in a darkened room, facing a luminous frame which surrounded a moveable luminous rod. When the frame was tilted at various angles, the subject was required to bring the moveable rod to an upright position, in line with the gravitational pull of gravity. This required that the subject isolate the rod from its tilted background by relying on gravitational cues. Witkin found reliable individual differences in perception on this task. He describes subjects who are free of error on this task as "field-independent," meaning that they have the ability to differentiate themselves from the environment. Tasks which require subjects to select an embedded figure in a picture which has been constructed to mask or camouflage it have also demonstrated that persons vary in this perceptual ability. Those who are adept are said to be field-independent while those who are poor are referred to as field-dependent.

Some persons tend to accentuate differences between stimuli while others tend to minimize the differences. Holzman and Klein (1954) labeled the former sharpeners and the latter levelers. This classification was based on their findings of having subjects judge the size of objects projected onto a screen. Although not directly comparable, the research of Petrie (1967) has identified two related kinds of persons—the reducer and the augment-er—who differ from one another in the ways of processing their experience of the environment. Using tests of pain tolerance and kinesthetic aftereffect, Petrie reported that reducers tend to subjectively decrease what is perceived whereas the augmenter increases what is perceived. This perceptual type will be discussed more fully in Chapter 15.

To summarize, people perceive objects and events quite differently. Moreover, there are a variety of factors which influence perception. But more significantly, people perceive in reliably consistent ways, and various perceptual "types" have emerged from the extensive research on perception.

PERCEPTUAL-MOTOR BEHAVIOR

People behave in relation to their perceptions; motor behavior, then, is dependent to a great extent on the kind and amount of sensory information and the perceptions which this sensory input produces after being integrated and interpreted in the brain. Theoretically, the more proficient the sensory systems, the richer the information stored in memory about similar stimuli, the more likely the individual is to make effective and efficient movements. There is indeed a substantial body of literature which demonstrates that perceptual mechanisms are intricately related to the execution of skilled motor behavior.

In recent years, scholars from several academic fields have begun extensive study of the relationships between perceptual abilities and motor behavior. The term "perceptual-motor" behavior is now frequently used by these scholars to indicate their focus on the interactions of input and output on motor behavior. The concept of perceptual-motor behavior, then, refers to the extracting of more and more refined information to produce greater control over one's overt motor behavior. Research from this work emphasizing the perceptual bases for motor behavior has offered pertinent guidelines for improving instruction in motor skills of all types, as well as advancing basic knowledge about human behavior.

With the greater interest in perceptual-motor relationships, there has emerged a notion that because voluntary movement is in part dependent upon various perceptual abilities, all perceptual abilities can be improved by a special movement training program. Because of the concern for the large number of children with learning disabilities over the past decade, a number of perceptual-motor "treatment" programs have been developed which purport to remediate specific learning disabilities and other cognitive problems. While a number of these programs report success in enhancing intellectual and language skills, the empirical literature provides very weak support for their claims.

One "spin-off" of the popularity of these programs has been a bandwagon movement in physical education directed toward the use of physical education programs for the enhancement of school verbal-cognitive skills. Indeed, some elementary school physical educators have claimed that the major justification of their programs is that they improve academic achievement. Although movement tasks may produce perceptual learning, they should not be viewed as a panacea for enhancing all children's cognitive development. B. J. Cratty (1969), one of the foremost leaders in this field of study, notes, "It is believed that motor activities can be a helpful learning modality; but to best utilize movement tasks within schools one must carefully examine research findings rather than simply paying blind devotion to one of the popular 'movement messiahs.' " Based on present evidence, it is naive to expect that a program of motor activities will significantly alter the perceptual and intellectual function of an undifferentiated group of youngsters. This is not to suggest that a well designed program of motor activities will not enhance general perceptual and motor skills, for there is good evidence that it will.

12

Speed of Perception

There are a number of perceptual abilities that play important roles in the execution of effective and efficient motor behavior. One of the most important of these perceptual abilities is perceptual speed—the ability to react quickly to sensory stimulation. In addition to reacting quickly to a stimulus, the effective performer must also carry out movements quickly, if they are called for. Thus, speed of response is important in many types of motor behavior.

Probably no type of measurement is so well known in the field of human performance as speed of perception and speed of response measurements. The typical measurements for these components of motor behavior are reflex time, reaction time (RT), movement time (MT), and response time. In this chapter the focus will primarily be on reaction time, since this particular component of behavior is primarily a function of speed of perception. The various factors which affect reaction time and the relationship between reaction time and motor behavior are emphasized. It is generally accepted that muscular efficiency plays a primary role in movement time, so this topic will not be covered to any extent in this chapter.

DEFINITION OF TERMS

In the study of perceptual and response speed, several terms are commonly employed. Since these terms have very specific meanings, it seems appropriate that they be defined at this time to avoid misunderstandings in the content that follows.

231

A. REFLEX TIME

Nonvolitional responses to stimuli are referred to as reflexes, and the time from the application of a stimulus to the first measureable effects of a reflex response is called reflex time. The reflex time for the knee jerk reflex, for example, would be the time lapse between the striking of the patellar tendon and the beginning movement of the lower leg.

B. REACTION TIME (RT)

Reaction time is applied to reactions requiring a volitional response. The delay between the presentation of a stimulus and the initiation of a response to it is referred to as reaction time. For example, if a subject is seated before a display panel with a finger on a response key and is asked to release the key as soon as a light on the panel goes on, the time lapse between the time the light goes on and the key is released is the RT. RT is the interval during which neural impulses are being transmitted to the brain, processed there, and impulses transmitted to muscles.

C. MOVEMENT TIME (MT)

Movement time is the time taken to complete a task after it has been initiated. That is, MT begins when movement of the body is initiated (not when the stimulus is applied) and ends when the movement of the body terminates the task.

D. RESPONSE TIME

Response time is a term used to indicate the combined time of both RT and MT. It is the total time from presentation of the stimulus to the completion of the task (Fig. 12.1).

E. SPEED OF PERCEPTION AND RESPONSE AND SPORTS PERFORMANCE

The various components of perceptual and motor speed are clearly evident in many sports. In track races, from the firing of the starter's pistol until

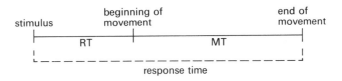

Fig. 12.1   Reaction time (RT), movement time (MT), and response time.

runners make their first movements in the blocks is the RT; the time from the first movement until runners break the tape is their MT; and the time from the firing of the starter's gun to the breaking of the tape (the time measured in track and most other timed sports events) is the response time.

SPEED OF PERCEPTION AND MOTOR BEHAVIOR

The performer in many sports must react to a variety of stimuli. Track and swimming athletes must react to the starter's pistol; in sports where a ball is used, the performers must make various reactions to the ball; many sports require fast reactions to opponents' maneuvers; and in team sports the actions of teammates must also be responded to. In sports such as basketball, soccer, field hockey, and volleyball a performer may have to react to 20 or 30 stimulus situations in less than a minute. In baseball the distance from the pitcher's rubber to home plate is 60'6" and if a ball travels the distance in 0.6 seconds (not unusual with a fastball pitcher), it is traveling about 10 feet every 0.1 second. If batters' RT is 0.2 seconds, they will be able to view the ball 10 feet longer than the person with a 0.3 second RT before they have to start their swings. This will, of course, give them a decided advantage in hitting over batters with a slower RT. One's efficiency in interacting with the environment in each of these cases is limited by the amount of time it takes to initiate movement.

Sports performers must, of course, do more than react to stimuli; typically they have to execute some movement pattern after the initial reaction, and the effectiveness of the movements determines the quality of the performance. Thus the total response—reaction time and movement time—determines the quality of a performance.

Poulton (1965) suggests that the best performer in fast ball games is not necessarily one with the best reaction times. He says, "The only certain generalization is that the man with the long reaction time will not be good at fast ball games . . . to be good demands more than simply a short reaction time."

THE STUDY OF REACTION TIME

The measurement of RT has had a long and rich history in the study of motor behavior. As early as 1868, Donders (1868) attempted to develop tasks to measure the time for such elementary operations as simple RT and choice reaction time (CRT). The pioneer experimental laboratories of Wundt in Germany and Cattell in the United States devoted a great deal of experimental work to RT studies in the latter years of the 19th century and the early years of this century. Speed of perception investigations continue to flow out of psychology and physical education laboratories today. The research designs of these studies become more sophisticated with each passing year.

A. THE COMPONENT PARTS OF REACTION TIME

RT is analyzable into component parts, based on neurophysiological function, and in research one goal is to ascertain which part of RT is related to the receptor, which part to afferent pathways, which part to central processing, which part to efferent pathways, and finally which part is related to muscle action. One technique which has been employed to achieve this goal is to fractionate RT. Some investigators have divided RT into a "premotor" part and a "motor" part. Premotor RT is the interval from the application of the stimulus until the first change in muscle action potential (measured by electromyographic recordings) in the acting muscle; motor RT is the interval from the first change in muscle action potential until movement is actually initiated (Botwinick and Thompson, 1966).

Other fractionations of RT have involved measuring the interval from the application of the stimulus until the first change in cortical activity in the brain (measured by electroencephalograph recordings). It has long been known that RT to auditory stimuli is faster than RT to visual stimuli by about 50 msec. Recently it has been discovered that auditory stimulus activity reaches the cerebral cortex 8–9 msec after stimulation while a visual stimulus takes 20–40 msec before reaching the cortex. Since both sensory pathways are about the same length, presumably the difference is a function of differences in transduction speed.

In all, RT is a function of the sensory transduction and afferent transmission to the brain, retrieval of the appropriate response from memory, the efferent transmission to the muscles, and the time for muscular response to be initiated. One of the most fascinating, but least understood, parts of RT is the retrieval of information drawn from memory for the appropriate response. E.E. Smith (1968) describes how the retrieval process may function in the sequence of stages between the presentation of a stimulus and the initiation of a response. First, the raw stimulus is "preprocessed" until a representation of it is formed. This representation then encounters memory representations of the possible stimulus alternative which were transferred to a rapid-access storage system in anticipation of the stimulus. On the basis of certain tests, or comparisons, between stimulus representations and the memory information, the stimulus is categorized as one of the possible alternatives. Given the categorization, an appropriate response is selected and the execution of the response is programmed.

B. USES OF KNOWLEDGE ABOUT SPEED OF PERCEPTION

Wherever speed of execution is important, knowledge about RT is useful, and, of course, there are innumerable places in the world of work and the world of recreation where speed of execution affects performance. Thus, the study of RT is of interest for the information it generates about individual differences and the factors which affect perceptual speed.

RT experiments are important or of interest not only because of the information they generate with regard to individual differences but also because of the information they generate about the functioning of the nervous system function, such as theories about attention, theories about perceptual processing capacity, theories about processing speed, etc.

MEASUREMENT OF REACTION TIME

Two of the most commonly used methods of ascertaining perceptual speed are RT experiments and tachistoscopic experiments. In the latter, printed matter or pictures of some kind are projected onto a screen for a very brief time (sometimes less than 1/100 sec) by a tachistoscope, which is basically a film slide projector which has been equipped with a very fast shutter speed; the slide is shown for just a brief instant. The tachistoscope was used extensively during World War II to train people to identify enemy airplanes from a brief exposure to their pictures or silhouettes. It is frequently employed today in teaching speed reading. It has also been employed extensively in speed of perception experiments.

Much more common, especially in motor behavior laboratories, are the RT experiments which employ response keys and chronoscopes. The apparatuses needed for measuring RT are:

1. A timer, usually a chronoscope, which records time in hundredths or thousandths of a second and which is activated by a stimulus (typically a buzzer or a light).

2. A reaction, or response, key that, when released (or depressed, depending upon the model), stops the time (Fig. 12.2 a and b).

Since movement time and response time are also frequently measured while doing RT research, the instruments for their measurement will be described. Instruments used to measure MT and response time also include response keys and chronoscopes, but they may include a photoelectric cell or microswitch and one or more additional timers as well (Figs. 12.2c and 12.3).

In a typical experiment in which RT, MT, and response time are all measured, a stimulus activates chronoscopes "A" and "B." Chronoscope "A" is

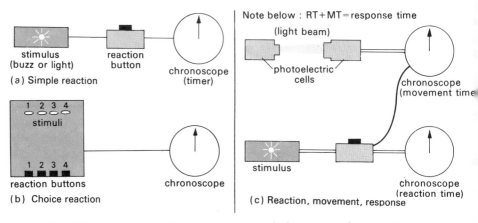

Fig. 12.2   Instruments for measuring speed of response characteristics.

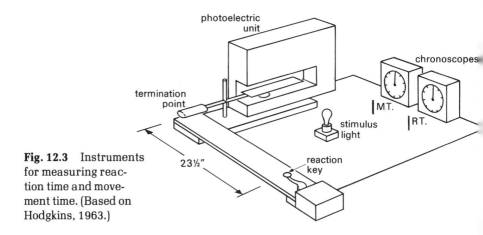

Fig. 12.3 Instruments for measuring reaction time and movement time. (Based on Hodgkins, 1963.)

stopped when the subject initiates movement (measuring RT). Chronoscope "B" terminates when a light beam of the photoelectric cell is broken by an arm, hand, or leg of the subject (indicating response time). To calculate MT, RT is subtracted from response time. Of course, chronoscope "B" can be wired to start when movement is initiated and stopped when movement ends. In this case, the time on chronoscope "B" will indicate MT. In this situation, the sum of the time recorded on the two chronoscopes provides the response time.

A third chronoscope may be used to start with the stimulus and terminate with movement through the photoelectric cell. This would record the response time on one chronoscope. In sports events that are started with a

gnal (usually a gunshot) and ended when the performer completes a re-
uired distance, the timer's stopwatch serves as a response time chrono-
:ope.

Many researchers have devised their own measuring instruments.
ome of the more sophisticated research designs concerned with speed of
erception and response characteristics have used as many as six or seven
ironoscopes.

ACTORS AFFECTING THE SPEED OF PERCEPTION

here are a number of factors which affect speed of perception. The speed
neural transmission limits reflex time, but RT is not as simple a phenome-
on, and various other factors in addition to neural transmission speed
ffect this variable. We shall examine the basic features of RT from two per-
pectives: (1) the nature of the stimulus; (2) the nature of the individual.

THE NATURE OF THE STIMULUS AND REACTION TIME

eaction time depends upon the external situation affecting the individual
nd on factors present in the individual at any given moment. The external
ctors are called stimulus variables, and in an experimental setting these
re controlled by the experimenter. Extensive research on stimulus vari-
bles and RT has been conducted and some rather clear-cut findings are evi-
ent.

Stimulus modality and reaction time

o we perceive and respond to various types of stimuli with the same speed?
here has been considerable research on the modality of stimulus and RT,
nd it has been found that RT varies with the particular sensory system re-
eiving the stimulus; in other words, the time required to react to a stimulus
modality specific. Stimuli resulting in the fastest RTs have been found to
ome in this order: auditory, tactual (touch), visual, pain, taste, and smell.

RT to a light stimulus is around 20 percent slower than for sound and
uch. Simple RT to auditory or tactual stimuli averages about 160 msec
hile RT to visual stimuli averages about 195 msec. The differences are
robably caused by delays in the photochemical processing which trans-
uces light energy into electrical energy. Davis (1957) noted that for an audi-
ory stimulus, impulses reach the cerebral cortex 8–9 msec after stimulation
hile signals from a visual stimulus do not reach the cortex for 20–40 msec.
his fact accounts for most of the difference in RT between these sensory
odalities. Additional difference may be a function of the brain mechanisms

responsible for retrieving and programming information from differei
modalities. There is no evidence that the efferent transmission speed is di
ferent, since the same muscles are being employed to bring about the initia
tion of a response.

With regard to RT to touch, the location of the stimulus is important.
site nearer the brain yields a faster RT; presumably this is because of tl
shorter neural conduction pathways.

Intraindividual correlations are rather high between RTs made to di
ferent modalities of stimuli. That is, individuals who react quickly to or
type of stimulus tend to react quickly to other modalities of stimulation. Fc
example, Wilkinson (1959) reported a modest but positive relationship b
tween RT to a kinesthetic stimulus and a visual stimulus. This seems to poii
to the presence of reaction time "quickness" in different degrees in diffe
ent individuals; however, this is apparently not a general "speed" trait, b
cause it does not correlate highly with movements requiring speed. In othe
words, the correlation between RT and MT is not high. This will be di
cussed later in this chapter.

The differences in RT to different modalities of stimuli must in son
way depend to a large extent upon different rates of the transducing proce:
in the various receptors. Since the sensory end organs have different way
of transducing the stimulus energy to electrical energy, and different stru
tures by which the stimuli are processed in the brain, it is not surprising tha
we find differences in RTs to stimuli in the various sense systems. There
also the possibility that central processing may partially account for the di
ferences, but it is doubtful that efferent transmission plays a role.

2. Stimulus intensity and reaction time

The intensity or strength of the stimulus has been found to be influential i
RT. Up to a point, the stronger the stimulus, the faster the RT, and a small ii
crease in intensity makes a marked difference in RT at low intensities (nea
the stimulus threshold), but there is proportionally less effect as intensity
increased. Teichner (1954), reviewing RT studies, reported that as intensi
of the stimulus was increased, the reaction time was shortened. He relate
that "people will react more quickly to a point, as the stimulus gets stronge
If the point is exceeded, the stimuli will tend to block performance becaus
of the stressful nature." Woodworth and Schlosberg (1954) and Vallerg
(1958), among others, report that RTs are shortened as the intensity of th
stimulus increases. It can be concluded that a bright light will elicit
quicker response than a dim light or a loud crack from a starter's gun wi
result in a faster reaction than a dull shot.

The speed and amplitude of a nerve inpulse are fixed characteristics (
a particular neuron, and the speed of transmission along a nerve fiber doe

ot vary with the intensity of a stimulus. Nevertheless, numerous studies report that RT is faster as the intensity of the stimulus increases. Although here are many variables which can account for this phenomenon in dynamic situations, in simple RT experiments it is probably a result of spatial summation. A low intensity stimulus excites a few, perhaps small, slow-conducting neurons, but a higher intensity stimulus activates the larger, faster-conducting neurons. The resultant effect is faster RT.

. Simultaneous or near simultaneous stimuli and reaction time

Mowbray and Rhoades (1959) found that RT was significantly faster when more than one of the senses were stimulated simultaneously. RT is faster with binocular stimulation than with monocular stimulation with the same ight. Also similar effects are produced with auditory stimuli when the same sound is presented to both ears rather than just to one ear.

Much greater theoretical and empirical interest has been shown in RT o stimuli which are presented in close sequential order than to the simultaneous presentation of stimuli because the results of the sequential stimulation have raised some interesting questions about the information processing capabilities of the nervous system. Telford (1931) provided the earliest description of RT performance under sequential stimulation. Inspired by the discovery of the physiological refractory period in a single neuron, he was curious about whether the brain as a whole showed similar characteristics. He discovered that when subjects had to respond to two stimuli that were presented in close sequential order when the interstimulus interval (ISI), the time between the presentation of the first stimulus (S_1) and the presentation of the second stimulus (S_2), was reduced to ½ second (500 msec) or less, RTs o S_2 increased considerably, compared with those with longer ISIs (Fig. 2.4). He concluded that this phenomenon was a general refractoriness of the nervous system and called it the "psychological refractory period" (PRP) Fig. 12.5). It was not until after World War II that a thorough analysis of the PRP and its implications was undertaken. With the advancements in computer technology accompanied by the development of cybernetic and information theory, concepts and research methods from these endeavors began to find their way into human psychological study. And these theoretical and methodological advances suggested that human nervous system functions could be analyzed in information and cybernetic theory terms. One information theory term that was applied to nervous system function is the single channel hypothesis. The single channel hypothesis suggests that a person may be conceived as a single channel operator—that is, one cannot perform two functions absolutely simultaneously, both of which require conscious attention. The notion here is that one signal in the brain has to be cleared and dealt with before another can be processed.

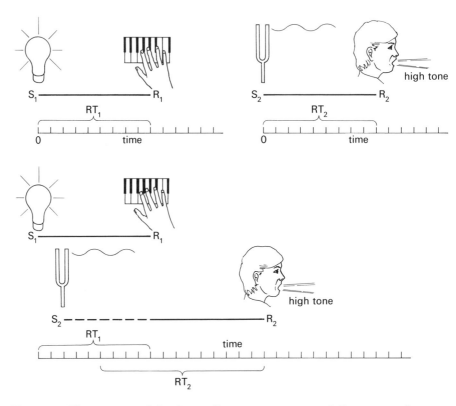

Fig. 12.4 The top part of the figure illustrates RT to two different stimuli iso-lated from each other in time. The bottom figure illustrates the delay in process-ing one stimulus when it is presented during the processing time of another stimulus. (Based on Keele, 1973.)

Employing information theory to explain the psychological refractory period, it is suggested that the brain has a single information-processing channel for tasks which require conscious attention, and the second stimulus has to be "stored" while the channel is busy processing the first stimulus; when the channel is cleared again the "waiting" period for S_2 ends and it now may be processed. In essence, then, the notion is that the PRP is due to a limited capacity of the brain to process information and therefore the information from the second stimulus is held in store until the central mechanisms are free.

In 1948 Craik (1948) proposed that the delay to a second stimulus is caused by a computing process that links the stimulus to a response. Accordingly, a stimulus that arrives while the "processor" is occupied presumably has to wait for attendance, which superficially makes the nervous system refractory. It was Welford (1952, 1959) who described the single-channel

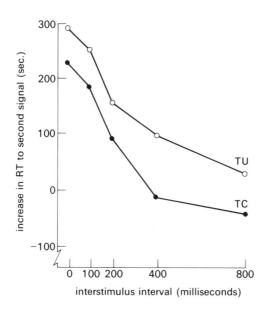

Fig. 12.5   The increase in reaction time to the second of two signals as a function of the intervals between stimuli. The open circles represent a condition in which the intervals varied from trial to trial (temporal uncertainty—TU) and the closed circles represent intervals which were fixed for a block of trials (temporal certainty—TC). These curves illustrate the psychological refractory period (PRP). (Based on Creamer, 1963.)

theory in more detail and who referred to the central computing system as the single-channel decision mechanism. He suggested that response execution is to some extent monitored by the single-channel, and that a minimum feedback from the responding action, indicating that it has begun or ended, is essential to clear the channel for the next stimulus. Finally, with regard to the PRP phenomenon, Lykken (1968) says, "It is natural to think of some sort of scanning operation here; the attention channel may open briefly at regular intervals so that S_1 must wait until the next 'opening' and S_2 must wait its turn until the first 'opening' after S_1 has been processed and the attention channel is released to accept a new input."

In the course of extensive research on the PRP several additional aspects of this phenomenon have been discovered. Even if the subject is not required to respond to S_1 at all, the effect on RT to S_2 is nearly as great as if the subject did react to S_1. Davis (1959) suggested that most of the delay arises "as a result of paying attention to the first signal, rather than the performance of any overt response to it."

The PRP persists with practice despite attempts to eliminate it. Gottsdanker and Stelmach (1971) tested one subject over 87 days but were not able to eliminate psychological refractoriness. Thus, it appears that psychological refractoriness is a stable aspect of one's performance.

The first stimulus and second may be in different modalities without changing the effect of the PRP. For example a subject will show a PRP if S_1 is visual and S_2 is auditory, or vice versa (Davis, 1959).

Telford's (1931) original suggestion that the PRP was a result of a general refractoriness of the nervous system has been found to be incorrect on both theoretical and empirical grounds. It is clear that the refractoriness does not stem from the same neurological process as that of neuronal refractory periods. Information processing theory concepts, as briefly described above, provides the most complete explanation of the PRP at the present time.

4. Forewarning cues and reaction time

It is well established that RT is faster when a stimulus is preceded by a warning signal than when it is not. This fact is used in several sports where the performers are given "on your mark, get set" cues before the starting signal. The warning presumably enables performers to maximize their state of readiness and thus lowers their threshold for responding. Keele (1973) notes, "People may be more efficient in processing information if they have prior warning of imminent events."

Typically, lights, sounds, and electrical shocks are used as forewarning cues in experiments, and, up to a point, more intense forewarning cues produce faster RTs. Oral cues such as "attention" spoken in a loud and commanding voice are more effective than oral cues given in a low, soft, and uncommanding tone. The more intense stimulus probably facilitates greater portions of the nervous system and mobilizes more neurons which are ready to fire when the stimulus signal occurs.

If one knows exactly the length of the forewarning periods, and thus when the stimulus will occur, RT can be reduced to zero. Of course, when the foreperiod is of a constant length we no longer have a true RT task but a problem in coincidence–anticipation timing. In this type of situation, the anticipation of when the stimulus will occur is involved, and since the foreperiod is of a constant duration, performers can get their response under way before actual occurrence of the stimulus, with the result that their RT is better than the optimal value that would be expected had they waited for the stimulus to occur and then responded. Practice with a constant foreperiod can result in RTs of zero or just a few milliseconds.

The longer the constant foreperiods, the slower the RTs and the greater the number of errors, that is, responding before the stimulus occurs. Jumping the gun in track is an example of an error in anticipation. Increasing RTs to increasing constant foreperiods is probably a function of the inaccurate time-keeping ability of neural central mechanisms.

The length of the forewarning period may be varied from trial to trial; that is, the period of time between the forewarning signal, such as "set," and the stimulus signal may be varied from fractions of a second to many seconds. The RT to all types of stimuli is slowed if the stimuli are complicated by this temporal uncertainty. When temporal uncertainty is introduced into RT experiments, RT becomes slower because the response cannot be anticipated in advance but must be initiated by the stimulus. Nevertheless, the RTs are faster than they are with no forewarning.

Several investigators report that the shortest RTs occur when the forewarning period (the period from the preparatory cut to the initiation of the stimulus signal) is between 1.0 and 1.5 seconds. On the other hand, Munro (1951) reported that the best interval between the warning period and the stimulus is two seconds. However, the length of RT is affected not only by the immediate forewarning period but also by earlier forewarning periods, when RT experiments are carried out as a series.

When foreperiod intervals are varied (say between 0.05 sec and 5.0 sec) within a series of trials, RT varies as a function of the position of a foreperiod interval within a range of foreperiod intervals. Rothstein (1973) and others who have worked with ranges of foreperiods of less than five seconds have found that as the foreperiod interval becomes longer, with regard to other foreperiod intervals in the range, RT is faster; e.g., if the foreperiod intervals are 1.0, 2.0, 3.0 seconds for a series of trials, RT will be faster to the 3.0 foreperiod. To summarize, if variable foreperiods are used so that subjects are uncertain about where the stimulus will occur, they generally show optimal performance near the end of the foreperiod.

Temporal expectancy is the term employed in explaining this phenomenon. Temporal expectancy is an increasing readiness to respond to events that occur over time. As readiness increases, RT decreases. At the neural level this readiness is represented by facilitation of appropriate neurons, producing increased arousal and attention. One implication for coaches training athletes is that if the coach practices the athletes with shorter intervals between the "get set" and "go" cues, their expectancy should be higher and RT faster at the meets, when the intervals are longer.

RT for a given trial in a series of RTs is also affected by the length of the foreperiod immediately preceding it. In general, a short foreperiod following a long foreperiod results in slower RTs than a long foreperiod following a short foreperiod. When a short foreperiod follows a longer one, the subject seems to be "surprised" by the stimulus and is not in an optimal state of readiness to respond to it. On the other hand, the temporal expectancy concept may be employed when a long foreperiod follows a short one; here there is an increasing readiness to respond to the stimulus over time.

On the basis of what has been said about forewarning cues and temporal uncertainty, numerous implications for games and sports situations can probably be imagined. For example, batters in baseball can time their swing much better against a pitcher who consistently throws pitches of the same speed. Batters can use the release of the ball as a cue as to when the ball will reach the plate, and they can adjust their swing to coincide with the arrival of the ball at home plate. The baseball pitcher who uses the same rhythmic wind-up before delivering the pitch makes it easier for the batter to anticipate when the ball will be thrown. Good strategy in many sports requires the manipulation of forewarning cues to keep opponents guessing as to when they will have to respond. In football, the quarterback varies the count on which the center snap is made to prevent the defense from anticipating it, and uses nonrhythmical counts to further confound the defense.

5. Choice reaction time

If an individual must make choices as to which stimuli to respond to or which response to make to a stimulus, RT is slower than to simple RT situations. The first demonstration that the time necessary to make a decision depends upon the number of alternative stimuli and responses that occur in a situation was made by Donders (1868) over a century ago. Carrying the observations of Donders forward, in 1885 Merkel (1885) found that choice reaction time (CRT) increased as the number of stimuli and responses increased—that is, CRT was found to be an increasing function of the number of available choices. However, each increase in the number of choices does not cause the same increase in RT. The increase caused by adding alternatives is larger when there are fewer alternatives than when there are many.

More recently with the advent of information theory, more mathematically precise descriptions have been made of the relationship of RT to alternatives. Hick (1952) proposed what has become known as Hick's Law: CRT increases at a constant rate as the amount of information conveyed by a stimulus increases. The amount of information, in information theory terms, increases as a logarithmic function (negatively accelerated) of the number of alternatives, each with a specific response demand, which constitute the task. Thus CRT should increase as a function of the number of alternative stimuli, and this is what Merkel and Hick's data show, and Hyman (1953), and Brown (1960) have confirmed Hick's Law (Fig. 12.6).

Although Hick's Law holds true over a wide variety of situations, when the stimulus–response relationships are familiar or compatible or the performers are well practiced, CRT tends to remain constant, rather than increasing, as the number of alternatives increases. In numeral-naming tasks, several investigators have found CRT to be unrelated to number of choices (Mowbray, 1960) (Fig. 12.7). Similarly, when stimuli were tactual vibrations of the fingers and the required response consisted of a depression of the stimulated finger, Leonard (1959) found that the number of alternatives, from two to eight, had no effect on CRT; that is, that after practice RT with

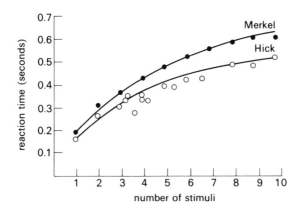

Fig. 12.6 Choice reaction time and the number of possible stimuli: the findings of Merkel and Hick. The experimental procedure involved a motor response, pressing the appropriate key, to a visual stimulus—in Merkel's case, to a Roman or Arabic numeral presented on a screen in front of the subject, while in Hick's case, there was an illumination of one of 10 lamps in a circular display. (Based on Hick, 1952.)

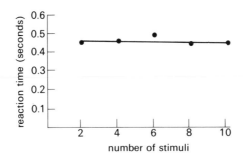

Fig. 12.7 Choice reaction time and the number of possible stimuli in a highly practiced task. The experimental procedure involved a vocal response, which was naming a numeral which appeared on a screen in front of the subject. The stimulus-response contingency was therefore a highly familiar one, and a practice period at the task was allowed before the data were recorded for analysis. (Based on Mowbray, 1960.)

eight alternatives was as short as RT with only two alternatives. Recent replications of Mowbray and Leonard's study have found that CRT was somewhat related to number of choices, but the relationship was small.

In addition to the number of alternatives, practice, and compatibility, several other variables such as the probability of occurrence of the different alternatives, sequential dependencies, and speed-accuracy trade-off affect CRT. RT becomes faster to the more frequently occurring stimulus within a set of stimuli (Fitts, Peterson, and Wolpe, 1963). In other words, in a three-choice task if one of the stimuli occurs 70 percent of the time and the other two stimuli each occur 15 percent of the time over a series of trials, RT to the most frequently occurring stimulus will become faster than RT to the other two (Fig. 12.8).

This is probably the result of the motor set. Thus, when two possible movements may be called for when the stimulus occurs, if, for each movement there is a corresponding internal motor program, or plan, which serves to control the movements, at the time of a forewarning cue, the threshold of either of these two motor programs can be altered by the performer. The most-likely-to-occur response may be placed in a motor set of very high availability. This notion suggests that the foreperiod involves a specific preparation of the responses as well as an increase in alertness. Although it is possible that such specific preparation involves an adjustment in muscle poten-

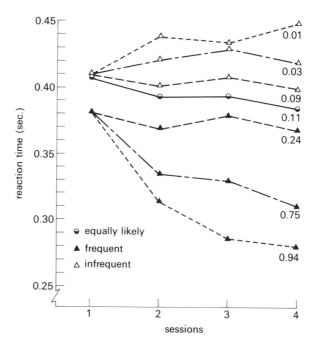

Fig. 12.8 Reaction time over four days of practice (top three curves) and to one frequent stimulus (bottom three curves). The middle curve represents a control condition in which all nine stimuli were of equal frequency. (Based on Fitts, Peterson, and Wolpe, 1963.)

tial, studies have shown that the forewarning cue reduced time between the stimulus and the muscle activation, not the time between muscle activation and the overt response.

Several studies have shown that when stimuli in a CRT task occur in a sequential order over a series of trials, the sequential dependencies can be learned, and RT reduced (Hyman, 1953; Shaffer and Hardwick, 1968). But just because sequential dependencies exist in a series of trials does not mean that a learner will recognize them easily. Keele (1967) reported that in a serial RT task subjects not instructed that a specific sequence was present did no better than subjects performing on a random sequence schedule. Instructions that describe the dependencies or techniques that emphasize the dependencies will vastly facilitate improved RTs.

In sequential dependencies, just as in CRT tasks where there are differences in the probability of the occurrence of stimuli, presumably a response has been retrieved and held in readiness in preparation for the stimulus. A probable stimulus will produce a response more quickly than an improbable one, since the retrieval from memory is biased toward a response that was considered probable during preparation. Such bias may be reorganized for each trial. Thus, if the stimuli alternate on successive trials, subjects will respond more quickly to the one they expect to occur.

Related to the sequential dependency findings is the finding that CRTs to stimuli that are immediately repeated, that is, repeated on the next presentation or trial, are faster than CRTs to "new" stimuli, that is, stimuli that are different from the immediately preceding one. This is called the "repetition effect" (Bertelson, 1961). This may be the result of facilitation of the neurons involved in the RT as well as the muscle action potential buildup in the responding limb. Both neural and muscle activity buildup takes some time to fade out.

When performing a CRT task, subjects are capable of trading off speed for accuracy, and this trade-off is a function of the instructional emphasis on speed or accuracy. If subjects are told to emphasize speed, the CRT will become faster, but they will commit many errors (that is, make the wrong response). On the other hand, if they are told to emphasize accuracy, CRT will become slower, but few errors will be committed (Fitts, 1966). It is probable that when speed is emphasized, the performer attempts to anticipate frequently which stimulus will occur and actually initiates the motor program that will be needed for that stimulus before it occurs. The football lineman that tries to get the jump on the offensive team's quarterback by anticipating which signal the ball will be centered on initiates the motor program before that signal is called and frequently finds himself charged with an offside penalty, because the quarterback has delayed the signal for snapping the ball.

Complex motor tasks in games and sports most frequently involve more than simple RT responses. The performer must make choices as to which response to make, many times to multiple stimuli, or which stimulus to respond to. With experience in these tasks, RT is reduced because the processing of this information is more rapid. Also the amount of processing may be reduced as irrelevant stimuli are ignored in the stimulus situation. Training and experience in the probability of occurrence of stimuli and the sequential dependencies of stimuli in different situations will also reduce RT for the sports performer.

B. THE NATURE OF THE INDIVIDUAL AND REACTION TIME

The present state of the individual at any given moment affects RT. In experimental situations, experimenters are not able to control these organismic variables as well as they can control stimulus variables. Indeed, it is impossible to even know all of the internal factors that may be affecting an individual's RT when the stimulus arrives. Nevertheless, some control over organismic variables can be maintained and a substantial body of information on this topic has been accumulated through research.

1. Activation, motivation, anxiety, and reaction time

Conceptually, the words activation, motivation, and anxiety have not been used in any consistent manner in the RT literature. Therefore, it is difficult to summarize the research findings with regard to these variables. For example, some investigators have applied electric shock to subjects and called it a motivational variable; others who have used electric shock treatment have considered it as an activation variable. With this problem in mind, we can examine the research on the relationship between these variables and RT.

Several investigators have reported that RTs are improved as a function of goal-related activation (Marteniuk, 1969b; and McGonnigal and Santa Maria, 1974). Electric shock treatment was used to enhance arousal, or activation. When shock was given only after an RT that was slower than the average which had been established by a subject in a previous set of RT trials, RT was significantly faster than when shock was given in a manner that was unrelated to RT performance. The RTs recorded by McGonnigal and Santa Maria (1974) enabled them to indicate that central nervous system processing was largely responsible for the faster RTs rather than processes which control impulse propagation in the periphery.

Motivational factors likewise improve RT. Several investigators have found that providing incentives to react faster produced improved RTs. Various incentives such as money, food, and verbal exhortations have been used in these studies. Competition has also been used as a "motivator." Church (1962) tested 92 subjects under normal and competitive conditions. The speed of simple RT and of CRT increased under the competitive conditions.

Farber and Spence (1956) conducted two experiments in an attempt to clarify the relations among manifest anxiety, experimentally induced stress, and various task variables on RT. Their results offered no evidence that variations in amount of anxiety affect RT. Similar results have been reported by others (Palermo, 1961).

2. Set and reaction time

There is evidence that performers can manipulate the relative emphasis which they place on sensory set and motor set and this emphasis affects RT. When performers must make quick reactions to a stimulus followed by a movement of some kind, if they consciously attend to the components of the movement response while waiting for the stimulus to occur, rather than to the stimulus which evokes the response, this is referred to as "motor set." Concentrating on the stimulus is called "sensory set." Henry (1960) and Christina (1973) demonstrated that consciously attending to the components of a movement response (motor set), instead of attending to the stimulus and allowing the movement response to take care of itself (sensory set) resulted in slower RTs than when the subjects performed under sensory set emphasis. Apparently, sensory set facilitates appropriate neural mechanisms more optimally than does motor set, at least in simple RT performance.

These findings suggest that in sports in which events are started with some kind of signal, such as a starter's gun, the performers can initiate movement faster by focusing their attention on the start signal after the instructions to "get set" have been given.

3. The various limbs and reaction time

Most RT studies employ fingers, hands, feet, or legs to provide the response, although responses involving other parts of the body have been studied. RTs for the two hands do not differ significantly from each other, nor do those of the feet. There is good correlation between RT of hands and RT of feet; that is, those who have fast hand RT tend to have fast foot RT (Lotter, 1960). RT is slightly faster for hands than it is for feet. This difference can probably be attributed to the difference in the distance of the limbs from the brain.

4. Age, sex, and reaction time

Goodenough (1935) and Hodgkins (1962, 1963) reported that males at most age levels have faster RTs than females, and training does not seem to change this situation (Fig. 12.9). Hodgkins found that males are superior to

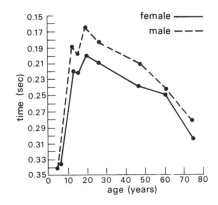

Fig. 12.9 Speed of reaction of males and females at various ages. (Based on Hodgkins, 1963.)

females in both RT and MT. These investigators report RT improvement from birth until the early twenties, with the fastest RTs recorded on subjects between 19 and 25 years of age. RT "peak" is reached at age nineteen, with very little change in the middle-age years, but a gradual increase in RT (meaning slower RT) in old age (Fig. 12.10). The various degenerative processes known to occur in the nervous system may account for the diminution of response efficiency.

5. Present condition and reaction time

Research on the effect of strenuous activity on RT is limited and inconclusive. Elbel (1940) reported that periods of varied intensity of stool-stepping followed by push-ups did not affect finger RT. Phillips (1963) found that RT was not influenced by either related or unrelated warm-ups continued to point of considerable fatigue. Similar findings were noted by Glidewell (1964) who reported that several different warm-up conditions failed to produce a significant change in RT of junior high school boys. Meyers *et al.*

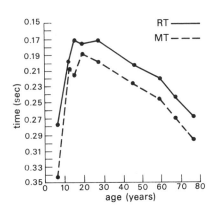

Fig. 12.10 Reaction time (RT) and movement time (MT) at various ages. (Based on Hodgkins, 1963.)

(1969) used a step test and assessed RTs before, immediately after, and four minutes after the stepping exercise. They failed to find any discernible effect of the stepping exercise upon RTs. On the other hand, Sorge (1960) found a significant decrease in RT after a step test, and RT decreased as the step test was intensified.

Simple RT was measured in all of the studies above. Levitt and Gutin (1971) assessed the influence of exercise at different levels of intensity on CRT. Exercise was induced by having subjects run on a motor-driven tread-mill with a CRT console mounted on it. CRT trials were administered at each of four levels of heart rate: rest, 115, 145, and 175 beats per minute (bpm). Fastest 5-CRT occurred at a heart rate of 115 bpm, and slowest occurred at a heart rate of 175 bpm. The investigators interpret their findings as show-ing that in tasks which require a great deal of perceptual processing, such as in this 5-choice task, optimal performance states are rather low. High de-mands on the physical state of the individual interfere with the ability to quickly make appropriate choices.

The limited research on the influence of the menstrual cycles of females suggests that RTs are not affected in any way. Genasci (1966) studied 44 college women to determine the effect of menstruation on total body RT. He concluded that the menstrual cycle does not affect total body RT. Similarly Loucks and Thompson (1968) reported no significant group results in RT measured on the 1st, 3rd, 6th, and 29th days of the menstrual cycle.

EFFECTS OF PRACTICE ON SPEED OF PERCEPTION

RT experiments have found that after a period of a few trials, very little im-provement occurs thereafter. Woodworth and Schlosberg (1954) report that subjects continue to improve for several hundred trials, but the change after the first 50 trials is very slight. Hodgkins (1963) found that RT was not sig-nificantly improved from the first through the tenth trial. Henry (1952) found no evidence of any appreciable improvement on RT due to practice during a practice period of 50 trials.

It would seem that many variables would account for differences one might find in RTs with practice. We have already reported that additional incentives may produce improved RT, and this holds even for well practiced subjects. Furthermore, RT improvement takes place rapidly if the task is simple, but very small improvement may continue for many trials if the movement following is complex. However, since simple RT involves a minimum of neural processing and is dependent primarily upon the trans-mission network, it is not surprising that little improvement results from practice.

Movement time, on the other hand, can be dramatically affected by practice. As a matter of fact, the best way to improve MT is through practice. The establishment of a movement pattern requires considerable neural processing, and when this movement pattern is repeated many times the efficiency of neural processing for the completion of a movement pattern increases. In addition a movement pattern requires the coordination of various muscles, which also develops with practice, and the overall effect is faster MT.

RELATIONSHIP OF REACTION TIME TO MOVEMENT TIME

It is commonly believed that individuals with fast reaction time also possess fast movement times. There is, however, considerable experimental evidence to disprove this belief, although a few studies have found high correlations between these two variables. Franklin Henry is the physical education researcher who has devoted the most effort to the study of the relationships between RT and MT. Henry, his associates, and graduate students have consistently obtained near-zero correlations between RT and MT in their studies. In a study on the RT and MT in four large-muscle movements, Smith (1961), who was an associate of Henry, concluded "that individual differences in ability to react quickly and ability to move quickly are almost entirely unrelated."

Insignificant relationships between these components of perception and response time in subjects ranging from age six to eighty-four were also reported by Hodgkins (1962). Henry (1960) has stated that "muscular force causes the speed of limb movement, whereas, latency reflects the time required for a premovement operation of a central nervous system program-switching mechanism." Guilford (1958) suggested that impulsion (rate of starting movements from a stationary position) is inherent or innate, whereas speed (the rate of movement after it has been initiated) seems to depend upon experience. It should be noted that despite the emphasis Guilford puts on experience developing speed, individuals have definite anatomical and physiological limitations.

Although statistically significant relationships between RT and MT were reported by Pierson and Rasch (1959) and Kerr (1966), the majority of research on this subject generally supports little or no relationship. The presumed reasons for this were discussed in the previous section.

In addition to the findings about the relationship of RT and MT, Henry and others (Henry and Rogers, 1960; Henry and Harrison, 1961; Norrie, 1967; Williams, 1971; Glencross, 1972, 1973) have found that RT is affected by the movement response which follows. The rather consistent finding is that when a movement response that follows the RT is complex, RT is slower than when the movement is simple.

Henry (1960) formulated a "memory drum" theory to account for this phenomenon. This theory states that a nonconscious mechanism uses stored information called motor memory to channel nerve impulses of afferent and CNS origin into appropriate neuromotor coordination centers, subcenters, and efferent neurons, producing the desired movement. According to Henry and Rogers (1960), "a more comprehensive program, i.e., a larger amount of stored information, will be needed and thus the neural impulses will require more time for coordination and direction into the eventual motorneurons and muscles." One of the theory's consequences is that a complex movement, with its more complex motor program, takes longer to organize, and this longer organization time is reflected in longer RTs for complex movements.

Norrie (1967) reported that the complex movement effects on RT can be partially attenuated with practice. Using a "complex movement group" and a "simple movement group," she reported that the former group showed a greater shortening of RT over 50 trials than the latter group. The complex movement group continued to show improvement in RT throughout the experiment while the simple movment group leveled off during the first 20 trials. Norrie suggests that this experiment supports the implication of Henry's theory, that the amount of motor program simplification and reorganization in learning of a simple movement is small and occurs early in the practice curve while that for a more complex movement is larger and requires more practice to reach the limits of simplification.

AMENDING AN INCORRECT MOVEMENT

How fast may movements be corrected, or modified? Motor tasks are rarely performed without at least occasional incorrect movements occurring. When an incorrect movement occurs which the performer must quickly amend in order to restore accuracy to the performance, a RT precedes the initiation of the correction. Presumably the speed with which one can correct movements voluntarily depends partially upon feedback processes; i.e., sensory feedback about the movement error, central interpretation and formulation of a new motor program, and motor signals to the muscles which correct the movement.

Klemmer (1957) reported that the lower limit of RT averages 0.200 msec when the stimulus occurrence cannot be anticipated. Keele and Posner

(1968) taught subjects to perform a movement at rates varying from 150 to 450 msec. On half the trials the room lights were extinguished immediately after the subject left a home position and remained off until he hit or missed the target. They found that the elimination of visual feedback affected accuracy of the movement only if it lasted more than about 200 msec. Thus, the minimum time for which the movement could be corrected by visual feedback was about 0.200 msec.

Other experiments in which movement correction was mediated via visual feedback rather consistently show the minimum time required by the performer to amend incorrect movements is between 200 and 250 msec. Apparently, however, it is possible for movements to be corrected more rapidly by kinesthetic feedback. Higgins and Angle (1970) have reported that the time to process kinesthetic feedback and initiate movement correction was between 110 and 160 msec.

The implication of the findings about the time required to amend an incorrect movement can be summarized by saying that in sports it pays to confuse or conceal your actions by doing what is unexpected, from the opponent's standpoint. This not only makes the stimulus input to the opposition less predictable and results in slower RTs but it also may get the opponent committed to an incorrect movement pattern. Under these conditions, valuable time on the opponent's part may be lost in initiating a movement and/or amending an incorrect response.

SPEED OF PERCEPTION IN GAMES AND SPORTS

In sports and games many movements are responses to signals, such as starting guns, movements of opponents, or flight of balls, and RT is important to performance. The track athlete or swimmer who can start faster, the baseball baserunner who can react faster to the pitcher's motion, the tennis player who can react faster to the opponent's shots, all have a clear advantage over other performers. It is not surprising then that numerous studies have been done on RT characteristics as they relate to games and sports.

A variety of studies have been done on RT and MT comparing skilled versus unskilled performers, athletes versus nonathletes, team sports participants versus individual sports performers, and individuals in team sports compared on the basis of their position played. In most cases, the results of the studies provided empirical verification of what most physical educators and coaches have long believed from observation.

Numerous investigations over many years on RT and MT indicate that the more skillful performers in physical education and athletics are superior to the less skillful in both of these components of time (Burpee and Stroll, 1936; Beise and Peaseley, 1937; Keller, 1942; Cureton, 1951; Youngen, 1959).

Athletes have consistently recorded faster RTs than nonathletes (Olsen, 1956; Wilkinson, 1959; Genasci, 1960; Considine, 1966; Matzl, 1966; P.E. Smith, 1968).

Significant differences in RT have been reported among various athletic participants. In general, members of team sports have faster RTs than participants in individual and dual sports (Cureton, 1951; Cooper, 1955; Wilkinson, 1959; Genasci, 1960).

Differences in RT within members of a sports team have been shown to exist in accordance with specific positions played, but the age of these studies makes any generalization about their findings highly questionable (Miles and Graves, 1931; Manolis, 1955; Westerland and Tuttle, 1931).

The unusually fast reactions which experienced athletes exhibit in game situations are probably not true RTs. Through experience with game situations, athletes probably learn certain cues which enable them to anticipate when a reaction is going to be called for, and they actually begin to respond before the occurrence of a stimulus which requires a fast reaction. Ryan (1969) reported that baseball players in his study did not exhibit faster reaction times on two laboratory choice reaction experiments but they did show significantly faster reaction times to a stimulus of a baseball hit off a tee.

In the first experiment the subject was required to strike a button located on his left when a light to his left came on, strike a button to his right when a light to his right came on, and strike a button located in the middle of the switch panel when a light directly in front of him came on. When the lights came on, one timer measured how long it took the subject to start after the light signal (RT) and a second timer measured how long it took the subject to strike the buttons once he had reacted (MT). In the second experiment a gun fired a plastic missile to the subject's left, right, or directly at him. The subject was to react just as before by striking the button in the direction of the stimulus. There was no significant difference in the reaction times of a group of college baseball players and a group of nonplayers in either of these experiments. In the third experiment a rubber tee was placed in a large gymnasium and a batter would hit a tennis ball off the tee to the subject's left, right, or directly at him. The batter was asked to conceal, as much as possible, the direction in which he was going to hit the ball. As in the other experiments, the subject would strike the button, depending upon the direction in which the ball was hit. In this experiment, there was a significant difference between the two groups, in RT, with the baseball players reacting faster than the nonplayers. Indeed, the RTs for the players was so fast that it appeared that they were beginning to react before the ball was hit. Thus, it seems that baseball-playing experience enabled the players to perceive cues from the batter prior to his hitting the ball which the nonplayers could not perceive.

13

Visual Perception and Motor Behavior

Visual perception is not just a copy of the image on the retina. Something more than reception of light stimuli by the eye must take place for the mass of sensory data to be organized into definite shapes, figures, and identifiable objects at variable distances from the body. In order to make effective use of visual information, an enormous amount of integration and interpretation must occur in the brain to give us visual perception. The image has only two dimensions, but our perceived visual world has three dimensions. We perceive our world as rightside up but the retinal image is upside down. Although there may be great disparities in the retinal image of an object when it is near or when it is far away, nevertheless we usually perceive the actual size of the object quite accurately. Finally, we receive an image with millions of separate cells in the retina, but we perceive a unified object in space.

Current knowledge of the integrative activity of the nervous system has not advanced far enough for more than only a very sketchy understanding of the neurophysiological basis of what we now call visual perception. As our understanding of integrative neural mechanisms increases, undoubtedly these complex phenomena will be clarified and we will be able to discuss in more detail the neural correlates of visual perception.

Vision and visual perception provide humans with a tool for processing environmental information in a rapid and precise fashion. These processes allow people to discriminate and identify objects in the environment and to make adaptive decisions necessary for survival and learning. Because of the obvious importance of vision in motor skills, researchers have attempted to correlate visual efficiency with excellence of performance in various movement tasks.

In order to perform effectively in many sports it is necessary to make precise judgments about moving objects in space, i.e., catching and striking balls, and about the spatial relationships of the body to other individuals or objects. These abilities depend upon visual perception. To take one example, depth perception is utilized extensively during motor performance. In all sports and games in which a ball is used, accuracy in judging the distance of the thrown or batted ball is necessary. Moreover, distance judgments about the location of teammates and opponents are essential for effective performance, and sports such as football, basketball, and baseball require distance judgments to be made simultaneously about the location of the ball, teammates, and opponents.

The subject of visual perception is complex and multidimensional. Only selected aspects of this topic will be examined here. As with other topics in this book, the focus will be on visual perceptual abilities which seem most closely related to motor behavior.

FOCUSING PROPERTIES OF VISION

Objects in space must be located and brought into clear focus if the eyes are to serve as an effective sensory system. Several mechanisms are responsible for the accomplishment of these tasks. Objects are located as the eyes move around in their sockets, and the extraocular muscles make this movement possible. Once an object has been located, reflex adjustments permit the object to be tracked if it moves or if the head is moved in relation to the object. In order to form a clear image of an object on the retina, the eye must refract the light rays so that they come to focus at the retina. Refraction begins as the light rays reach the cornea and occurs because light travels at varying speeds as it passes through substances that vary in density. Light waves entering the eye are first refracted as they pass through the cornea. Then the waves are further refracted as they enter the anterior surface of the lens, and as they pass through the posterior surface of this structure they are further refracted. Traditionally, the lens has been considered the primary refractive mechanism, but actually the cornea has about twice the refractory power of the lens. But the lens has the ability to change its convexity, which is even more important than just refraction, insofar as focusing is concerned. The change in lens convexity is brought about when the image on the retina is out of focus. An out-of-focus image triggers impulses from the brain to initiate a change in the contraction of the ciliary muscle; the neuromuscular mechanism adjusts the convexity of the lens to keep a clear image on the retina.

A. VISUAL ACUITY

Visual acuity is another term for sharpness of vision and implies the degree of detail the eye can discern in a stimulus object. It is the capacity to discriminate the fine details of objects in the field of vision. Good visual acuity implies that a person can discriminate fine detail; poor visual acuity implies that only gross features can be seen. When visual acuity is poor, fine details are blurred, and outlines and contours become indistinct.

There is an enormous number of physiological factors involved in visual acuity. One of the most important factors seems to be the "graininess" of the retina. This refers to the denseness of receptors in the retina. It has been suggested that when visual receptors are relatively far apart light might fall on nonsensitive parts of the retina, thus diminishing its resolving power. This position is supported by reference to visual acuity in different parts of the visual field. It is a fact that visual acuity is highest in the center visual field, that is, at the fovea. Here, the density of cones per square millimeter is greatest (about 147,000 per square millimeter) and the one-to-one type of cone projections allows separate paths for impulses due to light from different, small sources, such as two lines. Peripheral to the fovea, the density of cones diminishes, and so does visual acuity. This emphasizes the function of cones in visual acuity. Of course, another factor that is probably related to visual acuity is the increasing number of receptors, both rods and cones,

(a)   (b)

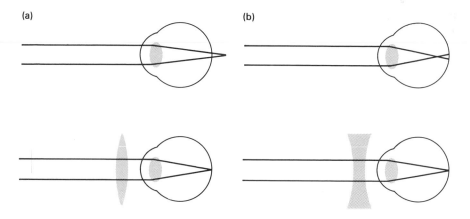

Fig. 13.1 Two common eye abnormalities. (a) Hypermetropia, or farsightedness. The eyeball is too short so the rays of light focus behind the retina. Convex lens in front of the eye brings the rays of light into focus on the retina. (b) Myopia, or nearsightedness. The eyeball is too long so the rays of light focus in front of the retina. Concave lens in front of the eye brings the rays of light into focus on the retina. (Based on DeCoursey, 1968.)

which converge on each bipolar cell as you go from the fovea to the edge of the retina.

Various abnormalities of the lens and cornea are common and they prevent correct focusing of the light rays on the retina. Hypermetropia, or farsightedness, myopia, or nearsightedness, and astigmatism are the most common visual abnormalities. These are all easily corrected by properly fitted artificial lenses (Fig. 13.1).

In addition to purely physiological properties of the eyes, visual acuity also depends upon various environmental factors: First, acuity becomes increasingly poorer as the stimulus object moves away from the center of the retina. Second, acuity improves with increased illumination. Third, acuity is better when the contrast between the object and its background is greater, but it is poorer if light of high intensity shines close to the direct line of vision.

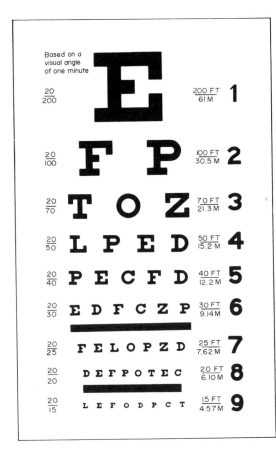

Fig. 13.2 A Snellen eye chart. With a full-sized chart, the subject with normal vision can read line 8 from a distance of 20 feet.

1. Measurement of visual acuity

The familiar Snellen Eye Chart is a frequently used method of testing visual acuity (Fig. 13.2). The chart consists of several lines of letters of different sizes. The smallest letters are on the bottom line and the largest, on the top line. Subjects stand twenty feet from the chart and if they can read the letters of the size that they should be able to read at twenty feet, they are said to have 20/20 vision, which is normal. If they can read only the lines above the 20/20 line, their visual acuity is below normal. On the other hand, if they can read letters on lines below the 20/20 lines, they have superior visual acuity.

More sophisticated instruments are used by optometrists and ophthalmologists, of course. The Keystone Telebinocular has frequently been used by motor behavior investigators. This is a precision-built testing instrument which can be used to assess various visual abilities, in addition to visual acuity. It is commonly used by state automobile license bureaus.

2. Development of visual acuity

The retina of the eye has not reached its mature development at birth; the cones in the fovea are short and poorly defined, suggesting that the infant has poor acuity. Moreover, the muscles that control the movements of the eyes are in such an underdeveloped state that the newborn cannot focus both eyes on the same object very well.

Visual acuity does not reach its maximum for children until about the age of eight or nine. This is due in a large part to the foreshortening of the eyeball which does not reach its most spheroidal form until about this age.

3. Dynamic visual acuity

Visual acuity for stationary objects is more properly called static visual acuity, and most acuity testing is for this type of visual efficiency. A second type of acuity is called dynamic visual acuity (DVA), and is the ability to discriminate an object where there is relative movement between the observer and the object. Dynamic visual acuity has interested researchers of motor behavior because the eyes commonly have to be used to see moving objects rather than stationary ones. For example, the speed of a baseball thrown by a pitcher, and observed from first or third base, travels at an angular velocity of about 100 degrees per second.

Acuity for a moving target deteriorates markedly and progressively as the angular velocity of the target increases (Fig. 13.3). This finding applies substantially whether the target movement is horizontal or vertical or whether the target is moving with the subject stationary or vice versa. DVA is, however, sensitive to illumination, and DVA performance can be improved through increasing target illumination.

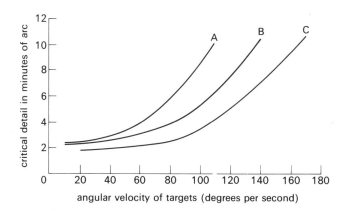

Fig. 13.3 Relation between visual acuity and the effective velocity of moving targets for each of three groups of observers A, B, and C. (Based on Ludvigh and Miller, 1958.)

Several techniques have been employed to test DVA. Two of the early researchers of DVA projected a C-shaped stimulus with a mirror arrangement so that the stimulus moved at various speeds across their subject's space field. The opening to the "C" was made to vary (left, right, up, down) and the subjects' task was to indicate in which direction the opening appeared as it quickly traversed the subjects' field of vision (Fig. 13.4) (Ludvigh and Miller, 1958).

There is little work on DVA development, but infants do show primitive pursuit movements in response to a moving object soon after birth. It appears that pursuit tracking ability and DVA are probably still developing up to late adolescence (Weymouth, 1963).

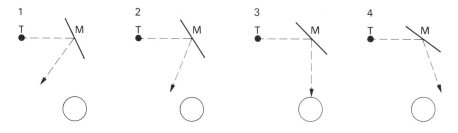

Fig. 13.4 A revolving mirror can pass the radiations from a target across the eye and thus produce the equivalent of a moving target. Each circle is the same eye but at a different instant. From left to right, the target is in effect approaching the eye. At third from left it is in full view; at the far right it has passed by. M is the revolving mirror. T is the target.

There has been a continuing controversy about the relationship between static visual acuity and DVA. Ludvigh and Miller (1958) found a very low correlation; on the other hand, Burg and Hulbert (1961) reported a significant relationship between the two types of acuity. Weissman and Freeburne's study (1965) suggests a reconciliation of the previous findings. They administered six speeds of DVA tests (20, 60, 90, 120, 150, and 180°/sec) and one static measure of visual acuity. Thresholds for the first four speeds were found to show a significant relationship with the static acuity thresholds, but the relationship disappeared at the two highest speeds. Thus, there appears to be a decreasing correlation between measures of static visual acuity and DVA, when the speed of the stimulus object in the latter tasks is increased.

Practice improves most perceptual abilities and DVA is no exception. In general, the effects of practice are more pronounced when target speed is rather high, i.e., 100 degrees per second, and slight or nonexistent at slower speeds. Moreover, whatever learning takes place is largely confined to the early practice trials (Miller and Ludvigh, 1962).

4. Visual acuity and motor behavior

Since deficiencies in visual acuity are so easily remedied with corrective lenses, very little investigation has gone into the effects of visual acuity on motor performance. Undoubtedly, poor visual acuity would adversely affect motor performance in many sports, especially the ones which require tracking and intercepting balls and those which require hitting a distant target, if performers did not have access to optical aids. Martin (1970), an optometrist who has tested hundreds of athletes for visual acuity, reported that about 22 percent of them had defective visual acuity. He suggests that many coaches and trainers may unknowingly have top athletes sitting on the sidelines because of poor vision.

There is some evidence that visual acuity can change as a result of exercise. Graybiel, Jokl, and Trapp (1955) reviewed visual perception studies which were first reported at the 1952 Olympic Games in Helsinki, Finland. The studies were conducted in Russia and are reported in a book by Kresltovnikov. He found that following a 1,000-meter race the visual acuity of 27 percent of the performers remained unchanged but that of the remaining 73 percent acuity was increased by as much as 45 percent. More recently, Whiting and Sanderson (1972) utilized a simulated table-tennis task and reported improved visual acuity in a group of subjects after a playing period of 10 minutes.

The enhancement of visual acuity with exercise may be interpreted in terms of peripheral effects, such as increased blood supply to the retina, or to a central effect of arousal. When persons exercise, this is accompanied by increased muscle tension, which is related to increased arousal levels, because muscular activity stimulates the reticular formation. An increase in arousal enhances the efficiency of the sensory systems.

FIELD OF VISION AND PERIPHERAL VISION

Field of vision refers to the entire extent of the environment which can be seen without a change in the fixation of the eye. Temporal field of vision is the area seen to the temporal or lateral side of the head; the more commonly used term for this latter aspect of vision is peripheral vision. Motor behavior laboratories have more often just measured peripheral vision rather than making the laborious field-of-vision assessment.

A. MEASUREMENT OF FIELD OF VISION AND PERIPHERAL VISION

A technique known as perimetry is used to measure the field of vision for each eye. The subject closes one eye and focuses the other eye on a small dot directly in front of the eye. Then a small dot (white or colored) or a light is moved inward along a meridian. Subjects indicate when they can see the dot, or light, and when they cannot. This is repeated for each meridian, and a chart is made showing the areas in which the subjects report seeing the dot, or light, and the areas in which they cannot see it (Fig. 13.5).

At approximately fifteen degrees lateral to the central point of vision, the blind spot will show up on perimetry charts because of the absence of rods and cones. Blind spots may show up in other parts of the field of vision

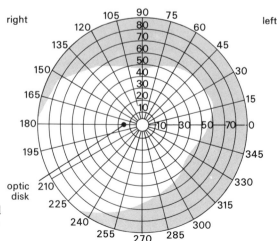

Fig. 13.5 A normal visual field of the right eye. (Based on Guyton, 1964.)

due to diseases such as retinitis pigmentosa which is caused by retina degeneration and buildup of melanin pigment in the degenerated areas. Initially, this disease usually affects the peripheral field of vision and then gradually the central areas. Actually, damage through disease or injury to the visual system, from the eye to the visual cortex, may cause loss of vision in areas of the field of vision.

The perimeter, of course, may also be used for simple tests of peripheral vision, but psychologists, physical educators, and automobile-driver training instructors have typically used simpler instruments than the more complex field-of-vision perimetry tests.

Normal peripheral vision is about 170° for the two eyes, while vertical vision is approximately 47° above the midline and 65° below the midline. Normally, peripheral vision fields are wider for white than for any other color. Blue is next, then red, and the smallest fields are measured for green. Detection of movement is more sensitive in the peripheral parts of the visual field than in the central portions. Since many animal species show this same characteristic, it has been suggested that it serves as a defensive mechanism to alert the individual to danger more quickly.

There is evidence that peripheral vision can be affected by tasks that the individual is performing; several investigators have reported that the detectability of a peripheral stimulus is reduced as the complexity or confusability of a central task being executed is increased (Liebowitz, 1969; Weltman and Egstrom, 1966).

B. DEVELOPMENT OF FIELD OF VISION

Unlike other visual perceptual abilities, the development of field of vision has not interested investigators to any extent. Awareness of movement in the periphery appears to occur at a very early age, and head turning movements designed to bring the eye-focusing mechanisms on a moving object in the periphery have been observed in infants soon after birth. Age does not alter the size of the field of vision until after 40 years of age, and then there is only a slight diminution in this perceptual ability.

C. EFFECTS OF PRACTICE AND EXERCISE ON PERIPHERAL VISION

Several rather old studies first indicated that peripheral visual acuity could be improved with systematic training (Holson and Henderson, 1941; Low, 1946). In his tests of peripheral acuity, Low found that peripheral acuity could be significantly improved with a 25-hour training program, and subsequent research has substantiated Low's findings (Johnson, 1952).

Graybiel et al. (1955) reported that Kresltovnikov measured peripheral vision before and immediately after motor performances and found a post-exercise increase in peripheral vision. As with other aspects of this work, there was no mention of how long the improved visual efficiency persisted.

D. PERIPHERAL VISION AND MOTOR BEHAVIOR

Reaction time to a stimulus in the periphery has been studied by several investigators. Studies of reaction time in the peripheral field of vision require that the subject recognize an object accurately and indicate this recognition by some overt action. Slater-Hammel (1955) reported that reaction time improved as the distance of the visual signal increased from the line of direct vision. Peripheral visual reaction time has been found to be superior for athletes by several investigators, and it is improvable with a specified training program (Buckfellow, 1954; Gill, 1955; Young and Skemp, 1955).

Looking directly at a target has obvious focusing advantages, but what are the effects of trying to hit a target when using peripheral vision? Sills and Troutman (1966) attempted to answer this question by having subjects shoot baskets using peripheral vision. They reported that as the number of degrees of peripheral sighting increased, accuracy in shooting decreased. The old coaching axiom "keep your eye on the target" seems well founded.

Apparently peripheral vision is important to certain kinds of motor performance. In one of Kresltovnikov's studies (Graybiel *et al.,* 1955) peripheral vision was excluded or the total vision was blocked on highly skilled javelin and discus throwers, and he found that their performances were much poorer. The movements of javelin throwers with peripheral vision excluded became clumsy and the distances of the throws were much shorter. The performances of discus throwers were very poor when their peripheral vision was blocked. On the other hand, Cobb (1969) reported no significant difference in performance when throwing for accuracy when the subject's vision was restricted.

That athletes possess superior abilities over nonathletes has been reported for numerous perceptual abilities including peripheral vision. Several investigators have reported that the peripheral vision of athletes is better than that of nonathletes. Stroup (1957) hypothesized that since basketball players relied upon visual cues from the peripheral areas of the retina, there would be a relationship between peripheral vision and basketball ability. He found a significant difference between the field of motion perception of college basketball players and nonbasketball players, with varsity players having the greater field of motion. Ridini (1968) investigated the relationship between visual abilities and selected sports skills of junior high school boys. He employed three tests of peripheral vision, as well as other tests, and found that the athletic group was significantly better than the nonathletic group. Williams and Thirer (1975) investigated the differences between college athletes and nonathletes on vertical and horizontal vision. Both the vertical and horizontal fields of vision were superior for athletes as compared to nonathletes (Fig. 13.6).

variable	horizontal	vertical	high vertical	low vertical
male athletes	186.55	119.90	50.11	69.79
female athletes	182.83	126.93	57.31	69.62
male nonathletes	167.32	108.36	47.36	61.00
female nonathletes	169.32	114.76	52.04	62.72
athletes	185.23	122.38	52.64	69.72
nonathletes	168.32	111.56	49.70	61.86
males	180.38	116.19	49.21	66.97
females	176.57	121.29	54.87	66.42

Fig. 13.6 Horizontal, vertical, high vertical, and low vertical means for four groups. (Based on Williams and Thirer, 1975.)

VISUAL PERCEPTION OF DEPTH

"In the world of the blind, the one-eyed man is king," for even a person with a single eye can witness the marvels of sight; among these is the ability to perceive depth. Our visual world is normally three-dimensional; this characteristic provides an aspect of vision that is at once richly esthetic and critically functional. One needs only to cover one eye to realize how different the world looks without three-dimensional sight.

The ability of the visual system to perceptually organize depth is one of the wonders of nature. Structurally, the retina does not have a means for achieving three-dimensional perception. Optically, the retina functions as a two-dimensional surface, but the visual world is perceived as three-dimensional, not flat like a photograph. We are able to take the flat image from one eye and combine it with another flat image from the other eye and construct a perception with the quality of depth.

A. BINOCULAR VISION

Binocular vision is the coordinated employment of the two eyes in order to produce a single mental impression, and provides the basis for depth perception. This ability to judge the distance of objects from the eye is one of the most critical functions the eye performs, and one of the classical mysteries of visual perception is how the brain and the eyes produce perception of depth. Although a vast amount of neurophysiological research has gone into the topic, the neural correlates of this phenomenon are only beginning to be unraveled, but that information, along with "cues" on which depth perception is known to depend, provides considerable insight into depth perceptual ability.

Traditionally, the sources of cues for depth perception have been organized into two classifications: monocular cues and binocular cues. Monocular cues are those that are utilized by a single eye and binocular cues are those which are derived from the simultaneous use of both eyes.

1. Monocular cues to depth

Monocular cues are those that are available to a single eye and binocular cues are those which are derived from the simultaneous activity of both eyes. Normally, both types of cues are used by the individual. Some of the more important monocular cues are proximal size, brightness, partial overlap, shading, texture, linear perspective, movement parallax, and accommodation (Fig. 13.7).

When an object moves away from an individual the image which the object casts on the retina decreases in size. This proximal size of an object serves as a cue to its distance from the observer. Also, when the size of an object is known, the size of the image that is cast on the retina serves as a depth cue. Finally, the sizes of known objects in the visual field can serve as cues to the size of an unknown object.

Brightness serves as a cue which can be correlated with depth. Normally, the brighter the object, the closer it appears to be. As with size, this relation exists only when the object is identifiable.

Partial overlap refers to the partial obscuring of a more distant object by a nearer object. Thus, when two objects are at a variable distance from the observer and the view of one object is partially blocked by the other, obviously the nearer object is the one blocking the view of the farther object.

Shading provides an important cue to depth because shadows cast by the contours of an object upon the object itself and shadows which are cast by objects can be used for depth perception. The distribution of light and shadow on two-dimensional pictures gives the appearance of depth.

All of the cues above apply to a single object or two overlapping objects without taking into account the other parts of the visual field. But surfaces and objects within the visual field have a powerful influence on depth perception. One powerful cue to depth perception which is normally within the visual field but not the focal point is the texture of objects. When there is any regular marking or visible texture on surfaces within the visual field, this texture on these surfaces becomes gradually denser to the eye as the distance of the surface extends away from the observer. There is said to be

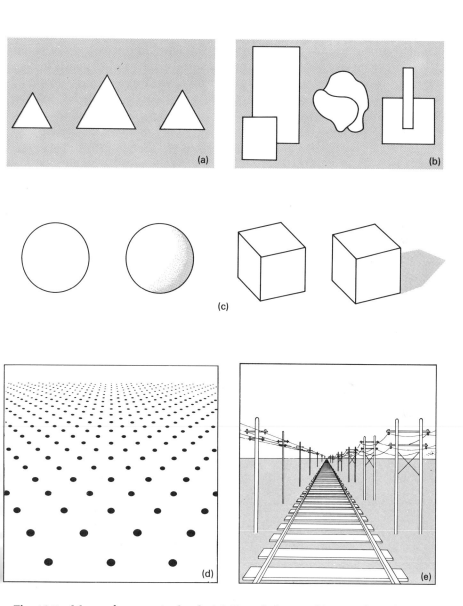

Fig. 13.7 Monocular cues to depth. (a) Size of objects. (b) Partial overlap. (c) Shading. (d) Texture. (e) Linear perspective.

a texture gradient which involves compression of the elements composing the surface of an object as it extends away from the observer. The grain and irregularities in near-space are clear and large in the nearer parts and diminish proportionally with distance? The units into which the surface is divided become smaller with distance. The retinal size of the units becomes smaller; the number of units per unit of retinal area becomes greater. As the distance increases, the angle subtended by small units falls below the limits of visual acuity and the amount of detail one can discern decreases. Far objects retain only gross structure.

Linear perspective refers to the tendency of objects which are parallel to converge on the retina as they become more distant from the observer. A familiar example of this is railroad tracks when viewed from in between the two tracks. Artists make extensive use of linear perspective to convey distance.

Parallax refers to the geometrical fact that the direction of a stationary object from an observer changes if the observer changes locations, and that the direction of the object changes less for a distant than for a near object. In movement parallax, objects which are close to an observer in motion seem to move faster than distant objects because they seem to move farther than distant objects in the same time period. When the head is moved, images of objects which are close move more rapidly across the retina than do distant objects. Thus, if the head is moved a short distance, an object that is very close to the eye will move almost completely across the retina, but an object at a great distance will not move to any extent on the retina. For example, when one is riding in a car, the fence posts beside the highway seem to be moving much faster than the fence posts in the distance. This phenomenon also causes the nearer object to seem to be moving faster when two objects are moving in the same direction and at the same speed.

The lens system of the eye focuses light rays coming from an object onto the retina. This accommodation for objects at various distances is accomplished by the contraction of the ciliary muscles. When focusing on a distant object the lens is in its normal flattened state, with little contraction of the ciliary muscles, but when focusing on a nearby object the lens must be made more convex; this is accomplished by ciliary muscle contraction. Proprioceptive sensations from these muscles are believed to provide cues to the distance of objects. Since there are only slight changes in the amount of accommodation beyond a few feet from the observer, monocular accommodation cues to distance are effective for short distances only.

2. Binocular cues to depth

The functioning of two eyes rather than just one adds several significant sources of information about depth. The first binocular cue is the differential feedback from eye muscles from accommodation and convergence on objects at different distances. The second is retinal disparity cues. A third is binocular parallax.

Accommodation by the lens of the eye operates in binocular vision essentially the same way it functions in monocular vision; as with monocular vision, accommodation is one of the least effective of the binocular cues. The convergence of the two eyes which is necessary to bring the focused image of an object onto the retina is brought about by the extraocular muscles. Their contraction due to variation in the distance of a stimulus serves as a cue to depth, and is much more effective than accommodation, but it is most effective only at short distance, just as with accommodation. An object that is far away causes the line of sight to become almost parallel and there is, consequently, insignificant convergence. Thus, for judging the distance of objects beyond twenty yards or so, convergence is not very effective as a depth perception cue.

The location of objects in the third dimension is possible, in part, because of the differential selective activity of neurons in the primary visual cortex, which responds to input from both eyes. The bilateral projection of nerve fibers, a part of the fibers from each eye going to each side of the visual cortex, and the presence of an interhemispheric link through the corpus callosum, produce a retinal disparity between the two hemispheres, and are powerful neural correlates of depth perception.

Retinal disparity refers to the fact that each of our eyes provides a slightly different angle of view of our visual world. Thus, the image of an object on each retina is slightly different. This disparity allows us to see behind near objects. Although the eyes cannot see around near objects, they are able to see a complete far object because the left eye sees a bit behind the left side of the near object and the right eye sees a bit behind the right side of the object, so together they see the entire background. The impression that we receive from retinal disparity is that objects in space have roundness or depth (Fig. 13.8).

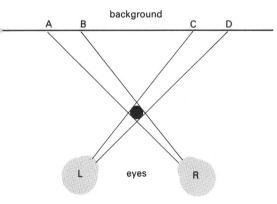

Fig. 13.8 Leonardo da Vinci's diagram illustrating that an object obscures the background from A to B for the right eye and from C to D for the left eye. Since AB and CD do not overlap, the two eyes together can see the entire background. (Based on Deese, 1967.)

From the principle of retinal disparity the appearance of depth can be obtained from a two-dimensional picture by the use of an instrument called a stereoscope. This instrument permits simultaneous viewing of two pictures which were taken simultaneously by cameras placed about as far apart as the distance between the eyes. As one views the pictures, convergence is controlled by keeping the pictures separate so that each eye sees a different image. The eyes then deliver to the same parts of the visual areas in the brain slightly different patterns of excitation. The brain integrates this information and contributes a third dimension, or depth, to the image.

Similar to retinal disparity is a phenomenon known as binocular parallax, which provides another cue for depth perception. Images of objects closer than the point of focus are seen as crossed while those beyond the focus point are seen as uncrossed. That is, if the eyes are focused on a near object, a far object is seen on the right by the right eye and on the left by the left eye. However, if the focus is moved to the far object, the near object is seen on the left by the right eye and on the right by the left eye (Fig. 13.9). These crossed and uncrossed images are normally suppressed and we are not conscious of them. One can become aware of this, though, by holding up an index finger about one foot from the eyes. Then by placing the other index finger between the eye and the first index finger and shifting the focus back and forth between the two fingers, one gets an idea of this situation.

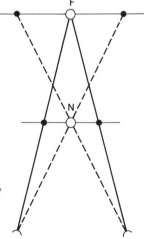

Fig. 13.9   Binocular parallax. When the eyes are focused on N, F is seen on the right eye and on the left by the left eye. When focus is changed to F, N is seen on the left by the right eye and on the right by the left eye. (Based on Woodworth, 1938.)

3. Nonvisual cues to depth

In visual perception of depth, or three-dimensional vision, apparently direct and nonvisual experiences are necessary for images to become symbols of the third dimension. When it is necessary to rely on two-dimensional images, which is what we must do because retinal images are two-dimensional, it seems that early tactile experiences are necessary for full development of three-dimensional perception in humans and some animals.

Held and Hein (1963) found that when kittens were required to remain passive while being moved through a visible environment they failed, when released, to display visual control of movement and showed greater deficits in depth perception than that displayed by kittens who had actively moved through the same environment (Fig. 13.10). Gregory and Wallace (1963) found considerable deficiency in three-dimensional perception among humans who had recovered from congenital or early blindness.

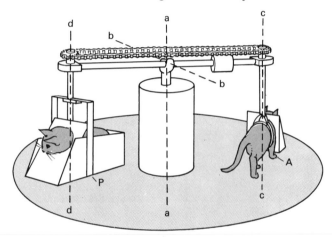

Fig. 13.10 Apparatus used by Held and Hein to equate motion and consequent visual feedback for an actively moving kitten (A) and a passively moved kitten (P). (Based on Held and Hein, 1963.)

Since it is not possible to use deprivation techniques with humans to ascertain the effects of touch and movement experiences on visual space perception, Held and his associates (White, Castle, and Held, 1964; White and Held, 1966) have enhanced motility and sight of the limbs and near objects with infants. They found that they could dramatically increase the rate of development of hand-eye coordination. In fact, they were able to advance the occurrence of visually guided prehension in human infants from an average age of five months to about three months.

4. Integration of depth cues

How the various visual depth cues influence one another and whether some are more important than others are largely unknown. The cues that are most important probably depend to a large extent on the situation. Certainly the richer a visual field is in depth cues, the more impressive the depth effect.

B. MEASUREMENT OF DEPTH PERCEPTION

Two general types of depth perception tests exist; one measures "real" depth and the other measures "apparent" depth. The Howard-Dolman apparatus has been the most commonly used test for real depth perception. The subject attempts to line up two black rods from a distance of twenty feet. One rod is stationary and the other is mounted on a moveable track. By pulling on a cord attached to the moveable rod, the subject attempts to bring this rod exactly next to the stationary rod (Fig. 13.11).

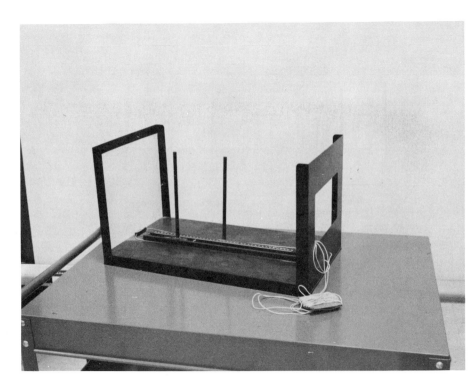

Fig. 13.11 Depth perception apparatus. The two rods are controlled by the string.

More sophisticated instruments are used by optometrists and ophthalmologists, but they usually measure apparent depth perception. These tests have been devised on the same basis as the stereoscope. On a picture viewed through a stereoscope, surfaces and elements stand out, as do figures—the consciousness of three-dimensionality of space is greatly enhanced. The observer views stereographic cards and indicates perceived distances.

C. DEVELOPMENT OF DEPTH PERCEPTION

Whether depth perception exists as an inherent ability of the individual or whether it is developed through learning experiences has interested scholars for many years. Although there is evidence on both sides of this question, there is mounting evidence that some depth perceptual ability is inherited. Fantz (1961) reported that one-month-old infants could discriminate between solid and flat objects, even when the objects were viewed monocularly. We have already reported (in Chapter 11) on experiments by Gibson and Walk (1960) with a "visual cliff" which show that the young of several species, including humans, display depth perception. These investigators demonstrated that human infants can discriminate depth as soon as they can crawl. Bower (1966) found that infants even younger have some perception of depth. He reported that infants as young as 6 to 8 weeks of age responded accurately to differences in size and distance of cubes placed before them. Thus, the infants were able to make gross distinctions between objects that were nearer versus those that were farther away from them.

D. EFFECTS OF PRACTICE AND EXERCISE ON DEPTH PERCEPTION

Although depth perception is believed to be an inherited trait which is not amenable to improvement, empirical evidence supports the notion that the ability to judge distances in specific situations can be improved. Gibson and Bergman (1954) report that subjects improved their distance judgments in a short training period.

An improvement in certain types of visual perception has been reported during and/or immediately after exercise, i.e., visual acuity and peripheral vision; but apparently exercise does not affect depth perception. Schwartz (1968) reported no significant differences between depth perception scores of a group receiving an increasing intensity of exercise and a nonexercised control group. Moreover, there were no differences in initial and final depth perception scores for the two groups. Drowatzky and Schwartz (1971) reported similar findings. Their subjects pedalled a bicycle ergometer under conditions of increasing work loads until a heart rate of 170 beats per minute was reached, or until the subjects were unable to pedal as required. The depth perception scores and heart rate were recorded simultaneously at preselected intervals. A control group did not exercise. There were no significant differences between depth perception of the two groups, and no significant changes in depth perception during the exercise period.

E. DEPTH PERCEPTION AND MOTOR BEHAVIOR

In many motor activities the ability to make distance judgments is essential to effective and efficient performance. The passer and receiver in football, baseball, and basketball athletes, the golfer on the fairway, all must make important depth discriminations to perform well.

Several investigators have assessed the depth perception of athletic and nonathletic groups and, in general, the results suggest that athletic groups possess superior depth perception. In one of the earliest studies, Montebello (1953) reported better depth perception for baseball players versus nonplayers, but there were no significant correlations with batting averages of the baseball athletes. In one of the more comprehensive studies, Olsen (1956) found that college athletes and intermediate athletes (nonlettermen who either participated in the university's intramural program, were members of a junior varsity squad, or participated in other recreation programs) had better depth perception than the nonathletes. In a similar study, Ridini (1968) used five tests of psychological function, including a depth perception test, and divided his subjects into athletic and nonathletic groups. He reported that the athletic group was significantly better than the nonathletic group. Miller (1960) studied visual abilities of champion, near champion, and low-skilled performers. She reported that depth perception was one of the major factors differentiating highly skilled performers from low-skilled.

Not all investigations have found relationships between depth perception and motor performance; several have found little or no relationship. For example, Dickson (1953), using five tests of depth perception on three different groups of college men (classified as skilled, semiskilled, and unskilled), found no relationship between depth perception and basketball shooting ability. Tomlin (1966) reported that correlations between depth perception tests and a badminton wall volley test, a softball repeated throws test, and a tennis wall volley test were not significant. Heimerer (1968) employed two tests of depth perception and reported little relationship between these tests and a test of tennis-playing ability. Shick (1971) also administered two depth perception tests to college female subjects. She then compared their basketball free-throw shooting scores with depth perception scores. There were no significant relationships between free-throw records and either measure of depth perception.

It should be noted that one of the differences between this latter set of studies and the previous set is that the subjects in the first group who show superior depth perception are athletes. In the latter set of studies, subjects were drawn from a nonathlete population. Another point needs to be made with regard to the athlete groups: the research designs that were used in these studies makes it impossible to ascertain whether the superior depth perception displayed by athletes is a result of innate visual abilities or whether depth perceptual abilities were enhanced via the sports experiences.

One aspect of depth perception and motor behavior for which there is little research is whether there is a relationship between *learning* motor skills and depth perception. One study suggests there is. Mail (1965) found that some aspects of depth perception are positively related to proficiency in learning tennis.

COLOR VISION

The visual system reacts to specific wavelengths of radiant energy and this information is processed into the subjective experience of color. The phenomenon of color vision is very complex and will not be given more than a limited treatment here. Almost three centuries have passed since Isaac Newton speculated on how colors are perceived, and yet the process of seeing color is still not clearly understood.

In the human retina there are three light-sensitive pigments which are found in three different kinds of cones. One pigment has its greatest sensitivity in the wavelength for blue light and is called cyanolabe (the blue catcher), one in the spectrum for green light is called chlorolabe (the green catcher), and one for sensing red light waves, which is called erythrolabe (the red catcher). The chemistry of these pigments is very similar to that of rhodopsin, except that the protein portions, the opsins, which are called photopsins in the cones, are different from the scotopsin of the rods. Furthermore, the individual cones contain one, and only one, of these pigments. These data have provided strong support to the component theory of trichromatic (three-color) vision. The basic premise of this theory is that the retina contains three color receptors and that light entering the eye with different wavelengths causes a differential excitation of the various cones which then signal the chromaticity of the stimulus (Brown and Wald, 1964).

All of the colors of the visible spectrum can be formed from three basic colors, i.e., red, green, blue (or violet). If two or more wavelengths fall upon the retina simultaneously, the result is a color fusion and the sensation is a different color from that of any single wavelength. For example, wavelengths for red and green give rise to the color sensation of yellow or orange; the fusion of blue and red produces a perception of purple.

Color perception, then, is produced by different wavelengths, and color is the interpretation by the brain of certain wavelengths, projected onto the retina. The perception of color possesses three important qualities:

1. *Hue, or tone.* This is a function of the wavelength of the radiant energy. Wavelengths of about 750 nanometers are seen as red; those of about 400 nanometers are seen as blue (or violet). Each of the other hues of the

visual spectrum has its own wavelength, which is located somewhere between these two extremes.

2. *Brightness.* Brightness depends upon the intensity of the light energy. Therefore, any particular hue, such as blue, may have a wide range of brightness. The human eye is most sensitive to the yellow-green section of the spectrum (550 nanometers), thus, when the amount of radiant energy is equal, the human eye sees yellow-green as much brighter than either red or blue.

3. *Saturation, or purity.* This quality of a color depends upon the white light which is combined with a particular hue. The less white light that is combined with a hue, the greater the saturation, or purity, of that hue. The degree of saturation decreases as white light is combined with a hue.

A. MEASUREMENT OF COLOR PERCEPTION

There are several methods of testing for color defects, but they tend to have certain limitations, some owing to their length, some to their inability to deal with the various kinds of defects, and some to the differences between them and the everyday conditions in which color deficiency is significant.

One form of test is the so-called pseudoisochromatic plate test. The plates are covered with various colored dots arranged in random relations except for certain dots that form given figures within the dot field. Subjects with normal color vision see the figures. Persons with certain color defects see the figures in some plates but not in others. There are several tests of this type.

Another type of test uses Munsell colored chips arranged in order of hue and is called the 100-Hue test. It is somewhat similar to the old Holmgren yarn test, which consisted of sorting yarn strips into groups according to hue.

Of course, more precise color discrimination may be determined by instrumentation. Optometrists and ophthalmologists have rather elaborate means of assessing color perception.

B. DEVELOPMENT OF COLOR PERCEPTION

It appears that little color perception exists in the infant. Fantz (1961) demonstrated that visual attention is attracted earlier to pattern than to color differences. Even three- and four-year-old children give preference to form or shape for identification and classification of objects rather than to the color of the objects. By age six or seven color is important in classifying and discriminating among and between objects.

Color preferences change with age, and the role of a specific variable, such as color, appears to be highly fluid, depending upon content. Thus, color preferences demonstrated in an abstract setting may not reliably predict usage of colored objects (Gramza and Witt, 1969). Hopson *et al.* (1971) reported that both background colors and amount of illumination affect color preferences of young adults.

C. COLOR PERCEPTION AND MOTOR BEHAVIOR

The effects of color perception on motor behavior have attracted very few investigators. Cobb (1967) assessed color recognition in the peripheral vision of athletes in several sports and reported that there were significant differences with regard to color; red and blue were recognized more readily than green or white. He suggested that it may be more beneficial for a team to wear blue or red uniforms, if it is desirable to have the team members easily recognized as they compete. Unfortunately very few coaches have an opportunity to select colors for their teams, since color combinations are part of an institution's tradition.

The effect of three ball colors and two background colors upon the catching performance of elementary school children was studied by Morris (1974). He found that ball color affected the performance of the elementary school children; blue and yellow balls produced significantly higher catching scores than did white balls, and blue balls against white backgrounds and yellow balls against black backgrounds seemed to influence positively the catching performance.

Few people today remember that basketball rims used to be black. Research conducted in the early 1950s by the National Basketball Coaches Association found that field goal shooting was better with an orange rim than with a black rim, and a rule was made that basketball rims had to be painted bright orange; the rule has been in effect over 20 years.

Periodic efforts have been made to change the color of balls used in several sports, with mixed success. Typically, these efforts have come from persons who just had a personal preference for a color which they wished to see used or from sporting goods manufacturers who stood to gain financially if a new colored ball was adopted.

FIGURE–GROUND PERCEPTION

Perception is characterized by organization. We exhibit several fundamental visual–space organization characteristics with regard to organizing figures in space, but we shall be concerned with only one of these characteristics here: figure–ground perception.

The figure–ground phenomenon is considered to be one of the basic spatial organizing components of perception. The visible environment is more than an array of unrelated and integrated bits of sensory data. Instead, it consists of figures separated from their backgrounds. This is referred to as the figure–ground principle (Fig. 13.12). Rubin (1958) presented seven classic differences between figure and ground:

1. If two fields have a common border, the figure seems to have shape while the ground does not.
2. The ground seems to extend behind the figure and not to be interrupted by the figure.
3. The figure appears to be a "thing," to be object-like (even though it may be an abstract form) while the ground seems like unformed material.
4. The color of the figure seems brighter and more solid than that of the ground.
5. The figure tends to be perceived as closer to the observer than the ground, even though both are at the same distance.
6. The figure is more impressive and tends to be better remembered.
7. The figure is more apt to suggest meaning. A common border between figure and ground is called a contour, and the contour is "shape producing," i.e., when the field is divided by a contour into a figure and ground, the contour shapes only the figure; the ground seems shapeless.

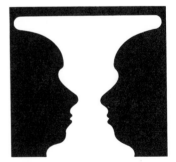

Fig. 13.12   A reversible figure—goblet or profiles. Illustrates the figure-ground relationship.

A. MEASUREMENT OF FIGURE–GROUND PERCEPTION

The two principal methods for assessing figure–ground ability are the Rod and Frame Test (RFT) and embedded figures tests. The RFT consists of a luminous square frame on which a luminous straight rod is suspended. Both the rod and the frame may be rotated independently. The apparatus must be placed in a completely darkened room while a subject is being tested. The subject stands 15 to 20 feet away from the rod and frame with a remote switch for controlling the position of the rod. During testing the frame is rotated so that it is not upright, then the rod is rotated so that it is not vertical. The object for the subject is to return the rod to a perfectly vertical position. This is done by remote electrical control of the rod. The subject's response is recorded in degrees of deviation from the vertical (Fig. 13.13).

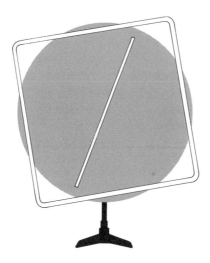

Fig. 13.13   Rod and frame apparatus.

Some subjects are able to make accurate adjustments of the rod, others are not. In other words, some subjects seem to be influenced most by context, the ground represented by the frame, whereas others are influenced most by figure, the luminous rod, when making judgments about verticality. The former are said to be "field dependent" while the latter are said to be "field independent."

There are several embedded figures tests. Basically, they are very similar, consisting of a series of pairs of figures and the subject's task is to find the simple figure of each pair within the much more complex figure of the two (Fig. 13.14).

B. DEVELOPMENT OF FIGURE–GROUND PERCEPTION

As with some other visual perceptual abilities, a primitive form of figure–ground ability must exist from birth because newborn infants respond differentially to figures (Fantz, 1961). Witkin (1954) found significant developmental trends in figure–ground perception. In general, children are

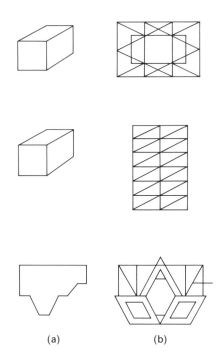

(a)   (b)

Fig. 13.14   Embedded figures used by Gottschaldt. The subject's task is to find the (a) pattern on the left in the (b) pattern on the right. (Based on Ellis, 1938.)

more ground than figure oriented up until the age of 10. Between 10 and 13 the greatest growth in field independence takes place and the individual remains essentially figure oriented until the age of 18, when ground orientation begins to appear again. Since no children under eight were tested by Witkin, no information on the development of figure–ground early in life is available.

Males are more field independent than females at all ages but the difference increases with age. Witkin (1954) noted that the increased figure orientation which occurs between 10 and 13 parallels the traditional differences in organized play between males and females.

C. EFFECTS OF PRACTICE ON FIGURE–GROUND PERCEPTION

There is little information about the effects of practice or specific experiences on figure–ground perception. The finding that males exceed females at all ages on field independence suggests two interpretations: One, that males for some as yet unknown reason are innately more figure-oriented than females. Two, figure–ground ability is enhanced with practice, and the experiences which males have produces field independence tendencies.

There is some direct evidence that practice affects figure–ground ability and indirect evidence that suggests experiences that males typically have which females do not may stimulate field independence orientation. Several investigators have reported that practice was effective at improving subjects' ability to find embedded figures, not only when the same designs were repeated, but also that there was transfer of practice to searching for new designs (Hanawalt, 1942; Kolers and Zink, 1962). As noted above, Witkin (1954) suggests that since the increase in field independence in males coincides with increased experiences in organized games, many of which involve the use of balls and making other figure–ground distinctions, the motor activities may be producing improved figure–ground ability. Traditionally females have withdrawn from these same activities as they reached adolescence. Thus, they were not experiencing activities which might enhance field independence.

D. FIGURE–GROUND PERCEPTION AND MOTOR BEHAVIOR

Perhaps one of the most important and persistent figure–ground problems occurs in motor activities in which there is a ball or other object which must be tracked and hit or caught. In these situations, the ball must be identified quickly and accurately as the figure, with the rest of the visual array perceived as the ground. Due to the color of the balls and the backgrounds on which they are superimposed, it is frequently difficult for them to be identified. Thus, in sports like baseball, football, and soccer, the ball may get visually "lost" in the background of the crowd, and sometimes even highly skilled athletes miss the ball because it cannot be differentiated from the background.

Although there is little empirical support at the present time, it would appear that persons who tend to be field dependent might have more difficulty in sports in which they must catch or hit a ball, since they tend to be poor at distinguishing figures from ground. Hunt (1964) hypothesized that the lower figure skill of females may account for their general inability to catch behind a bat or to strike moving objects accurately. Meek (1970) classified female subjects into highly skilled or poorly skilled performers on the basis of a variety of motor activities, then the two groups were administered the Rod and Frame Test. The highly skilled performer group was significantly more field independent than the group of poorly skilled performers.

Familiarity with the background in a given area seems to aid figure–ground perception at that site. Guidance cues seem to arise from the background that help the performers, even though they are not consciously aware of them. Perhaps one of the advantages to be gained from a day or two of practice at a strange sport area is the improved figure–ground perception for that environment.

VISUAL TRACKING

While seeing a stationary object clearly and judging its distance are important factors in motor activities, in many motor tasks objects are moving and must be caught or hit for appropriate task performance. Indeed, there are many sports and games where performance proficiency depends to a large extent upon catching and striking ability, and one of the universal axioms in these activities is "keep your eyes on the ball."

The main purpose of watching the ball is to obtain information about its flight characteristics so that appropriate responses to it may be made. Information about the position, direction, and velocity of a ball is necessary to predict future flight. Poulton (1957) suggests that the objective of a performer of a pursuit tracking task is to gain enough information about the characteristics of the ball in its initial flight to be able to predict when it will be within hitting or catching range and where it will be in space at that moment.

Monitoring an object in flight and then intercepting it is a complex perceptual-motor task. First, the object must be seen; the eyes are used to obtain information which will enable the performer to anticipate future flight. Second, anticipation and prediction must occur, and these are complex functions based upon current information and stored memories about flight characteristics. Finally, appropriate motor programs must be mobilized to bring about accurate responses for interception to be made. Alderson (1972) has made a component analysis of the task of catching or striking objects in flight (Fig. 13.15).

A. EYE MOVEMENTS

Movements of the eyes are exquisitely coordinated when tracking a moving object. The system regulating eye movements consists of a complex of brain pathways and motorneurons of cranial nerves III, IV, and VI innervating the extraocular muscles and is known as the oculomotor system. Each of these three sets of extraocular muscles is reciprocally innervated so that contraction of each pair synchronizes with relaxation of the other muscles.

The oculomotor system has important subsystems. One is the saccadic system which regulates saccadic movements which the eyes use to fixate on new objects in the environment. Saccadic movements are the quick flicks of

1	2	3
pursuit tracking task	prediction of where the ball will be in a reaction time + a movement time	catching or striking movement
predominantly perceptual analysis	central decision	predominantly motor response
covert processes		overt response

Fig. 13.15 Component analysis of the task of catching or hitting a ball in flight. (Based on Alderson, 1972.)

eye shifts as they move from one point to another. These flicks are so fast that vision is momentarily impaired while the movement takes place. A second subsystem is the smooth pursuit system which is used in pursuing a moving object. The smooth pursuit system attempts to maintain a clear image of the moving object by matching target velocity with eye velocity. The purpose of smooth eye movement is to permit the visual system to maintain the moving object in a stationary position on the retina in order to make perception of the object easier. The cerebral cortex and the superior colliculi are intimately integrated in function in order to make the pursuit system work. A third system, the vestibular system, monitors and evaluates the movements of the head and then, via a complex network of reflexes, stimulates the extraocular muscles to move the eyes to compensate for head movements.

Without any volitional effort the eyes can follow a moving object. This involuntary fixation mechanism is involved with locking the eyes upon an object once it is located, and these automatic movements are mediated by reflex pathways from retina to primary visual cortex to association areas and then to the superior colliculus, from which motor signals are relayed over the cranial nerves back to the eye.

B. MEASUREMENT OF VISUAL TRACKING

Visual pursuit tracking is rarely tested in motor behavior laboratories. Professional eye care specialists must use refined instrumentation to make assessments to this type. When pursuit tracking is measured in motor behavior laboratories, it is typically done in conjunction with a catching or striking task. Thus, the subject must visually track and intercept an object. Of course, there are many factors which influence the ability to intercept balls in flight, only one of which is the eye movements in tracking the ball.

C. DEVELOPMENT OF VISUAL TRACKING

As with other visual abilities, it appears that a primitive visual tracking ability exists from birth because newborn infants can follow a figure with their eyes as it is moved across a homogeneous ground. Haith (1966) reported that an infant as young as 24 hours old will respond to movement of a visual stimulus. At one month of age an infant can follow a dangling ring through an arc of 90 degrees. At these young ages the extraocular muscles are still developing so the pursuit movements are far from precise.

Visual pursuit tracking follows a progressive developmental sequence throughout infancy and childhood and becomes intimately related to hand movements. By eight or nine years of age, children are able to make rather precise judgments of speed and direction of a moving object and rarely overshoot or lag behind in their tracking of objects, but pursuit tracking ability continues to improve into early adolescence (Williams, 1973a).

There is no evidence that there is any inherited ability to anticipate and judge flight characteristics. It seems that this ability is acquired through numerous experiences with moving objects. Kay (1957) describes the response to a ball thrown to a child:

If we throw a ball for a young child to catch, he is invariably too late in positioning his hands and lets the ball hit him on the chest. We say that he doesn't anticipate the flight of the ball; he doesn't know where it will go but only where it is.

D. VISUAL TRACKING AND MOTOR BEHAVIOR

It has been traditionally assumed that keeping the eyes on the ball is essential for effective performance in ball skills, but there are a number of issues that may be raised with this dictum: Why is it necessary? How long can visual information be useful? Is that what skilled performers do?

If a performer is to intercept a ball in flight by either catching or hitting it, it is necessary to begin to position the hands or striking implement (bat, tennis racket, etc.) before the ball arrives; otherwise he will be like the young child who "lets the ball hit him on the chest." The purpose of watching the flight of the ball is to use this information for anticipating and predicting the future flight, thereby beginning interception responses well before the ball arrives. Kay (1957) discusses this function in watching the ball.

We may compare this situation with the case of someone trying to estimate the future position of a moving object say . . . the trajectory of a ball from a limited observation of its initial stages . . . . Let us imagine the situation is such that our . . . subject's head is fixed and he can only observe the trajectory of the ball by successive fixation. Thus we have the trajectory divided into a series of segments which one might think of as events a, b, c, and so on. An individual through his experience of watching how objects travel in space learns about the probable order and temporal relations of these events. Thus, given events a, b, c, he predicts the future position: and the skilled person is the one who can predict accurately on the fewest possible initial events. Once this is achieved the remaining events in the series are redundant or at the most confirmatory. So much for the popular dictum about "keeping your eye on the ball"!

Kay makes two salient points: First, with experience performers become very accurate at predicting future flight from initial flight information, and second, it may not be necessary to watch the ball up to the point of interception. With regard to these two points, there is both informal observational as well as empirical data which is confirmatory. Casual observation of skilled performers in ball sports verifies that they seem to need to watch less of the ball flight than beginners in making their responses to the ball; they seem to be able to take their eyes off the ball and observe teammates or opponents while the ball is in flight and they seem to have "all the time in the world" to organize their response.

A number of years ago Hubbard and Seng (1954) photographed over 25 professional baseball players in batting practice to ascertain their visual habits while batting. Their evidence conclusively showed that eye movements did not continue up to the point of bat contact with the ball, indicating that either the hitters were unable to visually track the ball as it approached the plate or that tracking stopped at a point where it could contribute no additional data that could be used for the swing. The investigators had this to say about the fact that eye focus did not continue up to bat contact with the ball:

. . . either the tracking was broken off at some point beyond which the additional information would have been superfluous since the bat was on its way, or was broken off because the visual apparatus broke down—became incapable of tracking at the very high relative velocity of a pitched ball near the plate—or both.

Although there was evidence that the batters' eyes were not focused on the ball at contact, some of the batters stated that they saw the bat meet the ball. Of course, just because the eyes are not focused on the ball does not mean that it was out of the field of vision. Indeed, the ball and bat may have been seen with peripheral vision.

Whiting and his colleagues in England have conducted a series of investigations designed to study the ability to intercept balls in flight. In one study, Whiting (1968) constructed an instrument that consisted of a miniature-type tetherball, which enabled a ball to be swung around a pole. The ball could be lit in various quadrants of its flight by a light within a metal screen while remaining in darkness for the remainder of its trajectory. Thus, the ball could be illuminated during parts of its trajectory or during its entire course. The amount of visual information necessary for ball catching was studied as well as the effects of practice (Fig. 13.16).

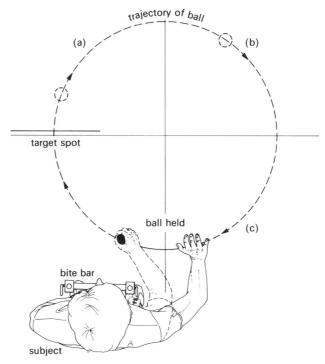

Fig. 13.16 Apparatus table showing quadrants in which ball could be illuminated, i.e., (a), (b), and (c). (Based on Whiting, 1968.)

Subjects were trained first in full light so that they could see the ball during its entire trajectory. Then they were required to perform the task under a series of restricted conditions, including total darkness. The results showed that once having had the opportunity to see the ball throughout its flight, similar performance could be maintained when opportunity to see the ball was restricted. Of course, the total darkness condition produced a significant decrement in performance, compared with the restricted light conditions.

Whiting's results indicate that the subjects learned to anticipate and predict the flight of the ball from information received near the beginning of the ball's flight. He suggested that this learning effect occurs during the acquisition of ball skills in sports—the experienced performers develop excellent anticipatory and judgment skills, and can predict ball trajectory from very brief inspection of the flight.

Although it may be unnecessary to view a ball over its entire flight in order to successfully intercept it, there is a positive relationship between catching or hitting success and the time which the ball is viewed by a performer. Whiting, Gill, and Stephenson (1970) constructed an apparatus which projected a ball through a trajectory with about 0.4 seconds flight time. The ball, made of perspex material, incorporated a bulb which could be illuminated over various parts of its flight in an otherwise blacked-out room. Times for lighting up the ball were for periods of 0.10, 0.15, 0.20, 0.25, and 0.30 seconds, and full light condition. The subject's task was simply to catch the ball with one hand. Catching ability improved as the time for which the ball was illuminated increased for each condition.

In a study designed to answer the same question, Nessler (1973) tested subjects who attempted to catch a tennis ball rebounding from a wall to which it was projected from a pitching machine. The ball flight took about 2.0 seconds. Subjects were positioned so that the ball could be caught without their having to move to catch it. The room was blacked-out when the ball was projected from the machine, but the room was illuminated at various predetermined times after the ball was in flight. Subjects were permitted to see the ball at the end of the flight for 0.50, 0.40, 0.30, 0.25, or 0.20 seconds. There were significant differences among each of the conditions, with increasing viewing time yielding increased catching success.

Finally, Whiting, Alderson, and Sanderson (1973) administered a ball-catching task in which tennis balls were projected over a standardized flight path. An electronic device enabled the investigators to extinguish the room lights at predetermined time intervals after the projection of the ball. Total ball flight took 500 milliseconds; the lights were extinguished at either 100, 150, 225, or 300 milliseconds after the ball was in flight. Results confirmed that opportunity to watch the ball for longer periods of time resulted in increased catching success.

These studies suggest that there is an advantage to be gained from watching a ball for as long as possible because this information provides useful data for predicting future flight pattern. This information is useful at least up to the point in flight after which central nervous system processing time and movement time preclude the use of further information for the organization of the appropriate response. For example, it appears that a baseball batter must make a swing on the basis of information which is available to the hitter prior to the last 300 milliseconds or so before the ball meets the bat. This estimation is based on the fact that visual reaction time is about 190 to 200 milliseconds and the swing takes about 100 milliseconds to bring the bat into the hitting zone. Assuming the ball is traveling at 10 feet per 100 milliseconds, which is quite possible for a good baseball pitcher, the batter must initiate the swing while the ball is still 30 feet away. Since the distance between the baseball pitcher's rubber and home plate is 60'6", the batter may only gain useful information about its flight during its first 30 feet.

There is some controversy in the literature as to whether or not reaction time is faster to a stimulus which is always present, such as a thrown ball, than to a stimulus which is suddenly presented, such as in a typical laboratory reaction-time study. Conceding that there are differences between a moving object that serves as a stimulus and a suddenly appearing stimulus, still there is an instant when the information about the flight pattern of the ball becomes a stimulus for a reaction and movement to intercept it. When that "instant" occurs, the processes which produce reaction latencies in laboratory RT work undoubtedly occur here, too. Thus, a latency of about 190 milliseconds presumably occurs between the time a batter decides to swing and the initiation of the movement.

Once initiated, how useful is visual information for altering the pattern of a ballistic movement, such as a bat swing? Evidence suggests that if the movement is completed in less than 200 to 250 milliseconds, visual information is useless for modifying the swing (Hick, 1949; Henry and Harrison, 1961). Noble (1969) reported that golfers could not alter their swing after the beginning of the downswing, which was about 100 to 120 milliseconds before impact. Hick (1949) employed an instrument which enabled him to trick subjects into executing an incorrect movement, and found that about 300 milliseconds elapsed before subjects could see their error and amend the movement. Thus, since an alteration cannot be made to an unexpected movement error before some 200 to 250 milliseconds, visual information about the moving object is of little use during the last 200 to 250 milliseconds. Watching the ball at this point would seem to make little difference. As Kay (1957) said: "So much for the popular dictum about 'keeping your eye on the ball.' " However, the delay in reacting to an unexpected movement error obtained via visual feedback might be slightly reduced if the performer could accurately anticipate the temporal occurrence of the error, the type of error, and the corrective movement that must be made to amend the error (Christina, 1970). Another reason for watching the ball is that eye direction may be effective because of its effect on bodily position or posture.

When the eyes are turned away, the shoulders and body tend to follow. Moreover, since there is no precise way of knowing when visual information becomes useless in a given sports situation, the instructional cue to "keep your eyes on the ball" seems appropriate.

EYE DOMINANCE

The human is a bilateral creature, and many structures come in twos, i.e., arms, legs, eyes, brain hemispheres, etc. As the individual grows and uses these structures, typically one of each pair comes to play a dominant role—we say that the person is left-handed or right-handed. In the case of the brain's hemispheres, since the left hemisphere has unique speech and language functions for over 90 percent of the population, it has become known as the "dominant" hemisphere. As with other structures, the eyes display this same characteristic. The dominant eye is the one that leads the other both in fixation and in attentive or perceptive function. It is the eye that is unconsciously and preferentially chosen to guide decision and action.

Although there is some consistency of dominance for individuals (right-handedness), this characteristic is far from perfect. Thus some persons are left-handed, and right-footed, and vice versa; some are right-eyed and left-handed; and some people show right-handedness for some tasks and left-handedness for other tasks.

A. MEASUREMENT OF EYE DOMINANCE

The two most commonly used eye dominance tests are the Alignment Test and the Hole-in-Card Test. For the Alignment Test, the subject is given a pencil and asked to hold it up at arm's length and, with both eyes open, to line it up with a black dot on a wall seven feet away. Subjects actually see two images of the pencil, but they automatically disregard one, and bring the pencil, the dot, and one of their eyes, into a straight line. Subjects are then asked to close each eye and then asked if the pencil is still lined up. The eye used to sight with (the eye that sees the pencil directly lined up with the dot) is considered the subject's dominant eye. To administer the Hole-in-Card Test, a piece of cardboard, 11" × 11", with a small hole (1/4 inch in diameter) in the center is held by the subject at arm's length with both hands directly in front of the body. The subject is asked to use both eyes and to look through a peephole at a white dot (1/2 inch in diameter) on a blackboard seven feet away. After the object has been located the subject is asked to close each eye and asked if the dot is still visible. The eye that sees the dot when the other is closed is considered the dominant eye.

B. DEVELOPMENT OF EYE DOMINANCE

Little is known about the eye dominance of infants, but by three years of age about 75 percent show eye dominance and by the age of five some 95 percent have become definitely right-eyed or left-eyed (Zagora, 1959). Once eye dominance is established, it is typically maintained throughout life.

C. EYE DOMINANCE AND MOTOR BEHAVIOR

In one of the pioneer studies of eye dominance, Lund (1932) reported superior performance on a target-aiming task when subjects used their dominant eye. Since then the majority of studies has indicated that unilaterals, meaning right-eyed and right-handed or left-eyed and left-handed, are better performers on a variety of motor activities than crossed-laterals, left-eyed and right-handed or vice versa. This has been demonstrated for sports skills such as bowling, swimming, and baseball (Fox, 1957; Sinclair and Smith, 1957; Adams, 1965) but no significant differences were found in basketball free throw shooting between unilaterals and crossed-laterals (Shick, 1971).

Adams (1965) indicated that there is a strong belief among baseball coaches that the batter of the crossed-lateral type has a definite advantage over the unilateral batter. The advantage, some claim, is due to the position of the batter's dominant eye in relation to the pitcher and the pitched ball. This notion claims that most right-handed batters cannot view the pitcher and pitched ball as well with their dominant eye if it is located on the right side; this is due to the unilateral's position in the batter's box. Often the batting stance is such that the right and dominant eye is partly obstructed from seeing the pitched ball by the bridge of the batter's nose. On the other hand, crossed-lateral batters do not have this problem regardless of the type of batting stance they use.

To test this theory, Adams determined the effect of eye dominance on baseball batting with collegiate baseball players. Comparisons were made on: on-base average, batting average, strikeouts, called strikeouts, and missed swings. The unilaterals scored better than the crossed-laterals in most batting categories, contradicting the hypothesis that crossed-laterals should be better.

In a similar study, Lakatos (1968) found that unilateral batters hit better against pitchers who threw with the same hand as the batters' batting hand than against pitchers who threw with the opposite hand. But crossed-lateral batters hit better against pitchers who threw with the hand opposite to the batters' batting hand than against pitchers who threw with the same hand. More recently, Llewellyn (1972), also using college baseball players, reported that handedness had a greater effect on hitting performance than whether the players were unilaterals or crossed-laterals. The right-handed batters were superior to left-hand hitters in his study.

The research on eye dominance and motor performance indicates that eye dominance seems to have some effect on certain aspects of motor behavior, and unilaterals tend to display superior performance on a variety of motor activities. However, there are crossed-laterals who perform quite well in these activities, and there is no compelling reason for switching a performer from a crossed-lateral to unilateral technique.

MOTOR LEARNING AND VISION

A series of experiments by Rock and Harris (1967) has shown rather decisively that the initial phase of motor skill learning is primarily under visual control. Traditionally, the sense of touch has been considered the primary source of information about the properties of objects, and it was presumed that touch educates vision. Rock and Harris have found that this traditional belief is incorrect. As a matter of fact, vision is completely dominant over touch (they include proprioception in their use of the word touch), and when touch and vision convey conflicting information, the visual information dominates.

Pew (1966) showed that after a period of practice subjects shifted from visual control of individual movements to the use of visual feedback for periodic correction, or modulation of the movement pattern. In Pew's study, the subject controlled the horizontal position of a target on an oscilloscope by alternately switching between two keys. When the left control key was depressed, the target accelerated to the left; when the right control key was depressed, the target accelerated to the right. The subject's task was to keep the target centered on the screen throughout each trial.

At first subjects made individual movements, visually analyzed the outcome, made a correction movement, analyzed the outcome, and so on. This resulted in their being off-target much of the time. As practice continued, however, the subjects changed their technique considerably. They began to make very rapid and regular alternating finger movements and then a single correction, or, as they began to drift off target, the alternating pattern was modulated so that one key was depressed slightly longer than the other during a series of movements. This finding suggests that with practice on a task, performers shift from visual control of component movements to the use of visual information for periodic modulation of the movement pattern.

14

Kinesthesis and Motor Behavior

The sensory receptors which reside in the muscles, tendons, joints, and vestibular apparatus signal information about the movement and amplitude of movement of body parts and the overall orientation of the body to gravity. These sensory receptors, collectively known as the proprioceptors, are constantly active and normally serve as an important source of information during motor behavior.

The perceptual experience that is presumed to arise from the proprioceptors is called kinesthesis. It is assumed by physical education instructors and coaches that kinesthesis is an important sensory modality for motor learning and performance. They frequently attempt to get students to use kinesthesis as a cue while learning and performing motor tasks. Students may be asked to concentrate on "getting the feel" of the correct movements as they perform. Or they may be placed in correct beginning or terminal positions for a given task and asked to "sense" the limb angulations and muscular contractions. In recent years, various weighted objects have been used in motor skill instruction in the belief that the kinesthetic perceptual illusions which occur when the normal weight objects are subsequently used in performing the task will produce improved performances. These various methods are examples of attempts to utilize kinesthesis as a learning and performance modality.

In this chapter we shall examine the neuropsychological dimensions of kinesthesis and review the findings with respect to the relationship between kinesthesis and motor behavior.

DEFINITION OF KINESTHESIS

Charles Sherrington (1906a), the English neurophysiologist, first defined proprioception to include the systems involved in the transmission of information from all the receptors located in the muscles, tendons, joints, and vestibular apparatus, and kinesthesis has commonly been used to denote the perceptual experiences which arise from this transmission. The term was originally generic, i.e., general, rather than specific and there have been frequent attempts to redefine proprioception, and hence kinesthesis, in more exact ways. Some have attempted to limit kinesthesis to information from the joint receptors (Smith, 1969), while others have suggested an extension rather than a restriction of the concept. For example, Gibson (1966) argues that kinesthesis should be viewed as "the obtaining of information about one's own action" regardless of the sensory modalities involved. He suggests that it is a fallacy to ascribe kinesthesis to proprioceptors because information concerned with movement may be obtained through many sensory systems.

In this text Sherrington's original definition of proprioception will be adopted as applying to kinesthesis, realizing that proprioception subsumes sensory systems with quite different physiological and functional properties, and also realizing that information from other somatosensory receptors may also mediate perceptual experiences we call kinesthesis, since they are so intricately associated with the proprioceptors anatomically and functionally. For our purposes, then, kinesthesis is the discrimination of the positions and movements of body parts based on information other than visual, auditory, or verbal. The immediate stimuli arise from changes in length and from tension, compression, and shear forces arising from the effects of gravity from relative movement of body parts, and from muscular contraction. It includes the discrimination of the position of body parts, the discrimination of movement and amplitude of movement of body parts, both passively and actively produced (Howard and Templeton, 1966).

KINESTHESIS AND NEURAL MECHANISMS

In spite of years of study and research, kinesthesis is not fully understood either physiologically or psychologically. Although the proprioceptors throughout the body are considered the mechanisms responsible for kinesthesis, and there is a fairly complete picture of their structures and transmission pathways, considerable confusion exists with regard to the exact role that each proprioceptor plays in kinesthetic perception.

As noted in Chapter 5, each of the proprioceptors is structurally differ-ent and responds to different types of stimuli. It is therefore rather obvious that each would have a different role in providing input to the brain for translation into perceptions.

A. MUSCLE SPINDLES AND KINESTHESIS

Muscle spindle afferents are stimulated by stretch, and the stretch may be applied externally by lengthening the entire muscle or internally via intra-fusal muscle contraction. The role of spindle afferents in kinesthesis is con-troversial. Rose and Mountcastle (1959) state: "There is...no evidence for and strong evidence against the notion that impulses provoked by stretch re-ceptors in muscles provide information for perception of movement or posi-tion of the joints." Gelfan and Carter (1967) stretched the muscles of sub-jects who were undergoing surgery for removal of growths, repair of in-juries, etc., by pulling on their exposed tendons with forceps, thus permitting activation of muscles stretch receptors and tendon end organs. These proce-dures failed to reveal any significant contribution by the signals from the spindle and Golgi tendon afferents to the awareness of position and move-ment of fingers, hand, or foot, since none of the subjects experienced any sensation referable to the muscles. The investigators concluded that "there is no muscle sense in man," meaning by this that there is no conscious awareness of muscle length or change of muscle length as a result of muscle afferent discharges.

For many years it was believed that spindle afferents could not play a role in kinesthetic perception because their signals did not reach the cerebral cortex. Experiments over the past 15 years have shown unequivo-cally that muscle afferents do in fact project to the somatosensory cortex in a number of related species and undoubtedly do also in humans (Oscarsson and Rosen, 1966; Albe-Fessard and Liebeskind, 1966). The fact that muscle afferents do provide input to the cortex does not prove that their signals give rise to conscious experiences, however.

Paillard and Brouchon (1968) have questioned the general assumption that muscle receptors serve no function in kinesthesis and have produced evidence that they are involved in the sense of active movement. Goodwin and his colleagues (1972), using a unique technique for exciting the spindle afferents, have produced evidence that the receptors do contribute to per-ception. Vibrating the belly of a muscle appears to stimulate the spindles, bringing about skeletal muscle contraction throughout the vibration. By having blindfolded subjects track the vibrated arm by keeping the nonvibrat-ed arm in alignment with it Goodwin et al. (1972) found that spindle afferent activity of the vibrated arm did influence movement in the other arm, thus throwing serious doubt on the current view that muscle afferent firing is without influence on perception. It is still perhaps premature to deny muscle afferents a role in perceptual experience.

Whether one wishes to classify certain reflex functions of the muscle afferents as "perceptual" or not is arbitrary, but they certainly are related to motor behavior. Two of the main functions of spindle activity appear to be that of contributing to the postural reflexes and the maintenance of muscle tone. Firing of the spindle afferent neurons reflexively excites motor units of the muscle in which the spindle lies, simultaneously facilitating synergists and inhibiting antagonists. When a muscle is stretched, spindle afferents fire a burst of impulses which cause a phasic contraction in the muscle; the knee jerk is an example. Because the shortening of the muscle relieves the original stretch, the spindle is "unloaded" so the spindle afferents cease firing.

For posture, the muscle spindle intrafusal fibers "set" the spindle at a length compatible with appropriate upright posture. Slow stretching of muscles due to the shifting of the center of gravity causes afferent response in the spindles and a contraction of the stretched extrafusal muscles which will correct the displacement. Postural adjustments mediated by the muscle spindle afferents go on continually in the living person.

The tonic function of spindle afferents has been mentioned by numerous neurophysiologists. Granit and Kaada (1952) found that gamma fibers continued to fire for some time after stimulation of the reticular formation, indicating that the gamma system, including the spindle afferents which it stimulates is suited for prolonged, tonic forms of activity. These investigators concluded that the gamma system is an important mechanism in the maintenance of muscle tone. The tonic discharge may be facilitated or inhibited from various central regions, including the cerebellum, known to be concerned with the regulation of muscle tonus.

Although it may be true that impulses from the muscle receptors do not contribute to "conscious" perception, they definitely do contribute to a number of important postural and tonic functions. Moreover, since the muscle afferents do project to the cerebral cortex, and it is believed that this afferent projection provides the cortex with information about the tone of muscles, this information may be used in adjustment of the voluntary motor signals to muscles. Thus, a spindle-to-cortex loop may exist whereby impulses travel from motor cortex to muscles (via both alpha and gamma motorneurons) and back to the cortex over the spindle afferents. Although information relayed over this loop probably provides crude and "low level" perception it probably does serve an important feedback function during voluntary motor activity. Eldred (1965) summarized the importance of the muscle afferents by saying that many of the finer attributes of sensitivity, restraint, and coordination which characterize muscular activity must be derived from feedback on the moment-to-moment status of muscles which is obtained by the muscle afferents.

B. JOINT RECEPTORS AND KINESTHESIS

Joint receptors are widely recognized as necessary for the perception of joint position and movement. Sense of position and movement of a joint are typically lost when the joint capsule is anesthetized. This evidence, and the fact that impulses arising in joint receptors are projected directly to the somatosensory cortex have led many neuroscientists to consider these receptors to be the major input source for kinesthesis, and indeed some claim that it is the sole mechanism for this form of perception (Merton, 1964; Smith, 1969).

It appears that there are, in fact, two basic functional types of joint receptors. One is considered to be responsible for the appreciation of final positions and their maintenance, since it has slow adaptation rates to the position of a joint but discharges in proportion to joint angle. These are called the "static-type" receptors, and they are capable of maintaining firing rates for over an hour without decline. The other type joint receptor is called "dynamic-type" because it is sensitive to the speed of angulation and speed of movement but adapts within a few seconds when movement stops.

Some joint receptors are so sensitive that a change of 2 degrees in joint angle is sufficient to alter the rate of firing. In any given position of a joint, some receptors are intensely stimulated, some are weakly stimulated, and others are unstimulated, but the receptors are located in such a way that there is no position in which all receptors are unstimulated.

Like the other proprioceptors, the joint receptors are involved with certain reflex activities. The head exerts important influences upon movements of the trunk and limbs, and neck reflexes arising from stimulation of joint receptors in the cervical spine are important in movement. The tonic neck reflex, present from birth, becomes subsumed under neck righting reflexes in infancy, and produces suitable adjustments in body and limb muscles to assure that the body follows the head. The TNR was discussed more fully in Chapter 8.

C. VESTIBULAR APPARATUS AND KINESTHESIS

In many respects the vestibular apparatus is a sensory system without a home. The receptors of this mechanism are usually not considered part of the exteroceptors (vision, hearing, taste, cutaneous) and many neuroscientists omit them from the proprioceptor category. Their major function, though, is undeniably concerned with motor control, so they are given a home here, and by many other writers, with the proprioceptors.

The major functions of the vestibular apparatus are carried out reflexively but its impulses do project into the cerebral cortex, thus suggesting a potential role in perception. Its reflex activity is helpful in maintaining balance and interpreting lateral, horizontal, and vertical movement.

The semicircular canals serve a major role in the maintenance of equilibrium during movement. Stimulation of the semicircular canals produces appropriate muscular responses for maintaining or regaining body balance either by causing movements of body segments to keep the center of gravity over the base of support or by changing the base of support to keep it under the center of gravity. The utricles are concerned with postural reflexes and in the differential distribution of muscle tone. Shortly after birth, reflexes arising from the utricles appear which are called tonic labyrinthine reflexes (TLR) and tonic righting reflexes. Stimulation produced by head movement or body position produces stereotyped adjustments. These reflexes were discussed in Chapter 8 and will not be repeated here.

As growth and development proceed the labyrinthine reflexes as well as the tonic neck reflexes discussed above become subordinated and voluntary motor control becomes more dominant. But these reflexes are not completely eradicated in the adult (Hellebrandt, Schade, and Carns, 1962; Hellebrandt and Waterland, 1962) and in fact may be used to facilitate muscular effort.

MEASUREMENT OF KINESTHESIS

During the past 100 years there have been varying degrees of scientific interest in kinesthesis. During the latter years of the 19th century and first few years of the 20th century interest in this topic reached a peak, then waned for several years. Advancements in electrical instrumentation in the past 25 years have spurred electrophysiological studies and a considerable body of information has been added to our understanding of kinesthesis.

In the latter years of the 19th century and the early years of this century, the investigators of kinesthesis studied primarily the psychophysical dimensions of this phenomenon. They attempted to determine minimum angular displacement and minimum velocity of movement thresholds for various parts of the body. One of the pioneers, Goldscheider (1889), measured joint thresholds, using himself as the subject, and reported that the shoulder and hip joints had the lowest thresholds for passive movements; thus, sensitivity in the proximal joints, such as the shoulder and hip, exceeds that of the distal joints, such as the fingers and toes. Subsequent psychophysical studies on joint thresholds have fairly consistently replicated Goldscheider's results. Cleghorn and Darcus (1952) have more recently made an extensive study of passive movement thresholds and reported that individuals (blind-folded for testing) detect movement of a joint more easily than they determine the direction of the movement. After moving the limbs 0.2 degrees per second, subjects reported that movement was taking place but they had to be moved at the rate of 1.8 degrees per second before their direction was perceived. Generally flexion movements were more easily detected than were extension movements.

A weakness in the studies that have established movement thresholds using passive movements is that active, or voluntary, movement may create a different pattern of kinesthetic information because of the greater tension and stretch on the proprioceptors. Lloyd and Caldwell (1965) have studied the difference between passive and active positioning movements on the lower leg. They found that active movements of the lower leg produced greater accuracy of positioning than passive movements in the middle ranges of movement (the full range was from full extension of the leg to 100 degrees of flexion), but not for the positioning near the extreme parts of the range.

In addition to the interest psychologists have shown in the psychophysical dimensions of kinesthesis, physical educators and human factors engineers have been quite interested in the precision with which individuals can position and move their bodies on the basis of kinesthetic perception. They have developed tests which attempt to measure kinesthesis from dimensions other than its psychophysical properties.

Tests of kinesthesis most frequently used in investigations by physical educators have been composed of tasks requiring the blindfolded subject to assume or reproduce a prescribed arm or leg position in the vertical or horizontal planes, make discriminations of balance and orientation of the body and its parts in space, and make discriminations of force and extent of muscular contraction (Fig. 14.1). For example, Scott's (1955) tests of kinesthesis include:

Lower leg flexion—Standing on one foot, knee pointing downward, flex lower leg of free foot until lower leg is horizontal (90°). Score = deviation from 90°.

Wrist flexion—Forearm supported on table, hand relaxed over edge. Extend wrist according to model (20°) flexion. Score = deviation from 20°.

Target pointing—Standing sideways to target, pointer in hand, eyes closed. Raise pointer to target. Score = deviation from center of target.

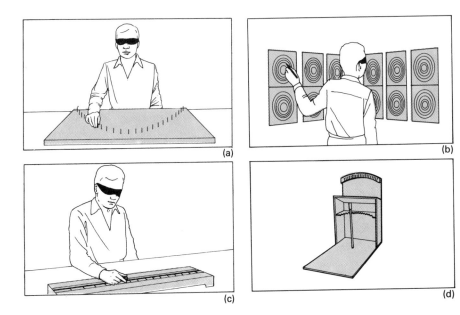

Fig. 14.1   Kinesthetic tests of accuracy of positioning movements. The tests require a blindfolded subject to (a) touch a certain peg or (b) mark a certain target, in response to verbal instructions. In tests (c) and (d), respectively, he reproduces certain movements with a knob or a stick control. (Based on Fleishman, 1958.)

Although there is a considerable body of literature on kinesthesis testing, there are very few established valid tests of kinesthesis. There have been considerable differences of opinion as to what exactly constitutes kinesthesis, and therefore what tests are appropriate. At one time, it was believed that kinesthesis was a general ability, but research of the past 20 years confirms conclusively that kinesthesis is certainly not a general ability; instead, it is composed of a number of specific abilities.

Wiebe (1954) obtained low intercorrelations on a 21-item kinesthesis test battery indicating that the various test items were not measuring the same quality. He concluded that there was no general kinesthetic sense. Rose and Glad (1974) also reported low intercorrelations between nine tests of kinesthesis which they used in testing. However, on the basis of a 28-item test battery which she administered to college women, Scott (1955) identified several specific abilities as those which determine kinesthesis. Recent factorial studies have identified static and dynamic arm positioning in the vertical and horizontal plane, thigh-leg positioning, awareness of force and extent of muscular contraction, and several movements for maintaining balance as among the best measures of kinesthesis.

A. FACTORS AFFECTING KINESTHESIS

Kinesthetic thresholds are influenced by several variables. How the limbs are held during testing periods has been found to influence threshold. For example, it has been found that sensitivity to weight is greatest when the shoulder is the fulcrum and is poorer when the weight is lifted from the wrist. Elbow-joint movement sensibility is lower when the joint is extended than when it is flexed. Kinesthetic sensitivity to movement is better in the upper limbs than in the lower limbs.

Kinesthetic perceptual accuracy of positioning seems to be better for more familiar movements. Lloyd and Caldwell (1965) found that the greatest accuracy of positioning coincided with the normal walking arc of the lower leg. These investigators suggested that kinesthetic perception of the limb position seems to be best in the range of movement which is used more frequently in daily activities. Phillips and Summers (1954) found that subjects performed significantly better on kinesthetic perception tasks with their preferred arm than they did with their nonpreferred arm.

Whether kinesthesis is improved with practice is still an open question. Meday (1952) found greater improvement for her experimental group following 12 practice periods on a scale press test and a target toss for direction than for the no-practice control group. Christina (1967) found that in most cases test performance on a side-arm positional test was more exact following practice. Several other investigators, on the other hand, have reported no significant improvement as a result of practice on various kinesthesis tests.

The question remains whether the improvement noted by some investigators is really an improvement in kinesthesis or whether improvement has occurred as a response to a specific situation. Practice may certainly lead to more precise specific responses but that does not establish improvement in kinesthesis of broad dimensions. Participation in a wide variety of motor activities will presumably result in some improved body positional control, balance, and movement control, but large general development of kinesthesis is probably impossible.

Kinesthesis probably plays an important role in awareness of a limb's position just prior to starting a movement pattern, and may be important in monitoring slow movements, but fast movements, once in progress, probably depend very little on kinesthesis. Angular velocities from 200 to 500 degrees per second have been recorded for hip and leg movements and up to 8000 degrees per second for joints in the upper limb, such as the wrist. Thus, once a fast movement pattern has been selected by brain centers and has been started, very little modification in this pattern can be brought about by kinesthesis. For example, a baseball swing or golf swing is difficult to modify once the head of the object has started through its arc. Noble (1966) found that golfers could not alter their swing to a stimulus which was applied just after the beginning of the downswing (0.10 to 0.12 sec. before impact).

Several other factors affecting kinesthesis have been studied and permit generalizations: Fatigue tends to decrease kinesthesis. Muscular tension affects tactual kinesthetic judgments of size. Motivational instructions do not enhance kinesthesis or kinesthetic learning.

DEVELOPMENT OF KINESTHESIS

From conception to birth and through the first two years of age the nervous system achieves most of its functional development. The proprioceptors, like the other sensory systems, undergo rapid growth and development during this period. At nine and one-half weeks after conception the limbs flex when they are stretched, meaning receptors in the muscles, tendons, and perhaps joints are functional. By 13 weeks there is a contralateral reaction of the limb on the opposite side of the body stimulated, and by the 25th week the knee jerk and Achilles tendon reflexes are elicitable, again demonstrating functional muscle spindle afferents.

For all intents, the newborn is a reflex animal, with all motor activity operating through subcortical influences. The most common reflexes are eli cited by cutaneous stimulation, such as the grasping reflex, Babinski reflex (extension of the big toe and extension and fanning of other toes when the sole of the foot is stroked), and rooting reflex (quick, jerky movements to bring the mouth toward the source of stimulation) but shortly after birth the tonic neck reflex and tonic labyrinthine reflex become prominent, indicating the function of muscle spindle and vestibular apparatus afferents.

It is beyond the scope of this text to detail the development of kines thetic perception through childhood and adolescence, but in general there is a gradual improvement of performance on kinesthesis. Balance tests have often been employed in motor ability testing but the subjects have often been allowed to use vision while performing, thus making these results useless for assessing kinesthesis under the definition commonly used. Age in preschool through elementary school children is a potent variable of balance perfor mance under blindfolded conditions. Older children perform better than younger children, and generally there are no sex differences, although dif ferences have been noted by some investigators (Haubenstricker and Milne 1974; Fleishman, 1964). During adolescence the findings on balance are equivocal; some investigators have found progressive improvement while others report no improvement.

Weight discrimination has also been found to change with age through out childhood, while performance on limb-positioning tasks has produced equivocal results (Haubenstricker and Milne, 1974; Witte, 1962).

The results of the studies of kinesthetic perceptual development suggest that some components of kinesthesis are undergoing developmental change throughout childhood, probably reaching their optimal state some time during adolescence. Whether these perceptual improvements are the result of maturation or experiences has not been determined by studies conducted thus far.

KINESTHESIS AND MOTOR LEARNING AND PERFORMANCE

The exact role that kinesthesis plays in motor learning and performance has generated a heated controversy in neuropsychology over the past 75 years. The classical position is that proprioceptive information is critical to motor behavior while a recently accelerating trend suggests that kinesthesis is less essential to both motor learning and performance.

A. MOTOR PERFORMANCE AND KINESTHESIS

An early theory of motor control suggested that each component of a movement pattern produces feedback via the proprioceptors. The feedback from one component of the movement was seen as being instrumental in triggering the next component in the pattern, and so on. This theory became known as the "S–R chaining" theory because according to it movement control was viewed as being a series of conditioned responses (Greenwald, 1970).

In addition to its intuitive appeal this theory also had empirical support from one of the most respected neurophysiologists of the early 20th century, Charles Sherrington. In 1895 Mott and Sherrington (1895) carried out a classic experiment. They deafferented* a single limb in each of a series of monkeys and found that although some random movements of the limb remained, no purposeful use was made of the limb. From these results they concluded that proprioceptive information is necessary for the performance of voluntary movement. This study was replicated by others over the next 25 years and the conclusions were in each case similar.

The notion that proprioceptive information was essential for movement evocation became an article of faith and, indeed, one psychologist made even conceptual learning largely dependent upon the S–R chaining of movement responses. Guthrie's (1935) learning theory proposed that thinking was done primarily by remembering minute movements of the vocal cords in the formation of word symbols and that perceiving was accomplished by establishing movement patterns in eye muscles. His one law of learning, from

---

*Deafferent means to remove or surgically interrupt sensory pathways, thus blocking certain afferent nerve impulses from reaching the brain.

which all else about learning was made comprehensible, was "a combination of stimuli which has accompanied a movement will on its recurrence tend to be followed by that movement."

Over the past twenty years the notion that proprioceptive feedback is essential to motor performance has come under increasing criticism. Motor performance has been demonstrated to be independent of proprioceptive feedback in insects, amphibia, and mammals (Wilson, 1961; Szekely, Czeh, and Voros, 1969; and Taub, Perrella, and Barro, 1973); in addition, many well-practiced human movements occur with such speed that there is no time for proprioceptive feedback to play any basic controlling role. Taub and Berman (1968) carried out a series of studies the purpose of which was to determine whether or not proprioceptive information is necessary for various types of learning and for the performance of various categories of movement. They deafferented sensation from the limbs of monkeys and then tested for the amount of movement and learning that was possible afterward. With one limb deafferented, they found, as had Mott and Sherrington, that no purposeful use was made of that limb. However, when the intact limb was immobilized, leaving the deafferented limb free, the animals did make purposeful movements demonstrating that purposeful movements could be made with deafferented limbs. Next they deafferented both forelimbs. After a recovery period of two to six months, the animals were able to use the limbs rhythmically and in excellent coordination with the hind limbs. Other workers, taking precautions to ensure that all kinesthetic feedback was eliminated, have confirmed Taub and Berman's studies (Bossom and Ommaya, 1968). Taub and Berman summarize their findings in this way:

...the most general conclusion that can be drawn from our research is that in mammals, once a motor program has been written into the CNS, the specified behavior, having been initiated, can be performed without any reference to or guidance from the periphery. Moreover, there does not appear to be any reason why the initiation, the trigger, cannot also be wholly central in nature.

It appears, therefore, that skilled movements do not completely depend on kinesthesis.

Although there is rather compelling documentation that motor performance can occur in the absence of kinesthetic information, there is, nevertheless, clinical and experimental evidence that kinesthesis may play a role in movement. In the disease tabes dorsalis the nerve pathways from the legs to the brain may be completely destroyed, while motor nerves from the brain to the legs remain intact. Tabes dorsalis victims, thus, will lack proprioceptive information from their legs while retaining motor control of them. In walking, the gait is uncertain and the movements of the legs are poorly coordinated, which results in stumbling and staggering, unless compensated for by visual monitoring. Another clinical situation was described by Lashley

(1917). He described a man who was unable to duplicate passive movement of the limbs and unable to appreciate that his leg had been moved, after a gunshot wound to the spinal cord which had eliminated all afferent pathways for the lower limbs. Laszlo (1966) used a nerve compression block to eliminate feedback from the arms of human subjects and found that tapping rates declined sharply.

In both Lashley's report and Laszlo's findings one factor remains disturbing to the conclusion that kinesthetic feedback is essential to performance. Lashley's gunshot victim could duplicate his own active movements within normal limits of accuracy, suggesting that while kinesthetic information may be necessary for the appreciation of passive movements, central control mechanisms can apparently mediate knowledge of active movements. Indeed, it has been shown that anesthetization of joint capsules abolishes perceptions of passive movement but does not diminish ability to duplicate voluntary movements (Browne, Lee, and Ring, 1954). When Laszlo's subjects were given a series of practice trials under nerve-block conditions, they almost completely recovered to pretest performance (Laszlo, 1967). The nerve compression block has been criticized on several counts, one of which is that there is some pain associated with its use (Keele, 1968; Kelso, Stelmach, and Wanamaker, 1974), and it is possible that this could account for the initial decline in performance which Laszlo (1966) reported.

To account for the mounting evidence that kinesthetic feedback is not essential for motor performance, "motor program" theories of motor control have been advanced. The concept of motor programs was introduced in Chapter 10 and, as you recall, this notion proposes that when a movement pattern is to be executed, neural impulses are transmitted to the appropriate muscles with the exact temporal and force characteristics necessary to carry out the action, and the neural impulses are largely uninfluenced by the resultant peripheral feedback. Many years ago Woodworth (1899) suggested that programs for simple motor responses are set up in advance of their beginning and are uninfluenced during their execution by any feedback, while complex responses may be preformed and initiated as a unit. His position now seems to be verified to a great extent.

Concepts about motor programs typically include considerations about skill acquisition, and thus the development of motor programs. This leads us to a consideration of the role of kinesthesis in motor learning.

B. KINESTHESIS AND MOTOR LEARNING

Although motor performance in the absence of kinesthetic feedback may be possible, it could not readily account for modifications in movement during performance nor for the acquisition of increased movement proficiency. To account for these processes various motor program models have been proposed which include a closed-loop mechanism. This notion was discussed in Chapter 11 and will be elaborated here. These models differ in many respects and each emphasizes a different aspect of motor control and skill acquisition via motor programs.

According to one model, the acquisition of a motor skill is accomplished by the learner initially cortically selecting motor programs, probably acquired while learning prior tasks, in an effort to produce the new movement pattern and modifying them by integrating feedback information. According to Adams (1971), as a learner practices, the feedback, one type of which may be proprioceptive, from the response begins to form a "perceptual trace" which represents the feedback consequences of the response just made. Over a number of trials the perceptual trace develops into an accurate representation of the feedback qualities of the correct response. When this occurs performers can compare the feedback from a given response with the perceptual trace to determine the correctness of the response. They have, in essence, developed an error detection mechanism for a given task which they can actually use to enable them to continue to learn even if other modes of feedback are withdrawn.

Support for Adams's notion of the development of an error detection mechanism was reported by Schmidt and White (1972) who showed that with practice, subjects developed an increasing capability for detecting errors in their responses. Subjects learned to move a slide a certain distance (9 inches) in a certain period of time (150 sec.). The subjects became increasingly sensitive to the direction and magnitude of their errors over the course of trials. This suggests that persons develop a capacity to determine their own errors on the basis of a learned internal error detection mechanism.

Experiments with animals with deafferented limbs who learn to make use of these limbs in the absence of vision raise a critical question: How can individuals without kinesthetic feedback and without vision learn movements, when by classical neuropsychological considerations they should not know where the limb is, whether it has moved, and if moved, in what way? Since the movement information could not have been signaled over sensory pathways, it must have been conveyed by some central-loop mechanism that does not involve the participation of the peripheral nervous system (Taub and Berman, 1968). Indeed, just such a mechanism has been proposed by several investigators in recent years.

A central loop, called "efference copy" by Von Holst (1954) and "corollary discharge" by Tauber (1964), has been suggested which carries information about the ongoing motor program, regardless of the overt results or sensory feedback concerning the movement. This notion proposes that some motor signals of the motor program go not only to the muscles but also form a copy of the command and it is these which may be compared against a central reference mechanism of the correct response. It is assumed that if movement error is detected motor programs can be altered for subsequent responses.

Assumptions concerning the neural basis of this central loop mechanism remain conjectural, but collaterals of the pyramidal tract have been identified at the cortical level, where recurrent collaterals start from pyramidal fibers, the subcortical level, where convergence of pyramidal axons has been demonstrated, and pyramidal and extrapyramidal tract fibers have been shown to play a role in the control of somatosensory afferents (Chang, 1955; Levitt, Carreras, Liu, and Chambers, 1964).

Although the mounting theoretical and empirical work over the past 20 years indicates that kinesthetic perception is not essential to motor behavior, this is not to suggest that kinesthetic feedback is unimportant. Keele (1973) has proposed four potentially important functions of feedback from the various senses, and in each case there is an implied role for kinesthesis.

According to Keele, the four functions of feedback are (1) It gives information relevant to starting position; (2) It is employed as a motor program monitor; (3) Motor programs evoke gross motor patterns, but a peripheral feedback loop is used to make fine adjustments; (4) Feedback is used in the acquisition of motor programs. The first function of feedback is to provide information about the position of the body to aid in the selection of the appropriate program or to determine the point in the program at which action should begin. Although it is recognized that it *is possible* for motor learning and performance to occur in the absence of kinesthetic feedback, a second function of feedback is that *normally* feedback from the proprioceptors serves to modify motor programs when there exists a conflict between the program and the actual position of body segments. Howard (1968) has pointed out the limitations of deafferented limb movements, especially their inability to compensate for changes in external load.

The third function of feedback proposed by Keele is related to the first and suggests that the proprioceptors are nicely designed for assisting with minute corrections in the motor program, especially through the gamma loop. It is suggested that motor program signals may activate both alpha and gamma motorneurons in such a way that they exactly nullify each other, so that there is no spindle afferent discharge. However, if a slight discrepancy occurs between the alpha and gamma motorneurons, the result will be a modification in spindle afferent discharge which will have the effect of increasing or decreasing neural activity at the alpha motorneurons and thus modifying extrafusal muscle contraction. This control of skeletal muscle activity via the spindle afferents is discussed in Chapter 5 and 8.

Keele's final function of feedback emphasizes that the full and complete development of motor programs for complex human motor performance is facilitated by feedback. Again, the notion is that while there is some empirical evidence for motor learning without kinesthetic information, presumably via a central-loop mechanism, this does not indicate that kinesthetic data play no role in learning. Indeed, it is likely that, normally, when developing a motor program, "a standard," or model, of the appropriate task performance is constantly being compared with feedback from the program which has just been employed. When there is a difference between the "standard" and the feedback, a different motor program is tried. Eventually a motor program emerges that brings about the desired performance—there is a motor program-standard match. This process is an integral part of recent models of motor learning (Adams, 1971).

C. RELATIONSHIP OF KINESTHESIS TO MOTOR PROFICIENCY

There does seem to be a general relationship between kinesthetic perceptual ability and motor proficiency, but considerable confusion exists in the literature with respect to this question. One of the sources of this confusion is surely the tests and measurements that have been used by the investigators. This problem was discussed earlier in this chapter.

Several investigators have reported a relationship between kinesthesis and motor learning (Phillips, 1940; Phillips and Summers, 1954; and Fleishman and Rich, 1963). Phillips and Summers found that there is a greater relationship between kinesthesis and task performance during the early stages of the learning process and that the role of kinesthesis decreases during learning, but most evidence supports the opposing point of view. Fleishman and Rich (1963) demonstrated that proprioceptive ability was of greater importance later in learning. They gave a Kinesthetic Sensitivity Test to a large group of subjects, then divided them into groups high and low on kinesthetic sensitivity. Then subjects learned a two-hand coordination task, in which they attempted to keep a target follower on a moving target with the left-right movement of the target follower controlled with one hand and movement toward and away from the body with the other. The two kinesthetic groups began at the same level but in the later stages, as kinesthetic ability apparently became more important, the kinesthetically superior group surpassed the other group.

The findings with regard to relationships between kinesthesis and various kinds of motor ability or motor performance on various motor skills have been equivocal. Roloff (1953) examined the relationship between the results of several tests of kinesthesis administered to 200 subjects and their scores on the Scott Motor Ability Test. She found a positive relationship between the two test batteries. Phillips and Summers (1954) found a positive relationship between positional tests of kinesthesis and bowling ability.

Mumby (1953) found that the kinesthetic ability to maintain a constant muscular pressure under a condition of irregular change in pressure was significantly related to wrestling ability. On the other hand, he found that kinesthetic ability to maintain a constant arm position against the irregular force created by the testing apparatus was unrelated to wrestling ability. Other investigators have found little relationship between motor skill and kinesthesis-test results. Wettstone (1938) and Young (1945) report low relationships between several kinesthetic tests and sports skills. Witte (1962) in a study of elementary school children found no relationship between their performance on tests of kinesthesis, which involved positional tasks and ball-rolling ability.

Investigations of the relationship between athletic ability and kinesthesis have generally found that athletes display superior kinesthesis, but there have been few studies of this type, and like the other studies which are reported above should be viewed with suspicion because they were done several years ago and/or the validity of the tests is questionable. Taylor (1933), in one of the pioneer studies on kinesthesis and motor skills, administered a battery of 14 tests to two groups of college basketball players. The results showed that the differences between "successful" (those who made the team) players in single tests were of little significance, but they were all, with one exception, in favor of the successful players. It was suggested that whereas the unit difference was of little significance, the cumulative differences were highly significant. In other words, boys who made the varsity basketball team scored better on the kinesthetic-test battery than did the unsuccessful candidates. Using 21 different tests to measure kinesthesis, Wiebe (1954) found significant differences in the scores made by varsity college athletes and nonathletes. LaBarba (1967) used high school students, undergraduate, and graduate college students and carried out a series of studies to investigate differential response sensitivity to kinesthetic and tactile stimuli. His hypothesis that different groups of individuals differ in response efficiency of these modalities of stimuli was only partially and minimally supported. He found no significant differences in modality efficiency between members of a high school football team and nonathletes.

KINESTHETIC AFTEREFFECTS

Kinesthetic aftereffects refer to a perceived modification in the shape, size, or weight of an object or to perceptual distortion of limb position, of movement, and/or of intensity of muscular contraction as a result of experience with a previous object. The baseball batter who swings several bats just before stepping to the plate, so that one bat will seem lighter, exemplifies the use of kinesthetic after-effect to produce an apparent change in weight of the bat. To use another example, running and jumping while wearing weighted shoes is usually followed by a perceived ability to run faster and jump higher after the heavy shoes are removed.

Kinesthetic aftereffects were first experimentally studied by Gibson (1933) in the early 1930s. In his original study, the subject passed one hand over a curved surface. After this experience it was found that a straight surface felt curved in the direction opposite to that of the exposure object. Numerous investigators have confirmed the existence of this phenomenon, but the whole field of aftereffects is relatively unstudied in the field of psychology. Most research on aftereffects has been done using vision as the sense modality.

Most studies of kinesthetic aftereffects have used tactile-manipulative tasks or fine motor tasks. In kinesthetic aftereffects experiments a stimulus object is first manipulated; this is called the I, or inspected object. Then a second stimulus object is presented; this is referred to as the T, or test object. In the case of Gibson's study referred to above, the curved surface was the I (inspection) object and the straight surface was the T (test) object. Petrie (1967) has developed a set of wood blocks that may be used to assess kinesthetic aftereffects. There are several blocks of different sizes which serve as inspection objects and there is one long tapered block of wood (tapering from 1/2 inch at its narrow end to 4 inches at its wide end) which serves as the test object. The blindfolded subject attempts to indicate the width of the inspection block, grasped in one hand, by moving the other hand to the same width on the test object, the tapered block. The Kinesthetic-Aftereffect Blocks have been used extensively in research on this modality of aftereffect.

Studies of kinesthetic aftereffect for gross motor movements are not plentiful, and those that have been done are usually concerned with the subject's motor performances after wearing or using heavy objects. A unique study by Cratty and Hutton (1964) demonstrated that locomotor activity under blindfolded conditions produced aftereffects. Subjects guided themselves ten times through pathways curved sharply to either the right or to the left. They were then placed in a straight test pathway. Aftereffects were evidenced by reports that the straight pathway was curved opposite to the direction of the curved pathway to which they had been exposed.

Several generalizations may be made on the basis of kinesthetic aftereffect studies: (1) There is a greater displacement, or aftereffect, with longer inspection time; (2) Aftereffects are maximal immediately after experience with the inspection object and then diminish gradually, leaving aftereffects that may be of long duration. Wertheimer and Leventhal (1958) found aftereffects remained for as long as six months; (3) The displacement tends to continue to diminish the longer the time delay between inspection and test; (4) Displacement may occur in one of two forms: assimilation or contrast. In assimilation the displacement of the test object is toward the inspection object; contrast is displacement of the test object away from the inspection object. Kinesthetic aftereffects usually produce contrast, but Petrie (1967) reported that subjects display either contrast or assimilation in a consistent manner; (5) When attention is distracted during the inspection test, the resulting aftereffects are reduced.

The underlying neural mechanisms responsible for kinesthetic aftereffects have been discussed by several scholars, but no definitive explanation has been formulated. The psychophysics of such explanations are complex but it seems that motor unit activity recruited for a given task, such as in manipulating a heavier-than-normal object, remains available and functioning when a lighter object is manipulated. The exact role of the neuromuscular mechanisms is not clear.

A. KINESTHETIC AFTEREFFECTS AND MOTOR PERFORMANCE

Kinesthetic aftereffect research has aroused the interest of coaches and athletes who have experienced the effects of this phenomenon in conjunction with "overload" training. One aspect of "overload" training that has become enormously popular in recent years is the use of weighted objects (i.e., weighted vest, anklets, shoes, balls, bats, etc.) to practice motor skills for a particular sport. These objects have been used with the expectations of improving performance (Fig. 14.2).

One theory underlying this technique is that the kinesthetic aftereffect experienced when these heavier-than-normal objects are removed actually produces better performance. A second theoretical proposition on which this technique is based is the so-called overload principle. This principle states that if muscles are forced to work against great resistance (overload), improved muscle strength, power, and speed of movement results.

In reviewing studies that have been done on this subject, we will direct our attention to the first theoretical premise, since the athletes report kinesthetic aftereffects. Nelson and Nofsinger (1965) measured the speed of elbow flexion just before and after applying various weights. They report no significant difference between pre-overload speed, although the subjects reported "feeling faster" during the post-overload trials. Lindeburg and Hewitt (1965) report that subjects who trained with an overweight and oversized basketball showed no significant difference from a control group on short shooting, foul shooting, or dribbling, but the experimental group did show significant improvement in passing. Gallon (1962), using weighted basketball shoes on subjects, and Winningham (1966), using ankle weights,

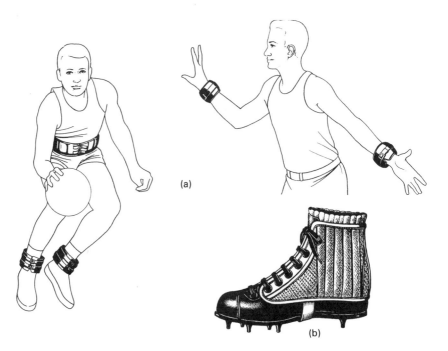

Fig. 14.2   (a) Weighted bands. (b) Weighted spat.

found that the control groups (those who practiced without weighted shoes) actually improved more on speed run tests than did the experimental groups.

Brose and Hanson (1967) report no significant differences in throwing speed among groups that trained by throwing weighted baseballs, throwing against pulley resistance, and throwing regulation baseballs. Also, none of their groups improved significantly in accuracy. Straub (1968) corroborated this finding. His subjects used weighted baseballs but the use of these balls resulted in no immediate or long-range improvement in throwing speed or in throwing accuracy. On the other hand, Van Huss *et al.* (1962) found that subjects who warmed up with a weighted baseball significantly improved their velocity of throwing regular-weight baseballs immediately following the "overload" warm-up, but there was no improvement in throwing accuracy under the same conditions. With a football, Hopek (1967) found no significant differences in accuracy between groups who trained with a regulation football and those he trained with a weighted ball.

Stockholm and Nelson (1965) investigated the immediate effects of overload upon vertical jumping performance. Three levels of overload (no overload, 5 percent, and 10 percent of the subject's weight) were used in the experiment. Subjects performed vertical jumps with a weighted vest, followed by jumps without the weights. They found no improvement in vertical jump performance after the overload practices. Boyd (1969) reported virtually identical results.

Most investigations, then, suggest that kinesthetic figural aftereffects are not accompanied by any measurable improvement in performance in the skills that have been practiced using the weighted objects. Any attempt to improve performance by utilizing objects that are slightly heavier than normal while practicing gross motor skills that will later be used in sports competition seems to be hardly worth the time spent and the money paid for the weighted objects.

Presumably the reason that the weighted objects do not enhance performance is that they do not bring about an increase in strength in the muscles involved. It is well established that strength development requires work against high resistance with few repetitions (Astrand and Rodahl, 1970). The overload provided by the weighted objects probably is not enough to achieve a "threshold" for strength development.

USING KINESTHETIC CUES IN TEACHING

The use of emphasizing kinesthetic cues as a teaching technique poses some rather serious difficulties. First, it is not at all clear to what extent kinesthesis is used, or is capable of being used, by the learner. Second, there is such a bewildering number of proprioceptive signals impinging upon the learner prior to, during execution, and immediately after execution of a movement pattern that it may be difficult to select the appropriate kinesthetic cues for attention during any of these periods. Third, there is no consistent body of research findings to indicate that an emphasis on kinesthetic cue utilization is an effective instructional method.

Given these problems, there are some techniques which have been tried in an effort to enhance motor learning through kinesthesis. In most cases they are intuitively appealing and none has proven to be detrimental to skill acquisition, so the enterprising teacher may wish to experiment with one or more of them.

One approach to enhancing skill acquisition through kinesthetic cue utilization has been to have learners practice the movement patterns with eyes closed or while blindfolded. One assumption behind this method is that learners have the potential of being aware of their movements through kinesthetic feedback without the aid of exterioceptive cues. Another assumption is that concentration will be on the movement rather than its outcome, and stimuli in the environment, which may be distracting, will be eliminated, thus making the learner aware of relatively ignored feedback. Espenschade (1958) and Dickinson (1968) both reported that removing visual information during the learning process enhanced learning rate. Durentini (1967) found no differences in improvement in basketball free-throw shooting between a group of subjects who practiced shooting while blindfolded and a group who practiced in the usual manner. The lack of visual cues apparently did not improve kinesthesis for that task. The effectiveness of this method has not been verified as a means of promoting learning from the scant literature currently available.

A second method of emphasizing kinesthesis in motor learning has been a manual manipulation technique in which learners relax as they are guided through the movement pattern. The assumption is that as learners are guided through the movement, the proprioceptors associated with the movement will be activated and will provide the learners with correct cues. Smith (1969) has suggested that manual assistance helps learners to "get the feeling of the proper movement" but there is little support for this claim and there is some reason to be suspicious of it, since the passive movement of body segments does not produce the same pattern of impulses as active movement and thus feedback is distorted. More research is needed to ascertain the effectiveness of this procedure.

A third technique which has been tried employs an emphasis on "feel." The learner is repeatedly told to "feel the position" or "feel the movement." Experimental support for this method is nonexistent. In one study an experimental group was taught bowling by the "kinesthetic-centered" method while a control group was taught without kinesthetic emphasis. Results showed no significant differences in bowling performance between groups (Haas, 1966).

There are a few limited situations in teaching sports skills which lend themselves to an emphasis on feel, such as the preliminary and terminal positions in the baseball, golf, and tennis swings, gymnastic stunts, and others. Since correct preliminary and terminal positions in these tasks are important to proper movement execution, it behooves learners to perfect these positions. They may be aided by learning the "feel" of these positions. Learners can attempt to achieve the correct preliminary and terminal "feel" and thus perhaps execute the movement correctly.

There are potential problems in asking either the novice or the expert to concentrate on feel. Beginners cannot benefit from the feel of a movement pattern because they cannot associate anything with a successful effort. To ask the highly skilled to experience the feel may result in "paralysis from analysis." This is exemplified in the following ditty.

A centipede was happy, quite
Until a frog in fun,
Said, "Pray which leg comes after which?"
Which raised her mind to such a pitch
She lay distracted in a ditch
Considering how to run!

15

Pain Perception
and
Motor Behavior

Pain is a perceptual response to a noxious or injurious stimulus. The obvious biological function of pain is to signal that damage is occurring to the body. It helps to protect the body from injury or insult, in a biological sense.

There are many facets to the study of pain. Psychologists and physiologists have studied it in the laboratory, while neurologists, anaesthesiologists, and neurosurgeons have studied it in clinics and hospitals. Each of these biological and medical specialties has made unique contributions to understanding pain phenomena but there is still no definitive understanding of the physiological and psychological aspects of pain perception. Indeed, neuroscientists still do not know to what extent pain is a specific modality and in what ways it interacts with other sense modalities. It is not clear, in fact, where the main sensory area for pain is located.

One thing that is clear with regard to pain is its tendency to take control of the individual's whole behavior, and even a weak pain stimulus tends to dominate over all other stimuli. It has been shown that pain interferes with motor learning not only by simple inhibition but also by severely interfering with and disarranging the motor control mechanisms. It is a daily experience of physical therapists and athletic coaches that the fear of pain alone inhibits motor performance considerably (McConnel, 1957).

Pain is a multidimensional experience which involves not only the capacity to identify the onset, duration, location, intensity, and physical characteristics of the stimulus but also includes the motivational, affective, and cognitive functions of pain, and the interpretation of the stimulus in terms of present and past experience (Casey, 1973). An enormous amount of research has been devoted to pain perception in the past two decades and what is emerging is a concept of pain that is quite different from the traditional views about pain. In this chapter we shall describe the current physiological and psychological views about pain perception and discuss the implications for motor behavior. We shall also review the limited research in pain perception of athletes.

PAIN AND SPORTS PERFORMANCE

The athlete experiences pain in two main contexts as a regular part of the sports experience—first in contact sports and second in endurance sports. Painful experience also frequently accompanies training and conditioning regimens of strength and endurance building. The ability to persist in an activity and the willingness to engage in and endure painful body contact, or both, are essential in the performance of many sports. Indeed, success and high performance in several sports appear to be partly determined by the ability to endure high amounts of pain.

In the world of sports, coaches and athletes commonly believe that the ability to tolerate pain and stress contributes to successful performances. Coaches often describe athletes by the way they respond to pain; football coaches talk of "hitters," meaning players who are willing to endure the pain of hard, violent blocks and tackles. Jim Counsilman, the swimming coach at the University of Indiana, is famous for this "hurt-pain-agony" formula which presumably differentiates champions from almost-champions from average athletes. According to him, athletes who will endure the highest intensities of agony typically become the best swimmers. The late champion distance runner, Steve Prefontaine, once said: "A lot of people run a race to see who is the fastest. I run to see who has the most guts, who can punish himself to an exhausting pace, and then at the end who can punish himself even more" (Putnam, 1972).

PAIN THRESHOLD, TOLERANCE, AND MEASUREMENT

People commonly use the terms pain threshold and pain tolerance as though they were synonymous, but they are not; indeed there are important distinctions in the two terms. Pain threshold is the lowest stimulus value at which a person reports feeling pain whereas pain tolerance refers to the highest intensity of stimulation which a person will endure.

Under precisely controlled laboratory settings, pain threshold is typically found to be about the same for normal persons, although it has been reported that there are ethnic differences in pain threshold (Hardy, Wolff, and Goodell, 1952). Although pain is perceived by normal persons at about the same degree of tissue damage, there are enormous differences in pain tolerance. Pain tolerance is a highly personal and variable experience which is affected by culture, the meaning of the situation, attention, motivation, and cognitive activities. Moreover, Sternback and Tursky (1965) found that the levels at which persons refuse to tolerate electric shock depends upon their ethnic origin. Other investigators have reported differences in pain tolerance between males and females, young and old, extroverts and introverts, high-anxious and low-anxious, and athletes and nonathletes. Finally, everyone has had the experience of personal variations in pain tolerance, depending upon the incentives under which the pain was to be tolerated.

A. TESTING PAIN THRESHOLD AND TOLERANCE

Tests of pain threshold and tolerance are of various types. Radiant heat has frequently been used to induce pain. This technique employs a 1000 watt light focused through a small hole which is directed toward a specific area of the body, usually the forehead. The person being tested controls the apparatus by turning a rheostat, which controls stimulus intensity, in accordance with directions, depending upon whether threshold or tolerance is being assessed.

Cold is another stimulus used in pain testing. In the cold-pressor technique, the hand or hand and forearm is immersed in ice water. The subject removes the limb when the pain can no longer be endured.

Several mechanical tests of pain have been employed to test threshold and tolerance. Pressure, applied by various methods, is usually the stimulus. In several studies a football cleat, secured to a curved plastic fiber plate, was placed against the anterior border of the tibia, midway between the ankle and the knee. The sleeve of a clinical sphygmomanometer* was used to secure the cleat in place. Cleat pressure against the tibia was obtained by inflating the sleeve. Pain tolerance was recorded in mm Hg (millimeters of mercury).

A condition in which blood flow is decreased is known as ischemia, and pain accompanies this condition. Ischemic pain is commonly assessed by inflating a blood-pressure cuff which has been wrapped around the upper-arm until the blood flow has been cut off. Then the subjects extend and clench their fingers at a rate of once-per-second until they can no longer endure the pain. The number of times the hand is opened and closed is recorded.

Many investigators have used electrical current as the pain stimulus. Typically an instrument with a rheostat to regulate electric current is used. As the rheostat dial is moved, electric current is increased. Subjects receiv-

---

* A sphygmomanometer is an instrument normally used for testing blood pressure. Pressure is measured in millimeters of mercury (mm Hg).

ing the electric current indicate when they perceive pain or when they cannot tolerate increased amounts of current, depending upon whether threshold or tolerance is being measured.

THE NEUROPHYSIOLOGICAL BASIS OF PAIN

Unlike the other major sensory systems, the neurophysiology of pain is relatively poorly understood. The two most prominant physiological theories of pain over the past hundred years have been the "specificity theory" and the "pattern theory."

The first of the modern "scientific" theories of pain was the specificity theory which was proposed in outline by Müller (1842) and more fully elaborated by Von Frey in the latter 19th century (Boring, 1942). In essence, the specificity theory of pain proposed that there are specific pain receptors which can be differentiated from other sensory receptors, i.e., pressure, heat, or cold. Associated with these pain receptors are specific nerve fibers over which the pain impulses travel to the spinal cord. In the cord is a specific spinal tract which carries the impulses to the brain. Finally, within the brain there is a pain control center that receives the pain signals.

Clinical, anatomical, and physiological evidence is overwhelmingly against this specificity of pain transmission. The notion, for example, of a pain center in the brain is completely rejected by Melzack (1973) who says, "The concept of a pain centre [in the brain]. . .is totally inadequate to account for the complexity of pain. Indeed, the concept is pure fiction, unless virtually the whole brain is considered to be the pain centre. . . ." It is true that there is a variety of distinct sensory receptors in the skin and other tissues, and in some cases there is a definite correlation between specialized receptors and some aspect of sensation, but such examples are rare, and it is not now possible to definitively identify a specific receptor uniquely associated with pain. It has been believed for many years that the free nerve endings were the pain receptors, but the majority of nerve endings in hairy skin are of this type, indicating that they must be involved with somatic sensations other than pain.

The second theory of pain is called the "pattern theory" but it is not a single theory; instead it is a group of theories which have evolved in opposition to the specificity theory and which have similar theoretical characteristics. Basically, this theory proposes that all receptors are alike and that the pattern of impulses produced by internal stimulation of nonspecific receptors produces pain. It is suggested that the integration and patterning take place primarily in the spinal cord and the variability of the spatiotemporal patterns of impulses produces pain.

The major weaknesses of this theory is that it considers only the sensory features or anatomy of impulse conduction and it ignores the fact of physiological specialization; it also fails to explain the motivational and cognitive aspect of pain perception. Moreover, recent evidence that intense stimulation of large, fast-conducting fibers of the somatosensory system does not result in pain confounds those who propose that pain is the result of overstimulation of any of the skin receptors.

Recently, a theory of pain has been advanced which overcomes most of the weaknesses of the older explanations and has a much sounder anatomical and physiological base. Melzack and Wall (1965) have proposed a "gate control" theory of pain, which is an effort to account for pain taking into consideration the anatomical and physiological factors in pain and recognizing that the notion that there are specific pain receptors in the body is not well supported and is inadequate to account for many pain phenomena.

The gate control theory is a way of accounting for the fact that perception of pain is not on a one-to-one relationship with the intensity of stimulation, i.e., weak stimuli sometimes produce extreme pain whereas very intense stimuli sometimes evoke little pain, and does not seem to be dependent upon specific pain receptors but can occur in any sense modality. There is considerable empirical support for the gate control theory, but it is tentative, and many details need to be worked out (Higgins et al., 1971; Melzack, 1973).

A. GATE CONTROL THEORY AND PAIN TRANSMISSION

According to the gate control theory of pain, noxious stimuli produce a coded pattern of nerve impulses which are transmitted over afferent neuron fibers of two different sizes, large diameter fibers and small diameter fibers. The large fibers tend to be myelinated, low-threshold, and fast conducting, whereas the small fibers are unmyelinated, higher-threshold, and slow conducting. The conduction velocities range from 80-100 m/sec for the large fibers (the fast fiber network) to 1–40 m/sec for the small fibers (slow fiber network).

Fibers of both large and small diameter enter the dorsal horn of the spinal cord and their presynaptic terminals form synapses with various neurons in the dorsal spinal cord. The terminals of the small fibers end on interneurons in the cord or on the second-order neuron whose axon crosses the cord and enters the spinothalamic tract, projecting directly to the thalamus while sending off collaterals to the large number of brainstem and reticular formation neurons. From the thalamus, impulses are transmitted to the cerebral cortex. The collaterals synapse in the reticular formation and brainstem where a complex network of neurons has ascending and descending axons with extensive connections in the spinal cord and higher brain centers.

The first-order neurons of the large afferent fibers enter the dorsal column of the cord and ascend without synapse to the brainstem, where they synapse on the second-order neurons in either the nucleus gracilis or the nucleus cuneatus. The axons of the second-order neurons cross the midline and ascend to the thalamus. Impulses from this system then ascend to the cerebral cortex. At the spinal cord level, the large fibers give off collaterals which synapse on interneurons in that segment of the cord (Fig. 15.1).

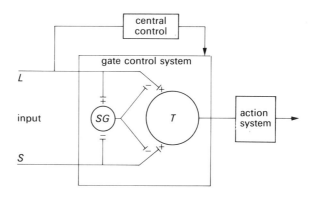

Fig. 15.1 Schematic diagram of the gate control theory of pain mechanisms: L, the large diameter fibers; S, the small diameter fibers. The fibers project to the substantia gelatinosa (SG) and first central transmission (T) cells. The inhibitory effect exerted by SG on the afferent fiber terminals is increased by activity in L fibers and decreased by activity in S fibers. The central control trigger is represented by a line running from the large-fiber system to the central control mechanisms; these mechanisms, in turn, project back to the gate control system. The T cells project to the entry cells of the action system. +, excitation; –, inhibition. (Based on Melzack and Wall, 1965.)

While pain signals from both the spinothalamic and dorsal column systems project to the thalamus and on to the cerebral cortex, the precise role that these parts of the brain play in pain perception is not clearly known. The initial conscious awareness of the crude aspects of pain are probably realized in the thalamus. Lesions in the thalamus often produce one of the most unbearable types of pathological pain. In some cases pain can be eliminated by extending the lesion into other parts of the thalamus; in fact, lesions in the medial thalamus and certain nuclei of this structure have provided relief from intractable pain (White and Sweet, 1969). So it appears that the thalamus is an important component of the pain process, but it would be unwise to conclude that this structure is the center for pain, as some have done.

As previously indicated, the cerebral cortex does not have a single pain center (Melzack, 1973). But cells responding to noxious stimuli have been found in the cortex and they are primarily in the somatosensory cortex (Carreras and Andersson, 1963). However, electrical stimulation of the cortex indicates that a very small proportion of cells in the cortex respond exclusively to noxious stimuli. In view of the paucity of pain perception from cortical stimulation, some neurologists have proposed that pain signals enter consciousness in the thalamus (Milner, 1970).

Now to return to the spinal level transmission. There is a dramatic difference in the physiological properties of neurons of the dorsal column compared with the spinothalamic tract. The dorsal column fibers and the brainstem neurons to which they project respond to light touch, and other gentle innocuous stimuli. Impulses are transmitted at high speed by this system from the body surface to the cerebral cortex; the system is organized for rapid transmission and is called the fast fiber network.

The spinothalamic tract is considered the classic "pain tract," since stimulation of neurons which make up this tract give rise to pain sensation, but this does not mean that it is exclusively for transmitting impulses involved in pain processes. Indeed, impulses for other somatic sensations use this tract. Furthermore, just because the dorsal column system transmits signals for touch does not prove that it does not play a role in pain transmission.

Both large and small afferent neuron populations respond to a variety of mechanical, chemical, and thermal stimuli. Anywhere from 15 to 50 percent of the large and small fibers respond primarily to noxious stimuli. The majority, however, respond to stimuli which are normally innocuous (Bessou and Perl, 1969; Burgess and Perl, 1967).

These sensory pathways to the brain, which include the spinothalamic and dorsal column systems, the thalamus, and the cerebral cortex, carry the specific, detailed, and topographically organized information from the site of the pain to the cortex and are the basic sensory-discriminative system for pain perception.

According to the gate control theory, both large and small diameter collateral fibers synapse on neurons in the gray matter of the spinal cord. Some of these spinal neurons are small interneurons and it is upon these that the afferent neurons send collaterals. This transmission serves to modulate the effectiveness of synaptic activity from the first-order neurons to the second-order neurons of the spinothalamic tract. These interneurons can therefore influence impulse transmission at the level of the first central synapse. The interneurons exert an influence on synaptic transmission, controlling the amount of sensory impulses that ascend in the spinothalamic tract; they are the "gatekeepers" over the sensory traffic at the spinal level (Casey, 1973).

Melzack and Wall (1965) have proposed that it is the small interneurons of the substantia gelatinosa* of the spinal cord which have a modulating effect on transmission from first-order neurons to second-order spinal neurons.

The smaller diameter fibers exert synaptic transmission on the inter neurons which *excites* the second-order neuron. Impulses via the large dia meter afferent neurons stimulate interneurons which in turn *inhibit* trans mission at the second-order neuron, thus opposing the effects of the small fiber system. The excitatory effects at the second-order neuron are there fore enhanced by small fiber impulses and inhibited by impulse activity in the large fibers.

According to Melzack and Wall (1965), it is the relative amount of neu ral activity of the two fiber networks that controls the perception of pain. Pain perception depends upon whether the small fiber network is dominant or whether the large fiber network is dominant. In the former, the gate is open and pain signals get to the brain; in the latter the gate is closed and sig nals are blocked.

It has been demonstrated that small fiber stimulation and large fiber stimulation evoke different experiences. When electrodes were placed into the slow fibers in an individual's spinal cord and stimulated, the individual experienced pain. But when the fast fibers were stimulated, the individual experienced no pain at all—even when the stimulation was intense. Indeed, if the individual was actually experiencing pain, stimulation of the indi vidual's fast fibers actually reduced the pain (Casey, 1973).

The gating of pain impulses at the second-order spinal neuron via the large fibers is only one source of several which exist. According to Melzack (1973), the gating mechanism is modulated by impulses descending from cor tical and subcortical neurons. These "central control" neurons are initially activated by the large, rapidly conducting fibers of the dorsal column sen sory system. These higher centers can close the gate just as effectively as can the large fiber firing at the spinal cord level. Under certain conditions the brain can "turn off" pain impulses by inhibiting the "spinal gate" action too.

The brainstem and the midbrain reticular formation areas exert a powerful inhibitory influence over the spinothalamic transmission network at the spinal cord level. When certain portions of the brainstem are electri cally stimulated, analgesia is produced in a widespread area of the body. Mayer, *et al.* (1971) reported that stimulation at various subcortical brain sites abolished responsiveness to intense pain. They note, "It seems plaus ible to us that the analgesia we have observed results from activation of a neural system in the brain which has an ultimate inhibitory action on sen

---

*A special variety of gray matter in the dorsal horn of the spinal cord which, in fresh condition, is gelatinous in appearance.

ory transmission in the spinal cord." The existence of such a system, a cen-
ral-control mechanism influencing the spinal "gate," provides neurophysi-
logical support for the powerful modulating effects psychological factors
re known to have on pain.

This inhibitory activity is carried out by descending fibers which im-
inge on the spinal gating mechanism. The decending inhibitory activity is it-
elf activated by the input from the large, fast-conducting fibers of the dor-
al column system. There are also projections from other sensory systems
nd in this way input from all parts of the body, as well as vision, audiation,
tc. is able to exert a modulating influence on transmission via the spino-
halamic tract (Melzack, 1973). Melzack has referred to the notion that the
eticular formation exerts an inhibitory influence on transmission at various
ynaptic levels of the somatic projection system, including the spinal cord,
s a central biasing mechanism, and suggests that it plays an important role
n the framework of the gate control theory of pain.

It is well established that neurons in the cerebral cortex can initiate
nhibition of synaptic transmission from somatosensory fibers at the spinal
ord level (Eccles, 1973, 1964). It is proposed that when you are highly moti-
ated to ignore pain signals, or when your attention is on other matters, you
re distracted from the pain signals, or when you are hypnotized, your brain
ends inhibitory impulses to the spinothalamic fiber system, and closes the
pinal gate.

These observations clearly indicate that cortical and lower brain neu-
ons can influence the activity of the sensory pathways and thus modify pain
erception.

SYCHOLOGICAL ASPECTS OF PAIN

ain is a highly complex physiopsychological event that is affected by many
actors. Melzack (1973) notes:

*he psychological evidence strongly supports the view of pain as a percep-
ual experience whose quality and intensity are influenced by the unique
ast history of the individual, by the meaning he gives to the pain-producing
ituation, and by his "state of mind" at the moment.*

Melzack has identified three psychological dimensions of pain percep-
ion; (1) Sensory-discriminative, (2) Motivational-affective, (3) Cognitive-
valuative. Each of these dimensions is subserved by physiological mech-
nisms in the nervous system.

The idea behind Melzack's classification is that pain is not merely a
ensory-discriminative experience, concerned only with the detection, loca-
ion, and intensity discrimination of pain, but also includes the motivational

qualities and emotional responses which impel the individual to tolerate
pain and the cognitive-evaluation made of the stimuli in terms of past experience and present context. Most investigators have treated pain as a purely
sensory phenomenon, largely ignoring its motivational, emotional, and cognitive aspects. This narrow perspective does little justice to a very complex
and critical function of the body.

A. SENSORY-DISCRIMINATIVE DIMENSION OF PAIN

In the previous section of this chapter, the sensory-discriminative dimension
of pain was discussed through an examination of the neural mechanisms
which subserve pain perception. These mechanisms, taken together, suggest
that dorsal column and spinothalamic systems, through their projections to
the subcortical and cortical projections, have the capacity to process information about the spatial, temporal, and intensity properties of noxious stimuli.

B. MOTIVATIONAL-AFFECTIVE DIMENSION OF PAIN

Melzack's argument for a motivational-affective dimension of pain seems
reasonable, for each of us can recognize that, in our personal experiences
with pain, emotional reactions frequently accompany the experience as well
as a drive to rid ourselves of the pain, or perhaps a drive to endure it, if survival is at stake.

There is considerable evidence that the reticular formation and certain
other subcortical structures which receive input from somatosensory pathways play a particularly important role in the motivational-affective aspect
of pain. Electrical stimulation of certain midbrain structures evokes escape
or other attempts to stop stimulation. Ablation of these and other structures
produces marked changes in affective behavior, including decreased responsiveness to noxious stimuli. This evidence indicates that brainstem and
midbrain structures provide a neural basis for the aversive drive and effect
that underlie the motivational dimension of pain.

C. COGNITIVE-EVALUATIVE DIMENSION OF PAIN

Stimulation of the sensory receptors does not mark the beginning of the pain
process because the noxious signals which enter the nervous system are
entering an active system that has a past history, anticipation, expectation,
anxiety, etc. These things, then, actually participate in the selection, interpretation, and synthesis of information from the total sensory input.

According to the gate control theory of pain, the early arriving information over the large, fast fiber system is evaluated, compared with other sen-

sory data, and interpreted in terms of past experience and present context in the cortex. These cortical events may now have a return effect on the sensory pathways which carry the slower impulses along the spinothalamic tract. Thus, the neural pathway carrying the slower information can be modulated by cortical events, markedly changing the input by the time it reaches higher pain areas of the brain. There is evidence that the frontal cortex can inhibit or modulate neural signals in the slow fiber spinothalamic system. Cortical events have been found to inhibit nerve impulses transmitted over the spinothalamic system, from the thalamus down to the dorsal horns of the spinal cord (Shimazu, Yanagisawa, and Garoutte, 1965; Hagbarth and Kerr, 1954).

Many cognitive factors influence the experience of pain: current context, prior experiences, attention, anxiety, expectations, etc. Such factors are usually considered to be mediated by the cortex.

People attach variable meanings to pain at a given time and thus influence the degree of pain they perceive. Beecher (1959) reported that severely wounded soldiers often indicated that they perceived little or no pain when brought to a field hospital and did not want medication to relieve it; presumably they were relieved just to be alive and out of the fighting zone. If someone hands you an expensive dish which is very hot, although you feel pain, you will probably tolerate the burning and have the "presence of mind" not to drop it. The knowledge of the social consequences of dropping the dish seems to override the pain and makes it tolerable.

Attention to stimuli contributes to the intensity of pain perceived. Football players, wrestlers, boxers, and other athletes often incur serious injuries during the contest without being aware that they have been injured. It appears that the cerebral cortex is able to block transmission in the pain pathway to the brain and so protect it from being bothered by stimuli that can be neglected. This is what happens when you are occupied, for example, in carrying out some action or in thinking. Under such situations you can be oblivious even to severe stimulation. For example, in the heat of combat or competitive sports severe injuries may be neglected.

Attention to pain stimuli may be diverted or masked through the stimulation of other sensory systems. An example of masking perception in one sense by stimulation of another is the apparent effectiveness of sound in reducing experienced pain (audioanalgesia) in dental treatments. Gardner and his colleagues (1960) reported that, for 65 percent of patients who previously required nitrous oxide or a local anesthetic, pain was completely eliminated by a combination of music and noise played through headphones. The investigators suggested a physiological mechanism to account for the effect; this mechanism involves an inhibitory effect by the auditory system on the painful stimuli.

One's understanding of the "pain situation" has much to do with the perception of pain. If we expect intense pain—anticipate it—the perception tends to verify our expectation. Clinical and experimental studies show that the mere anticipation of pain is sufficient to increase anxiety and thus the intensity of perceived pain (Evans, 1974). On the other hand, if individuals actually believe that they will not feel pain, or they feel capable of dealing with the conditions that produce it, or they are highly motivated to tolerate pain, anxiety is typically reduced and the pain perception is attenuated. Here, the cortex probably sends impulses to the "spinal gate" to suppress slow fiber firing.

Melzack (1973) has suggested that it is possible to explain the anaesthesis of hypnosis or of yoga by the cerebral pathways inhibiting the sensory pathways to the brain. In the case of acupuncture, the needle stimulation causes stimulation of afferent pathways that depress the pain pathways by inhibiting action at the various relays to the cortex.

PAIN PERCEPTION AND ATHLETES

Pain commonly accompanies competitive athletic experiences. The long-distance runner or swimmer experiences the effect of ischemia, while boxers, wrestlers, ice hockey, football, and rugby athletes experience violent body contact. In these sports, and in others as well, the ability to endure pain is one factor in successful performance—that is, high pain tolerance is important to excel in many sports. It might be expected, then, that the ability to withstand pain is related to participation in certain types of sports, and indeed to sports participation itself.

Although there is not an extensive literature concerned with pain perception of athletes, the limited research which has been done points to differences among sports groups and between athletes and nonathletes.

Puni (1965) reported differential pain tolerance among athletes who held their breath as long as possible under four different conditions. During the breath holding, the athletes were able to choose one of the following conditions: (1) think of anything they wish, (2) work out arithmetic problems, (3) concentrate on a frightening situation, such as drowning, (4) imagine a pleasant experience. The investigator found that the subjects who imagined a pleasant experience had the longest breath-holding performance.

Ryan and Kovacic (1966) tested three groups on pain threshold and tolerance: contact-sport athletes, noncontact sport athletes, and nonathletes. The contact-sport athletes were intercollegiate football players and wrestlers, the noncontact sport athletes were golfers and tennis players. Radiant heat was used to assess pain threshold. Pain threshold was measured by gross pressure and muscle ischemia. In the former, a football cleat was placed on the tibia and the sleeve of a clinic sphygmomanometer was used to secure the cleat in place. Cleat pressure was obtained by inflating the sleeve. Ischemia was produced by inflating a sphygmomanometer which was wrapped around the upper arm to 300 mm Hg.

In the pain threshold test the groups did not differ, but in the pain tolerance tests there were significant differences. The contact sport athletes demonstrated the highest pain tolerance levels, followed by the noncontact sport athletes, and the nonathletes endured the least pain. It seems, then, that pain tolerance is related to participation in certain types of sports and that athletes have higher tolerance than nonathletes.

Ryan and Foster (1967) repeated the Ryan and Kovacic study, using high school boys. They obtained similar results with the younger boys. In an effort to determine the reasons for differences in pain perception, they also measured the perceptual reduction and augmentation of the subjects. Petrie (1967) has indicated that certain individuals consistently reduce the intensity of their perceptions while others tend to augment their subjective perceptions. The reducers tend to have higher pain tolerance than augmentors. Petrie suggests that reducers tolerate more pain because of their tendency to reduce the perceptual intensity of the stimulation. Ryan and Foster found that the athletes with the higher pain tolerance were also "reducer" perceptual types.

Phillips (1972) tested groups of rugby players, cross-country runners, and nonathletes, using radiant heat to assess pain threshold and pain tolerance. He reported that the two athlete groups—the rugby players and cross-country runners—exhibited higher pain tolerance than the nonathlete group.

Ellison and Freischlag (1975) tested pain tolerance of intercollegiate athletic groups of basketball players, baseball players, football linemen, football backs, track distance runners, track field and sprint athletes, and nonathletes. Pain tolerance was measured by ability to continue protracted muscular contractions on a weighted trigger-like ergometer. Mean scores for track distance athletes were highest, followed by football linemen, and football backs; lowest mean scores were those of nonathletes.

Female intercollegiate basketball players were compared with nonathletes for pain tolerance by Walker (1971). She found that the athletes demonstrated a higher pain tolerance than nonathletes, and when the basketball groups was divided into two groups, members of the superior team (more highly skilled) had higher pain tolerance than the other group.

The question is still open whether the differences which have been demonstrated between athletes and nonathletes and between various athletic groups is a product of the sports experiences or whether persons with differences in pain tolerance are attracted to sports, even particular sports. The studies cited above provide no evidence to indicate whether athletes choose a type of sport because they have a high pain tolerance or whether they develop a high pain tolerance from engaging in their chosen sport. Morehouse and Rasch (1963) suggest that:

An inherent insensitivity to pain may be a quality which differentiates endurance athletes from those who stay away from events requiring discomfort of sustained performance.

ENHANCING PAIN TOLERANCE IN MOTOR ACTIVITIES

The notion of motivational and cognitive dimensions of pain suggests that there are numerous methods that instructors of physical activities might use to enhance the pain tolerance of those with whom they are working. First, since such cognitive factors as anxiety, expectation, and anticipation are so important in pain tolerance, it would seem that it would be wise to gradually introduce pain into the practice and competitive experience. It is well known that extremely painful or traumatic experiences often produce a phobia, a persistent fear of some object or stimulation in which the danger is magnified out of proportion. Morgan (1974) has described how an intensely painful experience of a track athlete produced a phobic effect, and the athlete was never able to duplicate his record performance.

Gradual painful experience allows individuals to develop cognitive constructs about the experience which probably enables them to anticipate less pain, and thus reduce anxiety, feel capable of controlling and enduring the pain, and even of accepting the pain. Morehouse and Rasch (1963) say:

The highly trained athlete in the peak of condition accepts pain as a regular part of the sport and knows that it will not injure him permanently. He realizes that it will disappear within a few moments after the event.

This gradual development of cognitive constructs to deal with pain probably produces modulation of the sensory transmission pathways for pain.

Another advantage of gradual introduction of pain is that since the cardiorespiratory system is responsible for getting oxygen to the cells and carrying away the waste products of muscular work, it is intimately involved with muscle ischemia. Ischemic pain results from lack of blood flow. This type of pain becomes delayed when training has produced physiological adaptation of the cardiorespiratory system—this system becomes more capable of carrying out its job of getting blood to the working muscles. A wise program of gradually increasing intensity brings about this adaptation of the cardiorespiratory system.

The evidence that pain is influenced by cultural factors suggests that young persons may be influenced by the attitudes of their parents about pain. Some families are overprotective and overrespond to their children's injuries while others show little sympathy or emotion to even serious injuries. It is undoubtedly true that the attitudes toward pain acquired early in life are carried into adolescence and adulthood. Since many individuals have been conditioned by overprotective parents to avoid pain or situations in which pain is present, instructors of motor activities may have to devote a good deal of time to changing the general attitudinal orientation of their charges. Their task, then, will be to modify the cognitive set under which their charges function in order to produce higher levels of pain tolerance.

As indicated in an earlier section of this chapter, motivation markedly influences pain tolerance. Incentives and needs control the motivation of individuals and thus the intensity of noxious stimuli which they will endure. Judicious use of incentives, keeping the performers' interests in mind, will probably produce higher amounts of pain tolerance.

16

Motor Skill Acquisition

It may seem curious to find this chapter entitled Motor Skill Acquisition when, in fact, parts of several previous chapters have been concerned with motor learning in some way, some quite directly and others indirectly. The title reflects a need to introduce certain topics about motor skill learning that simply were not convenient to introduce in previous chapters. By examining these topics at this time, the content in the following chapters is made more meaningful.

In this chapter, concepts which are frequently employed in motor skill acquisition research are defined and discussed. Then several general topics that are related to research data collection and analysis are examined.

TERMINOLOGY USED IN MOTOR SKILL LITERATURE

The literature on motor skill theory and research is replete with numerous terms, such as psychomotor skills, perceptual-motor skills, sensorimotor skills, etc. Why this bewildering array of terms? Do they define different domains of behavior? In some cases, it is merely by personal preference that an author uses one term instead of others. On the other hand, some writers use a certain term to emphasize a particular aspect of skill learning. For example, when the perceptual or integrative processes of motor tasks are studied, the term perceptual-motor is frequently used. When sensory cues influencing performance are to be emphasized, some writers use the term sensorimotor. But basically all movement behavior, other than simple reflexes and movements, involves the sensory, integrative, as well as the motor systems of the body. Although terms such as perceptual-motor learning may aid researchers in identifying specific areas of emphasis in skill acquisition,

335

it is not necessary to use the word "perceptual" in a general discussion of motor learning and performance. Indeed, if motor learning and performance are defined as behavior that is a result of experience, the word "perceptual" may be redundant.

A. A MOTOR SKILL

The phrase "a motor skill" has many different connotations and has been used in various different ways in the psychological and physical education literature. A motor skill consists of a number of perceptual and motor responses which have been acquired by learning. Possession of a motor skill enables an individual to accomplish a particular set of goals with precision and accuracy. Thus, the jump shot in basketball may be referred to as a motor skill, since it is a task made up of a series of perceptual and motor responses which are designed to bring about a specific goal—the ball going through the basket.

The acquisition of a motor skill is a process in which the learner develops a set of motor responses into an integrated and organized movement pattern. Thus a motor skill implies more than discrete responses in the service of a new goal. Each motor skill demands a new set of spatially and temporally organized muscular actions. By spatial organization we mean that the appropriate muscles must be selected while temporal organization refers to the fact that muscle contractions or relaxations must occur at the appropriate time.

B. SKILLED

Just as with the phrase "a motor skill," the word "skilled" has many connotations. Paillard (1960) gives a detailed description of what is meant by skilled:

We shall use it here to designate among motor activities a particular category of finely coordinated voluntary movements, generally engaging certain privileged parts of the musculature in the performance of various technical acts which have as common characteristics the delicacy of their adjustment, the economy of their execution, and the accuracy of their achievement.

Fitts (1964), a prominent motor skills investigator before his untimely death, said:

By a skilled response I shall mean one in which receptor-effector-feedback processes are highly organized, both spatially and temporally. . . . Spatial-temporal patterning, the interplay of receptor-effector-feedback processes, and such characteristics as timing, anticipation, and the graded response are thus seen as identifying characteristics of skill.

Operationally, definitions of "skilled" are usually given in terms of overt responses to controlled stimulation. The responses are scored on the basis of errors, correct responses, rates, and amplitudes. Stimuli are the energy inputs to the subject, which are generally expressed in units like frequency, length, time, and weight.

The word "skilled" may also be used to describe a relative level of proficiency; that is, for each motor task one is judged as being highly skilled, poorly skilled, or having average skill, depending upon the performance criteria standards for the task. "Level of skill" does not fluctuate much from one performance to the next. Of course, over many performances the skill level may change. For example, in learning a task an individual may go from a poorly skilled to a highly skilled level by regular practice.

1. Characteristics of skillful motor performance

A skilled performer is characterized as one who can produce a fast output of high quality, and this is the criterion of skillful performance with which most assessment is concerned. Skilled performance is also characterized by an appearance of ease, of smoothness of movement, an anticipation of variations in the stimulus situation before they arrive, and an ability to cope with these and other disturbances without disrupting the performance—indeed, increasing skill involves a widening of the range of possible disturbances that can be coped with without disturbing the performance. Novice tennis players stroke the ball in jerky movements while seeming to be involved in a frantic game in which they cannot quite keep up. They are caught unprepared by slightly unusual shots by their opponents. Skillful players, in contrast, seem to move with ease; they are in proper position sooner than the beginner, and they anticipate and react to situations with unhesitating movements. The skilled performer seems to "have all the time in the world," there are no surprises, in the sense that surprise involves a lack of readiness for the situation that has arisen.

Skilled motor performers are moving to accomplish a purpose, although their ultimate movement goal may not be discernible because many movements are performed to conceal the ultimate objective. For example, football running-backs who charge into the line after receiving a fake handoff from the quarterback keep their hands folded close to their stomachs to conceal the fact they they do not have the ball.

C. GROSS AND FINE MOTOR SKILLS

In the literature on motor behavior one frequently finds words used to denote the parts and the extent of the body involved in a movement pattern. Motor tasks are frequently described as "fine" or "gross" skills, but there is no standardized criterion on which to identify a skill as "fine" or "gross."

Cratty (1973) suggests that motor skills might be placed on a continuum, from the "fine" to the "gross," with a classification made "with reference to size of the muscle involved, the amount of force applied, or to the magnitude of space in which the movement is carried out."

Generally, movements that involve total body movement and multilimb movement, such as walking, jumping, swimming, shooting a basketball jump shot, or making a tennis serve are considered "gross" motor skills. Fine motor skills are performed by small muscles, especially of the fingers, hand, and forearm, and frequently involve eye-hand coordination. They involve the manipulation of tools and small objects or the control of machines. Tasks such as typing, sewing, handwriting, piloting an aircraft, or operating a rotary-pursuit apparatus in a psychological laboratory are considered fine motor skills. These latter tasks are also called manual or manipulative skills by some writers.

D. DISCRETE, SERIAL, AND CONTINUOUS SKILLS

Some skills are considered to be "discrete," others are "serial," and others are "continuous." Discrete tasks are characterized by a recognizable beginning and ending. They involve only a single exertion such as shooting an arrow or throwing a baseball. A task is serial in nature when the beginning and ending of components can be identified but events follow each other rapidly, such as in dribbling a basketball; in this task, the push of the ball to the floor repeatedly forms a sequence of movements. Continuous skills are repetitious movements with no clear beginning and ending; running and swimming would be examples.

E. OPEN AND CLOSED SKILLS

Several years ago the British pyschologist, E.C. Poulton (1957), suggested that human skills may be classified as either "open" or "closed," depending on the extent to which a performer must conform to a prescribed standard sequence of movement during execution and the extent to which effective performance depends upon environmental events, and the idea of a continuum from skills which are predominantly habitual through to skills which are predominantly perceptual was advanced by a British physical educator, Barbara Knapp (1961). "Closed" skills are those which require a consistency of movement pattern and are performed under an unchanging environment. A gymnastic routine, a platform dive, a shot put or discus throw is an example of a closed task. On the other hand, "open" skills are externally paced in the sense that they must be done under varying environmental conditions each time they are executed, so they require a flexibility of movement response. A shortstop's throw to the first baseman is always different because the shortstop always fields the ball from a different location on the field. The handball player is never able to use exactly the same movement pattern for two shots. Proficiency in open skills requires a diversification and versatility of movements to meet the demands of the particular task (Fig. 16.1).

sports in which closed skills dominate	sports in which open skills dominate
1. golf	1. soccer
2. diving	2. basketball
3. shot putting	3. baseball
4. gymnastics	4. hockey

Fig. 16.1   Examples of sports in which open or closed skills dominate.

MOTOR SKILL RESEARCH TASKS

There are many questions about motor behavior that are of interest to researchers as well as professionals such as physical educators and coaches. Questions like the effects of certain types of practice schedules, mental practice, incentives, etc. on learning rate or the effects of fatigue, certain drugs, or rewards on performance are some of the types of questions that interest the scholar and the professional. But how can objective answers be obtained? If one wishes to ascertain how certain factors affect motor learning and performance, one is immediately confronted with the problem of how to objectively investigate the question.

There are a number of strategies which could be used. One could ask the performers, but they are a poor source of objective information. One could ask the teachers or coaches, but they, too, are unreliable sources. The investigator could form opinions based on observation, but this, too, has many weaknesses. One could select two individuals or groups and study how the variable one had in mind is manifested as the individual or groups performed, but there is a multitude of factors which might account for any differences which might be observed (even if the observations are precisely qualified). For example: The two groups might have differed in initial skill. Practice trials and practice time might have differed. Environmental conditions might have differed and/or instructions might have differed (assuming instructions were not the variable which was being studied). It may be seen that in all of these situations one or more factors in the study may obscure the factor in which the investigator is interested or may give a distorted view of reality.

In order to make valid and reliable inferences from observations, the investigator must seek a better strategy than any of the above. At the heart of science is the experiment, and the major aspect of the experiment is controlled observation. Experiments in every discipline are typically carried out in a laboratory because the laboratory allows for good experimental control of subjects, good control of observations, and good control of important variables under study.

Systematic control, observation, and isolation of factors are the chief reasons why a great deal of motor learning and performance research is done in the laboratory. Ideally, motor behavior research findings from the laboratory should be verified in the sports settings—the gymnasium, athletic field, or the natatorium. Until this is done, however, principles which explain learning and performance in the laboratory may be extended to serve as guides to the teacher-coach of motor activities. Of course, it should be understood that motor behavior research should not always be expected to result in immediately applicable, practical, and specific implications for the teacher. The study of motor behavior is not just another name for "methods of teaching" although it often does and should play a supportive role.

In conducting controlled laboratory research on motor behavior, it is usually necessary to start the study with subjects who are at an unlearned level. Consequently, it is desirable to use unpracticed and unfamiliar tasks. Most typical sports activities are therefore inappropriate since they do not effectively satisfy the criteria of unpracticed and unfamiliar tasks. Virtually all adolescents and adults have had prior experience with these activities; thus, the movements have already been "learned" to some extent. Therefore, it is customary in the motor learning laboratory to employ so-called novel tasks—tasks that differ from those in the learner's usual repertoire of skills.

Motor behavior research that has employed lower animals as subjects has involved the use of cages or boxes to keep the animals from leaving the experimental area (Fig. 16.2). Mazes of all types have provided learning and performance tasks. Occasionally, animals are mounted in a restraining device which allows for only very restricted types of movements during the experiment. In many cases, the investigators have had to build special equipment for particular species of animal they were using and the particular variables under study.

Motor skill learning and performance research with human subjects has largely been confined to a few laboratory tasks. Some of the earliest and

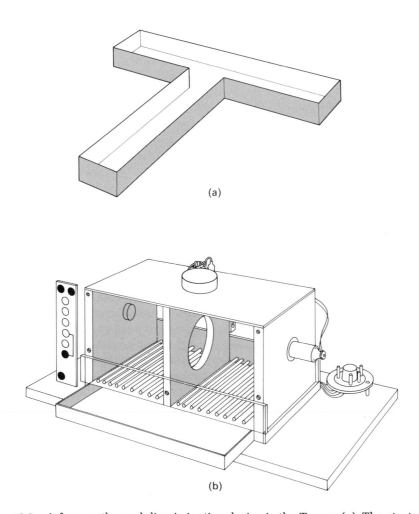

(a)

(b)

Fig. 16.2   A frequently used discrimination device is the T-maze (a). The start box is located at the base of the T, and there are two goal boxes located at the end of each arm. In a shuttle box (b), an animal may move between two compartments. When the cue (either light or sound) is turned on, the subject must move to the other compartment or receive an electric shock.

least sophisticated laboratory tasks which were used in motor behavior work were ball-tossing and juggling tasks. Probably, the most used instrument has been the rotary-pursuit apparatus (Fig. 16.3). This device consists of a turntable in which a round metal plug is embedded near the edge. The subject attempts to keep a metal stylus in contact with the metal plug as the

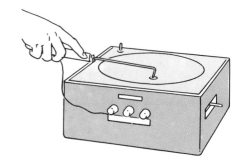

Fig. 16.3 A rotary-pursuit apparatus. The subject attempts to keep the metal stylus on the metal target on the turntable while it is revolving.

turntable rotates. An electric clock measures the amount of time that the stylus is in contact with the plug during a given time trial. As subjects learn to make the correct movements to maintain stylus contact with the plug, their time on target increases. New models of this instrument employ a turntable with a light as the target; the stylus is photosensitive, so when its tip is in contact with the light, the clock is operating. These more elaborate devices allow for automatic timing of the on- and off-target time, variable speed, and direction control of the turntable, and more complex orbital patterns of the target can be used.

Other instruments, such as mirror tracers, complex coordination timers, stabilometers, and the Bachman ladder-climbing apparatus have frequently been used by motor behavior researchers (Figs. 16.4, 16.5, and 16.6). An increasing trend is the use of computerized instrumentation for the conduct of motor behavior laboratory experimentation. The Selective Mathometer, originally designed by Clyde E. Noble in 1952, is now fully automatic. This apparatus is used in human selective learning experiments. All events are automatically recorded by counters and by a continuous, printout recorder (Fig. 16.7).

The highest forms of motor skill involve tasks in which one movement pattern is superimposed upon another pattern, such as shooting a basketball while moving, or throwing a football to a sprinting end. Performances of this kind are extraordinarily complex. Although it would be highly beneficial to study the learning factors of such behavior, only limited work of this kind has been done because of the bewildering technical difficulties involved in controlling and analyzing the stimulus and response variables involved in these situations. So there have been relatively few motor learning studies conducted in dynamic situations such as in the gymnasium, playing field, or swimming pool. Rather, studies have been more concerned with studying variables that cut across many motor tasks and identifying general principles that apply to many specific tasks. Variables such as practice, rest, feedback, motivation, and transfer are examples.

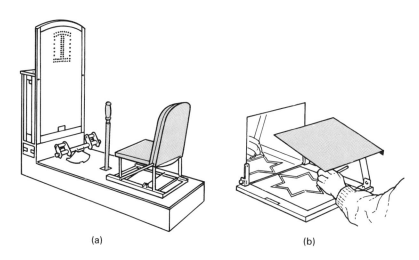

(a)   (b)

Fig. 16.4 (a) Complex coordination instrument. The stick and pedal controls are used by the subject to match a pattern of lights which are displayed to him on the panel. (b) Mirror tracing instrument. The subject traces the outline of a star while looking into the mirror. His hand is blocked from his view.

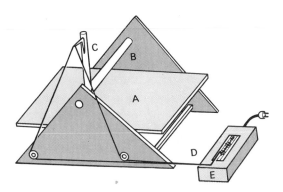

Fig. 16.5 Stabilometer. This instrument consists of a horizontally pivoted board (A) upon which a subject stands with his feet straddling the supporting axle (B). A lever arm (C) is attached to the platform and a cord extends from a needle (D) to a point under the rear pulley, around the rear pulley, to the lever arm where it is attached. A second cord runs from the lever arm around the near pulley and is also attached to the needle. The extent of movement of the platform is recorded on graph paper inserted in an electric kymograph. (Based on Singer, 1965.)

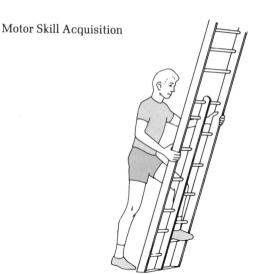

Fig. 16.6 This is a free-standing ladder. The subject climbs as high as possible on each trial until he topples over. Then he begins climbing again. Trials may be timed, i.e., 30 sec. or each attempt to climb may be counted as a trial. The score is the number of rungs climbed in a trial. (Based on Bachman, 1961.)

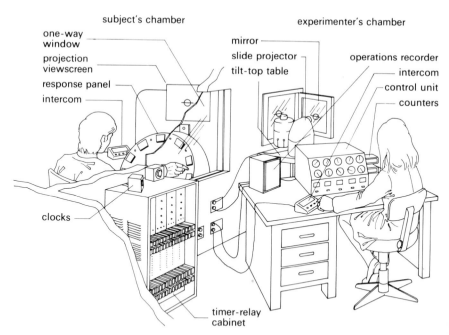

Fig. 16.7 The Selective Mathometer, an instrument for research in human selective learning. (Based on Noble, 1966.)

PERFORMANCE CURVES

The acquisition of a motor skill is typically accompanied by changes in performance, which is the achievement, or score, on a given event. These modifications in performance may be recorded by plotting on a graph the learner's achievement for each successive practice period. The graph is an illustrative method of depicting performance measures over a period of trials and is used to note the trend in performance. Performance curves help to illustrate the effects of such factors as practice, feedback, motivation, and other variables upon learning. These records of performances when published in the motor behavior literature are usually called "learning curves" but a more correct terminology is that of "performance curves," because performance variations do not necessarily reflect the individual's learned capabilities; performance can be affected by temporary conditions such as motivation, fatigue, or distracting environmental conditions.

On performance curve graphs, customarily the horizontal axis shows the units of practice (such as number of trials or the amount of time spent in practice). The vertical axis depicts the performance as measured by some index. These performance indexes may be classified into roughly three types, depending upon what aspect of performance is measured. One type of index is an error index. Here, performance is recorded by errors, and a decrease in the number of errors committed is plotted. A second type is a time index; the decreasing amount of time necessary to perform the task or the increasing time that correct performance occurs is plotted. A third type of index is an accuracy index; some measure of accuracy, such as hitting a target, is plotted. The scores may be recorded in actual scores or in percentage of success, according to a standard of some kind.

A. SHAPES OF PERFORMANCE CURVES

Performance curves which appear in journals or books usually represent scores of a large group of subjects whose performance on each trial has been averaged for the group. The curve formed by this method tends to be rather smooth. This gives the impression that skill acquisition progresses at a regular pace in a highly predictable manner, whereas, in fact, an individual's progress in learning a motor skill is erratic. Figure 16.8 shows a rather typical performance curve as an individual learns a motor skill.

When a large number of performances is averaged, the result is usually a smooth regular curve. Learning curves assume various shapes depending

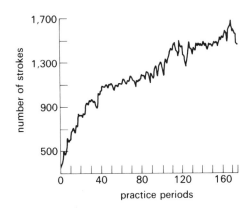

Fig. 16.8   The acquisition of typing skill by one subject. The curve represents 174 consecutive daily half-hour practice periods. The measure of progress in the skill was the total number of correct strokes made on the typewriter each practice session.

on such things as the complexity of the task, practice schedules, feedback, motivation, and other conditions present during the performance (Fig. 16.9). There is no single performance curve. A curve that shows rapid initial improvement, followed by decreasing gains from practice, is called a curve of decreasing returns, or a negatively accelerated curve. This kind of curve usually results when the task is relatively easy and mastery of the movements occurs rapidly. When a curve indicates little improvement initially, then a period of rapid improvement, it is called a curve of increasing returns, or a positively accelerated curve. This kind of curve is typical of a task requiring unique movements that take some time to learn, but once they are learned, performance improves quickly. An S-shaped curve shows little initial improvement followed by a period of rapid improvement and then a decreasing return curve. This S-shaped curve is most likely the continuation of a positively accelerated curve; i.e., practice continues until performance approaches its maximum potential. A linear curve is essentially a straight line. The curves described above refer to learning curves on which correct responses or accuracy are plotted, for they all indicate increasingly adept performances as learning continues. But a curve on which errors is plotted shows a declining characteristic.

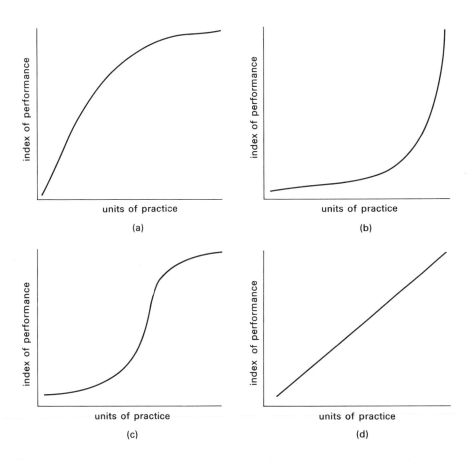

Fig. 16.9   Learning curves. (a) Negatively accelerated curve. (b) Positively accelerated curve. (c) S-shaped curve. (d) Linear curve.

B. PLATEAUS

A curious feature of performance curves that has been the subject of much discussion and debate is the so-called plateau. A plateau is a period during which relatively little improvement in performance takes place. Sometimes a learner reaches a certain level of performance and remains there for some time without much improvement, then again shows improvement. The notion that plateaus are an essential characteristic during skill acquisition was first proposed by Bryan and Harter (1899) in one of the pioneer studies on skill. In their experimental findings on learning to send and receive Morse Code as a function of practice, they discovered that as practice continued the performances seemed to show a "plateau," or level of performance where little or no improvement showed up on the performance curve over many trials. They explained plateaus in this way:

A plateau in the curve means that the lower-order habits are approaching their maximum development, but are not yet sufficiently automatic to leave the attention free to attack the higher-order habits.

The belief in the *essentiality* of plateaus, as proposed by Bryan and Harter, was widely accepted for many years. Even today one hears physical educators and coaches refer to the performance of their students as being "at a plateau." However, subsequent experimentation on the plateau has led some scholars to refer to this phenomenon as the "phantom plateau." In other words, they have not found plateaus to be an *essential* feature of learning. Keller (1958), on the basis of considerable evidence, concluded that a true plateau in skill learning does not exist, and that when such effects are reported they are artifacts of the measure of performance used or of some uncontrolled variable.

Other investigators have found that plateaus may occur during skill learning, under certain conditions. Kao (1937), after a comprehensive study of plateaus in motor learning, reported that plateaus may be due to fatigue, methodological changes adopted by the learner, or discrete changes in the environment, when learning simple skills, Kao suggested that, while learning complex skills, plateaus occur as individuals attempt to construct complex movements from simple patterns.

Plateaus are still a puzzling issue. Although they are definitely not *essential* features of skill learning, they may, and in fact do, occur under certain conditions. There are a variety of factors that result in periods during which there is little or no measurable improvement in performance.

MEASURING MOTOR LEARNING

Motor learning is typically defined as a relatively permanent modification in motor behavior which is a result of practice or experience, and not a result of maturational, motivational, or training factors. Many changes in behavior occur naturally as the individual grows and develops, and certainly behavior may be radically modified as a result of motivational states, but these types of behavioral change are not considered learning. Moreover, training, which involves systematic and progressive alterations in physiological systems that increase, or modify, behavioral capacities, such as strength and endurance, produces changes in behavior but these changes are not considered learning.

Learning cannot be observed directly; it can only be inferred by observing behavior, or performance. It is assumed, of course, that the modification in observable behavior is the result of some change in the nervous system—some biochemical and/or structural change—that now enables the individual to perform in a certain way.

Motor performance, as distinct from motor learning, is the achievement, or score, on a given trial practice period, game, etc. Performance, as everyone knows, can fluctuate due to such factors as motivation, fatigue, boredom, noise, and temperature. Thus, there are many transitory factors which affect performance. It may be seen, then, that learning and performance are not synonymous words. Therefore, distinct methods must be employed in measuring these two phenomena.

A performance curve allows one to make a subjective assessment about learning but other methods are more precise and permit statistical treatment within and between individuals and groups.

There is a variety of methods which have been developed for measuring learning. Each method has certain strengths and weaknesses, and there is currently an active controversy about the "best" method of measuring motor learning. Without going into details on this controversy or trying to suggest a one "best" method, three of the commonly used methods are listed below. All have been used in motor learning research.

Total learning score method.   This method consists of adding all performance scores on all trials, including the initial and final scores.

Difference in raw score method.   The difference in raw score is obtained by subtracting the initial score (typically scores on the first two or three trials) from the final score (typically scores on the last two or three trials). The formula is:

(Sum of last N trials) minus (Sum of first N trials).

N is an arbitrary number of trials, usually two or three.

Percent gain of possible gain method.   In this method, the learning score is computed by dividing the actual gain from the initial score to the final score by the possible gain from the initial to the highest possible score. The formula is:

$$\frac{\text{(Sum of last } N \text{ trials) minus (Sum of first } N \text{ trials).}}{\text{(Highest possible score on } N \text{ trials) minus (Sum of first } N \text{ trials)}}.$$

LIMITS OF MOTOR SKILL ACQUISITION

One topic that has been of considerable interest to motor learning investigators involves the limits of skills acquisition. Do motor skills continue to improve with practice? For how long? Although there are definite limits to the level of proficiency that one may achieve in any particular movement task, this limit is never known and proficiency approaches these limits so slowly that it is difficult to ascertain when individuals have reached their capacity for that task.

Usually several conditions affect the upper limits which one achieves on a motor skill. Frequent and intense practice is usually required in order to continue to improve performance levels; when practices are infrequent or short, performances remain static. Very high levels of skill are not achieved by repetitious, halfhearted practice either. Motivation is one of the most important factors limiting level of motor performance; when motivation wanes, performance is affected accordingly. Improvement in performance at high levels seems to be highly dependent on motivation of the performer. Champion athletes increase their skill because of their interest in their performance, whether for financial or personal reasons. There are certainly other factors which might be identified, such as aging, lack of feedback or standards of mastery, but practice schedules and motivation are certainly two of the most critical factors affecting ultimate skill level.

A. EVIDENCE FOR PROLONGED PERIODS OF SKILL IMPROVEMENT

Several investigators have shown that skills can be improved almost indefinitely. Snoddy (1926), using mirror drawing as the motor task, had subjects trace with a pencil a star-shaped path while watching their writing hand in a mirror. During the experiment, the subjects were given one trail a day for a period of 60 days, and the performance score was based on time and errors. Snoddy plotted the logarithm of performance against the logarithm of trials on a graph in order to show the relatively slow performance changes after protracted practice. The results clearly show that improvement in performance occurred during the entire experiment of 60 days of practice. The findings also showed that the rate of improvement declined over time (Fig. 16.10).

Even in simple motor tasks such as typing, telegraphy, and assembly line work, performance continues to improve, sometimes over millions of practice trials. Crossman (1959) found continued improvement of performance from subjects whose practice on a fine motor skill extended over several years. The subjects were operators of hand-operated, cigar-making machines. The speed of performance on this task improved for up to four years and only leveled off because the cycle time of the machine set a limit on the rate of work that was possible (Fig. 16.11). Crossman concluded that speed of performance in simple motor tasks increases gradually and continuously for many practice trials, providing that motivation for speed is maintained.

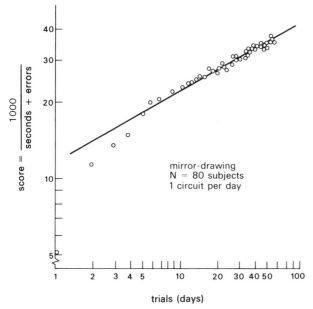

Fig. 16.10 Gradual improvement in mirror-tracing with long practice. (Based on Snoddy, 1926.)

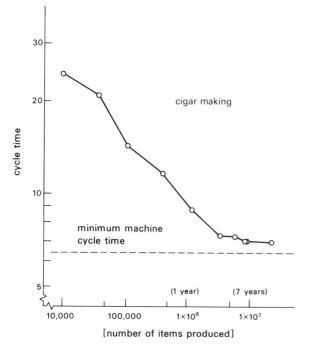

Fig. 16.11 Performance on a fine motor task over a prolonged period of time. (Based on Crossman, 1959.)

Further evidence for the continued improvement of performance in motor skills comes from case histories of championship performers in various sports. In order to reach performance levels to compete successfully in national or international sports events, many years of intensive practice are usually necessary. The typical Olympic figure skater, skier, or fencer has intensively practiced the sport for at least ten years. Professional golfers or bowlers have many years of amateur competition behind them before they can survive as professionals. The successful modern dancer or ballerina usually has been in constant practice since early childhood. When performance does level off, it seems to be due to loss of motivation, or in some cases, the effects of aging rather than the reaching of a true limit in capacity for further improvement (Fitts, 1964).

RETENTION AND FORGETTING

The distinction between acquisition and retention stages of motor learning is that the acquisition phase is the time or trials needed to attain a certain level of proficiency, while the retention is the "savings" of proficiency after a period of no practice. Retention is the persistence of proficiency on a skill following periods without practice, and what is retained is called memory. Typically, retention of motor skills is measured after considerable lapses of time between practice—anywhere from a day or so to several years—but retention intervals from a few seconds to minutes have been used in motor behavior laboratories.

Most motor skills, such as sports and industrial skills, are learned with the intention of performing them at a later time. Athletic contests and assembly line performance are examples of occasions in which the retention of skills learned during prior practice is demanded. Thus, instructors of motor skills, as well as learners, must be concerned with retention as well as acquisition during motor learning.

As noted in Chapter 9, memory of previous events, including verbal and motor skills, may be divided into short-term memory and long-term memory. The focus of the presentation in Chapter 9 was on short-term memory—its characteristics and processes. In this chapter our focus will be on long-term memory, which usually is examined under the conceptual rubric of retention. Whereas, most experimental designs for the study of short-term retention involve one or a very few trials, a brief period (fractions of a second to several seconds) of no practice, and then a "recall" of the task, studies of long-term memory retention typically involve considerable practice of the task until some proficiency has been obtained, then a period of no practice (the retention interval), and finally, recall of the task. Thus, long-term memory is concerned with well-learned tasks that presumably have become consolidated into structural changes in the nervous system.

A. MEASUREMENT OF RETENTION

There are two principal methods for measuring retention: recognition and recall. The recognition method is rarely used in motor skill retention studies but is frequently used in paper-and-pencil tests of verbal materials. The multiple-choice question is an example of the use of recognition to measure verbal retention. When recall is used for measuring retention, there are two techniques which have customarily been employed in motor skills work. The first is called the "percent-of-gain" technique. Here retention is assessed after a period of no practice and is recorded as a percentage of the proficiency level just before the retention interval. The proficiency level before the retention level is considered to be 100 percent and the proficiency after the no-practice period is a percentage of original learning. If performers were able to hit a target 10 times out of 10 tries before the retention interval and 8 times out of 10 tries after it, their retention was 80 percent.

A second technique for measuring recall retention is called the "savings" technique and it involves tabulating the number of trials the learner requires to reach a certain level of proficiency, the criterion level; then after the retention interval the number of trials is counted which are required for the learner to again reach the criterion level of proficiency. The difference between the original level and the retention trials is considered the retention "savings." Using this technique, if a learner required 100 trials to attain the criterion of 10 target hits out of 10 tries, and then required 40 trials after the retention interval, the savings is 60 trials, or 60 percent.

B. RETENTION OF MOTOR SKILLS

Numerous writers have noted that motor skills, once learned, are remarkably resistant to being forgotten. Once a person has learned to swim, ride a bicycle, or throw a ball, these skills can be performed again even after years without practice. Furthermore, although long intervals without practice may produce some decrement in performance, this can often be overcome with a few practice trials. Thus, it is commonly thought that motor skills are retained better than verbal tasks, but an exact comparison cannot be made between a motor task and a verbal task because it is virtually impossible to equate them for difficulty. Moreover, it is impossible to ascertain how much learning on one task corresponds to a certain level of learning on the other task. Thus, it is difficult to conclude that motor skills are remembered best, although the few studies that have attempted to ascertain this relationship found that memory for the motor tasks was better than for verbal or procedural tasks (Mengelkoch, Adams, and Gainer, 1971).

Motor skill retention has been the subject of numerous investigations over the years. Most studies report little or no forgetting even over extended intervals of no practice, and the small decreases in performance that did occur were regained rapidly. Although the motor skills used in many of these studies have been tracking or procedural skills, the sparse research on gross motor tasks corroborates the findings from these other tasks.

Jahnke and Duncan (1956) investigated retention, using a rotary-pursuit task, for intervals of time ranging from ten minutes to four weeks. They found no evidence whatever of forgetting; indeed, with some retention intervals there was improvement in performance. Fleishman and Parker (1962) studied retention on a complex tracking task for intervals from one to 14 months, and they reported "virtually no loss in skill regardless of the retention interval." Their findings support conclusions of other studies on motor skill retention.

Several investigations of gross motor skill retention have been reported. Purdy and Lockhart (1962) investigated retention on ball toss, foot volley, and bongo-board balance skills and found essentially the same pattern of retention as that reported for fine motor tasks. Ninety-four percent of the subjects' best performance was retained after one year, and rapid relearning occurred for those who showed retention deficits. Meyers (1967), using the Bachman ladder climbing task, found no significant loss in retention for layoff periods varying from 10 minutes to 13 weeks. Ryan (1962) found that retention was high for both rotary-pursuit and stabilometer tasks up to 20 days, although the pattern of retention was not the same for both skills. In a subsequent experiment, Ryan (1965) tested for retention on a stabilometer task after 3 months, 6 months, and 12 months. He found significant loss on the first trial of the retest by all three groups, with the 12-month group suffering the most loss of proficiency. Relearning was rapid, however, with the 12-month group requiring more trials to regain their initial proficiency. Melnick (1971) reported that each of four groups that had originally practiced to a criterion level of proficiency on the stabilometer "saved" over 50 percent of the trials they spent in attaining the learning criterion on retention trials one month after the original learning; a group that had considerably overlearned the task had a savings score of 97.5 percent.

Why are motor skills retained so well? Two explanations are usually proposed for this extremely good retention: First, motor skills are generally very well learned and therefore well retained. Many practice trials are often necessary to attain proficiency, and then each time the skill is used, this constitutes a practice trial. Thus, each time bicyclists ride their bicycles or tennis players serve, they are practicing the skill. Second, in the retention interval, very few new responses are developed that would interfere with the original skill. After bicyclists stop regular riding, they learn many things but few things that would directly interfere with the pedaling, balancing, and steering necessary to ride a bicycle. Thus, subsequent motor experiences typically do not interfere with a previously learned skill.

While there is an abundance of evidence that many motor skills are retained quite well even after prolonged periods of no practice, some investigators have found that certain motor skills are poorly retained (Adams and Hufford, 1962; Bilodeau and Levy, 1964; Lersten, 1969). Thus, when these latter findings are considered, there are wide differences in the retention characteristics of motor skills. Schmidt (1972) analyzed tasks which have been used in the motor retention studies and noted that those tasks which are well retained tend not to be dependent upon cognitive decisions concerning what to do but rather are concerned with making well-defined movements correctly and quickly. More recently, Schmidt (1975) has noted that:

. . . tasks that show the greatest retention are continuous tracking tasks and those that show the poorest retention are serial manipulative tasks; discrete tasks appear to be approximately intermediate in retention.

Several reasons have been advanced to explain why continuous tasks are retained better than serial or discrete: Continuous tasks are more highly overlearned than the other types, discrete tasks are similar to verbal tasks because they have a heavy cognitive component, memory traces for continuous tasks are typically more meaningful, allowing the learner to utilize principles and relationships from prior learnings (Schmidt, 1972; Stelmach, 1974).

C. EFFECT OF CERTAIN VARIABLES ON MOTOR SKILL RETENTION

Just as with skill acquisition, the amount of retention and its persistence are dependent on a variety of factors. Some of the most prominent are degree of proficiency attained during original learning, meaningfulness of the task, interval between original learning and retention measurement, nature of the task, practice schedule under which original learning occurred.

Several investigators have indicated that the most important factor in the retention of a motor skill is the level of proficiency achieved during the initial learning period. Fleishman and Parker (1962) found a near linear relationship between the degree of proficiency attained during initial learning and the amount of proficiency retention following intervals of 9 to 25 months of no practice. Purdy and Lockhart (1962) reported that the higher the initial level of skill on several gross motor skills, the greater the retention. They found that after one year of no practice as much as 94 percent of original proficiency was retained. As noted above, Melnick (1971) found some relationship between amount of overlearning and retention on the stabilometer.

For verbal tasks the interval between original learning and the retention testing is a powerful factor in retention; forgetting of verbal materials is most rapid immediately after the cessation of practice and then is less pronounced with time. Motor skill retention does not follow the same pattern. As noted above, in many cases there is little or no forgetting over long periods of time. Bilodeau (1969) summarized the findings on motor skill retention by saying:

In summarizing, over a period of several decades in the investigation of training and retraining of skills involving continuous responding, we find insufficient forgetting to cast up a forgetting curve.

Several studies have shown that meaningful tasks are remembered better than meaningless tasks. Naylor and Briggs (1961) found that motor tasks which were arranged in an organized sequence were remembered better than arbitrarily arranged tasks.

The effects of interference of competing skills seem to differ between verbal and motor skills. While interference seems to strongly influence verbal retention, it does not affect motor skill retention as dramatically. However, there have been very few motor skill studies in which potentially interfering variables in motor retention have been studied. At the present time the experimental literature is too incomplete to make any definitive statements.

A serial position effect on retention has been consistently found for verbal materials. When subjects learn a list of items in their correct order, typically the first few and the last few items are retained best, with the items in the middle of the list least retained. Little study of the serial position effect has been made with motor skills. Cratty (1963) reported findings that were similar to those of verbal studies but Singer (1968) failed to obtain the serial effect.

Research on the effects of distributed versus massed practice schedules on retention has yielded ambiguous results. Several investigators have reported retention effects to be better under distributed schedules, while others have found no retention differences in the two practice schedules. An occasional researcher has found retention to be better after massed schedules. Singer (1965) reported that massed and relatively massed practice conditions yielded significantly better retention results than the distributed condition one month after the last practice. It seems that the task and the specific research strategy which is used in a study must be important to retention when different practice schedules are compared, but distributed schedules have been found to be better for retention for most tasks.

Numerous other variables have been studied with regard to their effect on retention. This literature is too extensive to report here. None of the other variables has been demonstrated to have more unequivocal influence on retention than the variables discussed above. There is one old and interesting study that has never really been followed up but should be. Zeigarnik (1927, trans. 1938) found that whether or not a task had been completed appeared to influence its recall. She allowed her subjects to complete some of the assigned tasks while interrupting the completion of others and discovered that retention was better for the interrupted than the completed tasks. She argued that tensions set up during performances of a task persist if the task is uncompleted and therefore facilitate retention. This is called the "Zeigarnik effect."

B. THEORIES OF FORGETTING

One may ask the question: Why is there any forgetting at all? Why should not skills be retained at a certain level regardless of how much time intervenes between performances? The two basic theories of forgetting are the "trace decay" and the "interference" theories. The former assumes that passage of time causes a regression or weakening of memory traces; that is, if you do not practice basketball shooting, you will forget how just from lack of practice. The idea here is that whatever structural modifications occurred in the nervous system during learning decay when practice is not continued to maintain the modifications.

The most powerful opposition to the "trace decay" theory has come from "interference" theory, which has been and remains the most influential theory of forgetting. Interference theorists argue that forgetting occurs because of competition among responses. In other words, learning some things tends to make one forget others. For example, learning tennis skills might interfere with the movement patterns built up for basketball shooting skills. Basically, most of the behavioral research on interference is supported by data obtained in experiments on transfer of learning. Transfer is the effect of learning one task upon the learning of a second, and interference theory suggests that forgetting occurs as a result of interference from learning other things. The interfering activity can occur before the main task is learned in which case it is called proactive interference, or it can occur between learning the original task and the retention test, in which case it is called retroactive interference.

As noted earlier in this chapter, very few studies have explored the effects of interference on motor skill retention. It is not even clear whether the interference effects are similar for motor skill retention. There is some controversy on this issue (Schmidt, 1971).

REMINISCENCE

The passage of time does not always lead to a diminution of performance when practice is resumed; indeed, it may result in a higher level of performance than existed at the end of the last practice. This phenomenon of an increase in performance after a period of no practice is called reminiscence. Hilgard (1957) defined reminiscence as:

. . .a psychological term for the occasional rise in the curve of retention before it falls; that is, when under some circumstances more may be retained after an interval than immediately upon completion of learning.

Ballard (1911–1913) is usually given credit for first isolating reminiscence. He reported that children, while memorizing a poem, could recite more of the poem on the day following study of the poem than immediately after they had studied it. Since Ballard's report, reminiscence has been found on a wide variety of verbal and motor tasks, using rest intervals from a few minutes to up to a year after the last practice trial. In addition to the basic finding, these studies rather consistently show that reminiscence is inversely related to the degree of original learning. They also show that gross motor skills seem to yield greater reminiscence over longer intervals of time than verbal materials.

A. REMINISCENCE AND MOTOR SKILLS

The majority of investigations on reminiscence in motor learning have used the rotary-pursuit apparatus. Irion (1949), Ammons (1947), and Kimble (1949) are only a few investigators who have published studies showing reminiscence using the rotary pursuit.

Very few studies of reminiscence have been done in which the learning of sports skill was involved. Fox and Young (1962) studied reminiscence in two badminton skills (a wall volley and short-serve task) using nonpractice periods of six weeks and twelve weeks. Reminiscence did occur on one of the skills but did not occur on the other. Fox and Lamb (1962) tested for reminiscence of softball skills after five weeks of no practice (first retest) and 17 weeks after the first retest. There was no significant reminiscence for the first nonpractice interval but there was significant reminiscence for the second nonpractice interval. They concluded that for softball skills reminiscence did occur during a long interval without practice.

3. THEORIES OF REMINISCENCE

Several psychologists have presented a theoretical basis for reminiscence, but there is no unanimity of opinion with regard to its explanation. Reminiscence has been frequently interpreted in terms of Clark Hull's (1943) inhibition theory, which postulates two types of inhibition in every learning situation. The first of these is an inhibition (reactive inhibition) caused by a reluctance to repeat a response—an inhibition to further activity of the sort demanded by a specific task. And the greater the work demanded by a task, or the more often the task is continuously repeated, the greater the inhibition. A second type of inhibition (conditioned inhibition) is that which becomes conditioned to the stimuli associated with the task. For Hull, both types of inhibition restrict performance. Rest allows recovery from the first type of inhibition and this causes improved performance. A more extended discussion of inhibition theory is found in Chapter 19.

In an attempt to explain certain criticisms of inhibition theory as an explanation of reminiscence, Eysenck (1965) has proposed a revision and extension of it. The main feature of Eysenck's theory is the employment of consolidation memory theory. Eysenck suggests that improved performance results from a consolidation of previous learning and from the recovery of performance which has been depressed by the accumulation of inhibition. With regard to the consolidation theory, he proposes that performance sets up cortical events which, in order to become available to the performer as *learned behavior*, require a rest period during which they consolidate. Eysenck recognizes that the theory does not apply to well-learned tasks, where reactive inhibition may still theoretically be responsible for deterioration of performance and dissipation of inhibition for reminiscence. Moreover, he notes that it is possible for certain tasks to contain elements of both consolidation and inhibition, so that reminiscence could be partly due to consolidation and partly to inhibition, and that these parts could differ from person to person, depending on ability, degree of practice, arousal, etc.

17

Organizational Features and Phases of Motor Skill Acquisition

Motor skill acquisition involves the development of several organizational features, and learners typically go through several distinct phases as they acquire a motor skill. In this chapter we shall examine these organizational characteristics and the phases of motor skill acquisition.

ORGANIZATIONAL FEATURES OF MOTOR LEARNING

Although there are undoubtedly numerous subtle organizational processes, three general features are prominent: hierarchical organization, spatial organization, and temporal organization.

A. HIERARCHICAL ORGANIZATION

Skilled movement patterns are hierarchically organized. The word "hierarchy" implies that certain "higher" structures have "overall" responsibilities for the functions of the entire system, with other "lower" structures serving subordinant roles in carrying out specific functions. It has already been noted that the nervous system may be viewed as a hierarchical system, with the lowest levels in the peripheral and spinal cord areas and the higher centers in the brain. Each level may act independently of other levels, but this is normally not the case; thus, behavior initiated by the higher centers usually requires activity of the lower centers for its completion. There is, therefore, some anatomical support for the notion of hierarchical organization of motor skills.

Fitts and Posner (1967) suggest that hierarchical organization of motor skills may be viewed as analogous to programs which govern the operation of electronic computers. The operation of such systems is governed by an "executive" and subroutines. The executive provides overall logical and decision framework to the system, provides flexible and adaptive characteristics for it, and regulates the execution of subroutines. The subroutines of the executive are fixed sequences which may be utilized as units of the overall operation, and they may be repetitious until a given point is reached or until stopped by the controlling executive. Thus, in executing a motor task, the overall movement pattern is accomplished in the context of an overall plan. The purpose of the task may be viewed as the executive; and various component parts of the task, such as leg movements and arm or finger movements, make up the subroutines. Typically, skill learning consists of reorganizing and repatterning subroutines learned from prior experiences, and using them in the new task.

The hypothesized mechanism which actually produces the effector impulses to the muscles for a movement pattern is called a "motor program." This mechanism has been discussed extensively in other chapters; therefore, little will be said about it here. Once the executive, including the various subroutines, orders a motor program, it is executed faithfully. When the movement is finished, the consequences of the action are fed back to the executive for analysis of the effectiveness of the orders. This feedback information becomes the basis for future orders by the executive.

In the beginning of learning a motor skill, the executive relies heavily upon previously learned tasks in ordering the execution of motor commands. Orders tend to be brief and incomplete, making movements "jerky" and inefficient; but as the executive obtains feedback, motor programs tend to become more complete and appropriate for task accomplishment. These programs then produce smoother and more efficient and effective movement patterns. Since the executive commands become more elaborate, producing longer and longer movement sequences, the executive has only to occasionally monitor the actions, thus freeing itself to perform other tasks during movement.

The results of a study by Pew (1966) nicely illustrate the apparent development of hierarchical control of a task as learning occurs. In Pew's study, subjects were seated before a screen on which a moving dot was displayed. The subjects' task was to keep the dot centered on the screen. A button depressed by the right hand accelerated the dot to the right while the left-hand button, when depressed, accelerated the dot to the left. At first, subjects pressed one button or the other and waited for the dot to move so that they could see the displacement that was occurring; then they pressed the other button to correct the error. This strategy produced jerky movements and was largely unsuccessful in maintaining the dot in the center of the screen. As practice continued, the subjects adopted a new strategy. They pressed the buttons quite rapidly in alternation at a rate of about eight per second. The rate of pressing a single button seemed to be altered about every second, depending upon the location of the dot, suggesting that the subjects were emitting a motor program of about eight or so presses, then monitoring the error and correcting it with a new program.

Pew suggests that in the early learning the executive was fragmentary and corrected after each response. But in the later stages of learning, the executive programmed longer response sequences which had to be modified only after they had run off.

B. SPATIAL ORGANIZATION OF MOTOR LEARNING

Another organizational characteristic of learning a motor task is spatial organization. Spatial organization refers to the fact that the appropriate muscles must be selected to efficiently and effectively perform a motor skill. Skeletal muscles produce all of the voluntary movements of the body. A single muscle is made of thousands of individual muscle fibers. When stimulated by motorneurons, the muscle fibers contract, producing movement. Each muscle and each combination of muscles produces different movement effects when stimulated.

A motor skill is executed to accomplish a specific goal and in order for it to do this, specific muscles must contract while others relax or the correct movement pattern will not appear for task accomplishment. With practice, and the feedback which accompanies practice, an organization of correct muscular responses gradually emerges, making goal accomplishment possible. Thus, spatial organization is achieved.

C. TEMPORAL ORGANIZATION OF MOTOR LEARNING

Temporal organization refers to the fact that muscle contraction or relaxation must occur at the appropriate time. Skillful performance implies that there is a smoothness or "dovetailing" of connections from one component of a movement pattern to the next. For example, the components of a tennis serve must be executed in consecutive order with a certain timing for each for an effective serve. Movements of the legs, shoulders, arms, and wrist must be brought into play in a prescribed sequence and time. If they are not, an awkward, ineffective movement pattern results. Lashley (1951) very articulately described the importance of temporal organization in motor tasks in the following remark.

Temporal integration is not found exclusively in language; the coordination of leg movements in insects, the song of birds, the control of trotting and pacing in a gaited horse, the rat running a maze . . . and the carpenter sawing a board present a problem of sequences of action . . . .

Bartlett (1958) noted that the crucial point in the linkage of receptor and effector functions " . . . is the accurate timing of the constituent items within their series." Several investigators have demonstrated that timing is important in the learning of motor skills, particularly where serial muscle contractions or movement sequences are involved (Provins and Glencross, 1968; Glencross, 1970).

PHASES OF ACQUISITION OF MOTOR SKILL

Assuming that skill learning does depend on features of hierarchical, spatial, and temporal organization, we may now examine the phases of learning that tend to be involved in the acquisition of motor skills. But first it should be noted that skill learning is a continuous process and it is a mistake to assume independent and distinct phases in skill learning. There are gradual shifts in the movement patterns of skills, and in the nature of the processes employed, as learning progresses. The movement pattern is gradually organized into larger units and toward hierarchical organization. Thus, there are "general" changes during skill learning which may be identified. The typical changes which occur as one acquires a skill are a reduction in errors, improvement in accuracy, improvement in rate, reduction in overall muscular tension, smoothness of performance, greater consistency of performance, greater freedom from the effects of distractions, and a decreased feeling of effort.

Fitts (1965) identified three phases of skill learning: An early or cognitive phase, an intermediate or associative phase, and a final or autonomous phase. These phases were derived from a study by Alfred Smode, who interviewed physical educators and coaches and asked them questions about the acquisition of sports skills.

A. EARLY OR COGNITIVE PHASE IN MOTOR LEARNING

In most skill learning situations, Fitts asserts, the beginner must first come to "understand" the task and its demands. Three broad aspects of understanding are (1) The goal of the task, (2) The movements which will bring about accomplishment of the goal, and (3) The "strategy" which will work best to produce the desired movements. It may be seen, then, that the learning of a skill does not begin when actual practice starts but before with a cognitive understanding of the motor task.

The learner must construct an executive program, or cognitive map, for task accomplishment, based upon the goal. The notion that motor learning involves the formation of some cognitive plan or map has been proposed by several learning theorists. Tolman (1948) proposed the formation of cognitive maps while Miller and his colleagues (1960) used the word "plans" to refer to this initial cognitive structuring.

From a learning and teaching standpoint, the way in which the learner constructs a cognitive map or executive program is important, and learners who have difficulty forming an accurate plan of what is required will not be able to achieve the desired results, regardless of how much they practice. Many failures to learn are due to failures to perceive, or comprehend, what has to be learned, rather than any difficulty of registering or holding material in memory.

The cognitive phase of motor learning may be accomplished in a few moments or a few weeks, depending upon such factors as the complexity of the task, prior experience with similar tasks, perceptual abilities, frequency of practice, and so forth.

To summarize, in the cognitive phase the learner arrives at an overall understanding of the task and develops a cognitive map of the movements that are most likely to accomplish the goal. It is during this state that stimulus selection and discrimination are taking place and perceptual cues are being developed for that particular task. There is, then, a perceptual organization from which the elaboration of the "motor image" or representation of the movement proceeds, and the movement pattern is performed with more or less conscious attention to the details of the execution.

In this phase, learners seem to organize the new movement task by reference to similar patterns within their repertoire of prior learned skills, which usually produces a sequence of successive approximations starting with unnecessarily gross and effortful movements, many times involving the entire body. It is during this stage when various forms of instructions to the learners are most effective. Although an instructor may communicate the general strategy that should be used, it remains for the learners to supply the detailed tactics of using individual muscle groups for carrying out the "Plan" with their own muscles.

1. Instructional techniques

An instructor is certainly not necessary for an individual who wishes to learn a motor skill and, indeed, many motor skills which each of us has acquired have been learned without the presence of an instructor, usually in a laborious trial-and-error manner. However, skills can be learned more expediently with effective instruction, and one of the key contributions of a capable instructor is to enhance the learning rate and the ultimate proficiency level of a learner.

There are three basic means through which instruction in movement may be communicated to the learner: visually, auditorially, and manually (Lockhart, 1966). Each has unique contributions to make, and each may be more or less effective with different learners. Moreover, the task to be learned may lend itself to employment of one or the other of these communication channels.

It is generally accepted that some form of demonstration is the most direct and economical technique of communicating the task to the learner, although it is possible, of course, for many skills to be learned without demonstration, if verbal models are substituted. A demonstration provides a "visual model"—a model that can be internalized into a cognitive plan of action.

In some cases, a demonstration may be done through the use of loop films or videotapes. The amount of information can be controlled this way and the information can be repeated as often as the learner seems to need it. Observational learning studies have demonstrated that visual observation of another's performance facilitates the learning of skills (Bandura, 1965). These findings are most directly interpreted as indicating that visual images of performance acquired during the observation experience enhance subsequent performance.

Bandura and Walters (1963) found that more skillful demonstration models motivate increased imitation by learners as well as direct more attentional processes toward the model's behavior. They suggested that models who have demonstrated high competence, who are purported experts, who demonstrate a high level of ability, and who possess status-conferring symbols are more likely to command attention and serve as more influential sources of behavior than models who lack these qualities. In a recent study, Landers and Landers (1973) reported that a demonstration model does facilitate and enhance acquisition of behavior responses, particularly in the initial stage. It seems, then, that demonstrations should be performed as well as possible even though a beginner will not be able to perceive all of the details nor be able to imitate a demonstration in detail in the initial practice trials.

Although there is little experimental work on the speed, or tempo, at which a demonstration should be performed, many writers suggest that the demonstration should be given at performance speed. Robb (1972) suggests that if the objective of the demonstration is to show the sequence of the movement pattern, the demonstrator should emphasize that the learners "look for" this sequence. Slowing down the tempo of the demonstration may be helpful in this case. But when the spatial and temporal organization is being emphasized, a demonstration of normal speed seems appropriate.

In addition to the visual information supplied by the instructor, it appears that visual information provided by practice itself is a valuable modality for early learning. Fitts (1951) suggested that early motor learning is primarily under visual control. According to him, vision is the major error-correcting mechanism used by the individual; as errors in performance become smaller, the appropriate "feel" or proprioceptive cues may become more prominent for error correcting. Rock and Harris (1967) have shown rather decisively that the initial phase of motor skill learning is primarily under visual control. In a recent study by Stallings (1968) examining the relationship of visualization, visual-spatial orientation, and perceptual speed to performance of two gross motor tasks at successive stages of learning, visual-spatial orientation was related to the learning of a two-handed ball pass during the early learning stages. Earlier factor analytic studies by Fleishman and his colleagues, (Fleishman and Hempel, 1954; Fleishman and Rich, 1963), found that spatial orientation and visualization abilities were highly important in the initial stages of learning coordination tracking tasks. The researchers concluded that the learner with a greater capacity for utilizing visual information will make more rapid progress in the early learning stages.

Auditory communication with learners may be supplied by two sources: the instructor and the learners themselves. Verbalization of skills by instructors is perhaps the most used and abused mode for transmitting information, especially to the beginner. Lockhart (1966) asserts, "The beneficial effects of verbal directions decrease in proportion to the amount given!" Not only is there a tendency for instructors to overdo verbal descriptions but there is also some evidence that a great deal of the verbalization is not related to task objectives. Schwartz (1972) analyzed statements made by 15 teachers during instruction and found that only 1.3 percent of the more than 2000 statements made were related to the objective of the lesson.

While verbal description has a place in assisting the learner to develop a cognitive map, there is little evidence that it is very effective in facilitating learning. There are several factors that have to be considered with regard to the amount of verbalization, such as the complexity of the skill, maturity of the learners, and comprehension level of the learners. Nevertheless, verbalization is well suited for directing attention to specific aspects of the task, helping to establish a learning set, giving feedback, and motivating learning (Lockhart, 1966).

Motor skill learners may verbalize with themselves in several ways. They may actually describe what they are attempting to do before practicing, they may talk themselves through a performance, and they may verbally provide feedback to themselves after a performance. Adams (1971) indicates that the first practice trials in learning a task involve verbal-cognitive analysis. That is, the learners verbally discuss with themselves or aloud what they are to do and then verbalize what they have done. This allows the learners to arrive at a conceptualization, or plan, of the task to be learned. Lockhart (1966) summarized several studies which showed that various forms of learner verbalization tended to facilitate learning.

Manually guiding learners through a motor skill is a potential medium for helping them achieve a cognitive map of the task. This form of communication is called manual guidance. The few studies in which this technique has been employed are conflicting in their findings, but motor skill manuals are filled with various suggestions of where to employ this technique: only in the early learning stages, with slow learners rather than fast learners, with young students, etc. These suggestions are merely speculations rather than conclusions based on experimental findings.

Since there is no evidence that manual guidance actually *hinders* motor learning, perhaps the best generalization is that it may be used as a last resort when learners lack confidence to perform on their own, when they are having difficulty developing a cognitive map through other communication media, or when they are visually or auditorially restricted.

In addition to actually communicating with the learner, the instructor has the critical task during the initial stage of learning to direct the learner's attention to a limited and specific set of stimuli. If the learner's attention is not directed to appropriate stimuli, communication of any other kind will be ineffective. Thus, one of the requirements of good motor skills teachers is that they know which information within the sensory display is worth attending to. For example, they may instruct learners to "keep their eyes on the ball" because they think that this is the most important source of information in the display. If learners are instructed to attend to a certain stimulus, then their attention will tend to be directed toward it.

The typical motor learning environment—the gymnasium, playing field, swimming pool, etc.—has an enormous amount of distracting stimuli; with so many stimuli, it is not unusual for learners to have difficulty understanding directions and demonstrations by instructors. A major function for the instructor is to help the learners attend to the relevant information if they are to develop a cognitive map.

With regard to selective attention, then, it is the instructor's responsibility to reduce the amount of irrelevant stimuli in a learning situation so the student will be free to concentrate attention on the relevant stimuli. Then as skill improves, the number of irrelevant stimuli may be increased until the situation becomes quite natural, or gamelike. One technique which the instructor might use when it is not possible to reduce the irrelevant stimuli is to call the student's attention to what to look for—to point out which stimuli are relevant. It has been substantiated by Schlesinger (1954) that individuals vary in their abilities to distinguish the relevant from the irrelevant and maintain an attentive set. Individual differences of this kind, then, should be recognized by the instructor.

One method of directing attention and limiting stimuli is for instructors to present the general movement demands rather than the details of the movements in their initial communications to the learner. As the learner practices and becomes more adroit, the details of the task and the tactics associated with its use may be added gradually.

With practice, and as the executive program becomes more consolidated, less attention needs to be given to the movement pattern itself. Welford (1968) notes:

...*practice seems to enable the skilled performer to select from among the mass of data impinging on his sense organs so that he neglects much of what is, to an unskilled person, striking, and reacts strongly to data that a normal observer would fail to notice.*

As noted in earlier chapters, there is good evidence that learners have limited information-processing capabilities. Therefore, the amount and speed with which material is presented to learners should be carefully controlled. Otherwise they will be unable to process the instructional information. Beginners who are given an elaborate explanation on how to execute a skill and who are asked to watch the details of a demonstration at the same time may not process all the information simply because they are not capable of doing this.

To suggest that feedback is essential in the early stage of learning would be to state the obvious. The topic of feedback has appeared in several earlier chapters and will also be the subject of Chapter 20. Therefore, the only statement that needs to be made at this point is that the instructor who can motivate learners to practice diligently with the intention of improving will be enhancing the learning rate of the learner.

B. ASSOCIATED OR INTERMEDIATE PHASE OF MOTOR LEARNING

Fitts's (1965) second phase of skill learning is characterized as a period during which the movement pattern begins to fuse into a well-coordinated movement pattern. Spatial (correct body segments are employed for best mechanical advantage) and temporal organization becomes "fixed," and the executive program becomes more fully developed. Components of the movement pattern which were independent at first become fused and integrated as the temporal aspects of the task are refined. Extraneous movements are eliminated; gross errors gradually attenuated.

Bahrick, Nobel, and Fitts (1954) showed that proprioceptive feedback becomes increasingly important after extended motor learning and there is less reliance on visual cues as learning of a motor task progresses. As learning of a first task progressed, a second visual motor task had less and less interfering effects on the first task, providing the first task was highly coherent and highly overpracticed. Fleishman and Rich (1963) also found that kinesthetic sensitivity became increasingly important as learning a two-handed, target-tracking task progressed.

The length of time this phase lasts will vary considerably. In learning a skill such as serving a tennis ball, some novices may show rapid improvement while others flounder along without improvement for a long time before their performance improves appreciably. Such factors as prior experience with similar skills, complexity of the skill, practice schedules, teaching methods, feedback, and motivation of the learner will determine the length of this phase of skill learning.

1. Instructional techniques

The instructor should know enough about the component parts of the skill being taught to be able to identify movement errors and prescribe corrections. This role of "movement diagnostician" and "movement prescriptor" is at the heart of teaching motor activities, and the ability to correctly and precisely identify movement errors and communicate accurate instructions for corrective actions is the mark of a competent instructor.

Since the proficiency of a group of learners may become more heterogeneous as they practice, it behooves instructors to increasingly individualize their instruction. Close observation of individual learners will enable instructors to identify individual problems and prescribe corrections.

Tasks such as organizing practice schedules, providing feedback, and motivating learners are all important instructional tasks during this phase, and each will be discussed in later chapters.

The same communication media that were available and useful during the cognitive phase may be employed at this phase. Demonstrations are especially useful at this stage for showing tactics if the skill is to be used in a game. In addition, learners may serve as their own demonstrators via the replay of their performance on film or videotape.

As learning progresses, verbal description, analyses, and various verbal cues come to be more meaningful to learners because they have enough comprehension of the objectives of the task and its demands to utilize verbal information. Even the sounds associated with the execution of the skill—the "swish" of the tennis racket, the "click" of the golf club head against the ball—begin to provide meaningful auditory information to the learner.

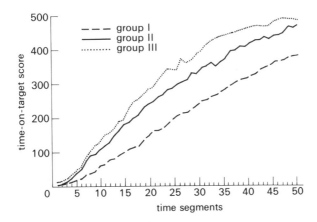

Fig. 17.1   The effects of instruction on learning a tracking task. The task required subjects to keep a dot in the center of an oscillograph display while at the
same time trying to keep a pointer centered on an instrument dial. (Based on Parker and Fleishman, 1961.)

The advantage of modifying verbal guidance as learning progresses
was nicely shown by Parker and Fleishman (1961). Three groups of subjects
learned a complex tracking task under different guidance methods. Group I
received no formal guidance at all, Group II received "commonsense" or
traditional guidance, and Group III received the same guidance as Group II
but also received special guidance at certain points in the learning process.
For Group III, the visual-spatial aspects of the task were emphasized in the
early learning, kinesthetic-coordination aspects of the task were emphasized later in the learning, and knowledge of various task components
was emphasized near the end of learning. Group III performed best throughout the study (Fig. 17.1). These results suggest that different verbal emphases may be more appropriate during different stages of learning.

Of course, motor learning takes place not so much from listening or observing as from moving, so regular practice with the intent to improve becomes one of the best instructional modes for the learner at this stage.

C. THE FINAL OR AUTONOMOUS PHASE IN MOTOR LEARNING

The final phase of motor skill learning, according to Fitts (1965), occurs as
the spatial and temporal aspects of the skill become highly organized and
component processes become increasingly autonomous. There is a development of units of increasing size which are translated into motor programs of

activity which then function with little or no "conscious" attention, allowing a state of readiness for coming movements. During this phase, the movement pattern is less directly subject to cognitive regulation, and less subject to interference from extraneous activities in the environment. The "old pro" is not bothered by distractions (except in golf and tennis where performers have come to expect no distractions). Ells (1969) and Salmoni (1973) have both demonstrated that as practice continues the movement becomes more automatic, freeing attention to be devoted to other stimuli in the display.

As the movement pattern becomes automatic, conscious introspection about the component parts of the pattern during this phase of learning often results in the so-called paralysis from analysis phenomenon. Of course, occasionally learners may have to use a component analysis of their movement pattern if they wish to further improve their proficiency or correct an error that has crept into their execution. Temporal organization tends to be the last organizational characteristic of skilled behavior to become mastered by learners and it is the most fragile and most easily disrupted. Timing is usually the first aspect of a skill to be impaired under stressful conditions.

In the later stages of learning a closed motor skill, the emphasis is on refinement of technique. For open skills, the emphasis is on adaptation of movements to the various environmental conditions. Higgins and Spaeth (1972) report that their research shows that movement patterns of open skills become more diversified in the later stages of practice while those of closed skills become more consistent.

In the case of athletics, as beginners develop into skilled sports performers they probably also modify their selective attention in order to discriminate more precisely between accurate and false information. Indeed, perceiving the appropriate stimuli while the opposition is attempting to confuse the display is critical for effective skillful performance in most sports. Also, with increased playing ability sports performers must learn how to deceive their opposition with false (or irrelevant) information. Carroll (1972) suggests that much of the art of competitive play consists of misleading the opposition by confounding the display. He says, "as beginners develop into competent game players, they also pass through another important stage—they learn both to deceive and to discriminate between accurate and false information."

1. Instructional techniques

Instructors of highly skilled performers serve to organize practice for skill maintenance and attempt to motivate for continued skill improvement. They also serve as movement diagnosticians and prescriptors, frequently suggesting variations in a movement pattern for greater proficiency. They also must detect errors which may be reducing performance effectiveness. Finally, in sports, instructors may serve as sources for strategy planning before competition and as tacticians during the contest.

A great deal of effective performance in sports depends upon the performers being able to anticipate environmental stimuli, especially the relevant stimuli. Thus, anything that instructors can do to assist their performers to direct their attention to the relevant cues and anticipate them will be beneficial to their performance. They may do this by providing performers with knowledge about typical tactics used by opponents and with knowledge about certain movements which precede certain actions by the opponents.

D. EFFECT OF PRIOR EXPERIENCE DURING THE PHASES OF MOTOR LEARNING

Except for the few reflexes with which we are born, all skilled movement patterns must be learned. After the first few years of life, an individual never begins the acquisition of a skill except from the background of many already existing and highly developed general and specific skills. For example, when one learns to swim, the skill is learned against a complex of existing movement patterns. Mednick (1964) says, "For example, when learning to swim, a person knows how to kick, to move his arms around, to breathe in and out, before he actually goes into the water." So motor skill acquisition involves building new movement patterns out of already existing skill patterns. Rarely is an entirely new skill learned; instead, it is "put together" out of an existing repertoire of skills, and the effects of these prior skills on the acquisition of new skills are evident in all three phases of motor skill acquisition.

In the cognitive phase, past experience provides the "raw material" out of which the learner comes to understand the new skill. The transfer of cognitive "sets," methods of performance, and appropriate strategies, which are a product of previously learned skills, are related to the new skill.

It is in the intermediate, or associative, phase that the effect of previously learned movement responses comes to affect the rate of learning of the new skill most markedly. If the new movement pattern requires a response opposite to a previously learned movement pattern when the stimulus situation is similar, the rate of learning may be slowed; there is a so-called negative transfer of skill, and a condition called proactive inhibition exists. That is, the learning of a new task is impaired by a previously learned task. But if the new skill requires similar motor responses to similar stimulus situation, rate of learning is enhanced, and positive transfer is said to occur.

The persistence of old habits is remarkably resistant to extinction. Therefore, even in the final, or autonomous, stage of learning, behavior that was part of a previously learned motor skill will occasionally reappear. This usually occurs during periods of stress. Swimmers who have recently changed their stroke and kick for greater efficiency frequently revert to their old movement pattern under the stress of competition. Basketball players who have recently changed their shooting movements for the jump shot may revert to their old shooting technique when confronted by a defensive player.

FACTORS AFFECTING ACQUISITION OF MOTOR SKILLS

From the information presented in this and the preceding chapter, one fact stands out very clearly concerning learning and performance of motor skills. That fact is that there are a great many variables which account for the speed with which motor learning occurs, the retention of skills, the skill level which can be achieved on a task, and the performance at any given time. Anyone who is responsible for improving effectiveness and efficiency in motor behavior should be familiar with these factors. The following chapters in this book will examine the current knowledge about a number of the more important factors that affect motor learning and performance.

18

Motor Abilities and Motor Behavior

The nature and development of human abilities have been of interest to psychologists for many years. Indeed, some have devoted their entire careers to devising and perfecting ability measurement instruments—the intelligence tests would be the most obvious example—while others have studied the relationship of certain kinds of ability to behavior. To use intelligence tests again as an example, many investigators have studied the relationship between intelligence, as measured by intelligence tests, and such things as scholastic achievement, occupational achievement, and so on.

Paralleling the interest in intellectual abilities, a few psychologists and many physical educators have been concerned with motor ability, its nature and development. Although numerous physical educators have been "interested" in the study of motor ability, very few have contributed to its theoretical or empirical literature. Nevertheless, there is a substantial body of knowledge on this topic. In this chapter we will examine the issues and problems that have been evident through the years and suggest some implications in light of the current state of the art.

DEFINITION OF MOTOR ABILITY

Ability is a general trait of an individual which is rather enduring and permanent after childhood. Biological forces are presumed to be primarily responsible for an individual's basic ability. Although the bodily structures and functions are similar for each individual, no two persons have *exactly* the same structural makeups, and bodily processes function a little differently for each person. Thus, there are differences in sensitivity of the sensory systems, making for individual differences in ability to detect and discriminate among stimuli; there are differences in actual number of muscle fibers and neuromuscular connections, which result in differences in potential for making motor responses. We could go on detailing the various structural and functional differences among individuals, but the point is that these differences which are genetic in origin play an essential part in determining basic abilities.

Of course, within biological limits, environment plays a significant role in the development of basic abilities. Research on the young of various species, including humans, indicates that early environment is critical for development of many basic abilities, especially motor abilities. Studies have shown rather conclusively that lower animal and human infants raised in environments which restrict sensory experiences or motor activity have a narrower range of motor abilities throughout their lives. It is, then, generally believed that the greater the variety of sensory and motor experiences individuals have during their early years, the fuller will be their motor ability repertoire, within the limitations set by their genetic heritage.

No complete and final list of human abilities has ever been compiled. Psychologists have discovered a bewildering number of basic human abilities, and new ones will probably be identified in the future. The most comprehensive study of human motor abilities and cataloguing of these abilities have been carried out by Edwin A. Fleishman. Using statistical techniques called correlation and factor analysis, he and his colleagues have investigated over 200 different tasks administered to thousands of subjects. From the statistical treatment, they have been able to account for performance on the numerous tasks by a relatively small number of abilities (Fleishman, 1966, 1972).

A. ABILITIES AND SKILLS

Ability and skill are not synonymous concepts. Abilities serve as the foundation stones for the development of skills, which are specific responses for the accomplishment of a task. A skill is learned through practice and depends upon the presence of underlying abilities. Balance, speed of reaction, and flexibility are examples of abilities which are important for the execution of a variety of skills, such as the tennis serve, the breaststroke, and the forward roll.

B. STATISTICAL TECHNIQUES COMMONLY USED IN MOTOR ABILITY ASSESSMENT

A brief description of correlation and factor analysis techniques will help the reader understand how various motor ability studies have been done and how their findings are used to advance our understanding of motor abilities. Correlation is one of the most frequently used measures of relations. A correlation coefficient is ascertained from scores from at least two tests which have been administered, and is expressed as some number between + 1.00 and − 1.00. Numbers between 0 and + 1.00 indicate a positive relationship, meaning high scorers on one test tend to be high scorers on the second test. Numbers between 0 and − 1.00 indicate a negative relationship; thus, high scorers on one test tend to be low scorers on the second test.

The magnitude, or strength, of the relationship between the test scores is indicated by the size of the correlation. Correlation coefficients that are near zero (0 to + 0.20 or 0 to − 0.20) indicate little or no relationship between the tests; in the latter, the relationship is said to be inverse; + 1.00 or − 1.00 correlations indicate a perfect association. Finally, correlations between + 0.80 and + 0.20 or − 0.80 and − 0.20 show moderate relationships, the strength of relationship depending upon how close to 0 or 1.0 they actually are.

Frequently, correlation techniques are used to determine whether or not two tests are measuring the same ability. If two motor tasks are administered to a set of subjects and the correlation coefficient is found to be + 0.95, it can be inferred that both tests are estimating the same motor ability. But if there is a + 0.08 correlation coefficient, it can be inferred that the two tests are not measuring the same ability or that the ability contributing to the performance on one task is not the same as that on the other task.

Coefficients of correlation are themselves subject to extensive and elaborate forms of analyses, one of which is factor analysis. Factor analysis is a statistical technique for identifying, on the basis of scores from a number of test items given to a large group of subjects, a relatively small number of common qualities. It tells us, in effect, which test items belong together—which ones measure virtually the same thing, in other words, and to what degree they do so. It reduces the number of variables, or tests, with which one must cope. It also helps to locate and identify unities of fundamental properties underlying tests and measures. For example, if 20 tests were administered to a group of individuals and the results showed that three of these tests intercorrelate highly with each other, then one factor is identified. Additionally, if three of the other tests correlate highly, but do not correlate with the first three tests, a second factor has been identified. Once the various factors emerge from the analysis, the experimenter subjectively names each factor by some descriptive statement.

The use that Fleishman and others have made of correlational and factor analytical techniques will be described throughout the remaining sections of this chapter. Suffice to say at this time that these techniques have served as the basic tools for unlocking the mysteries of motor abilities.

GENERAL MOTOR ABILITY

One of the most persistent bits of folklore of physical education and athletic coaching is the notion of a "general motor ability" (GMA)—a singular unifying motor ability which enables certain individuals to perform well or to acquire quickly a high proficiency on any motor task they undertake. Phrases such as "a natural athlete" or "an all-round athlete" characterize this so-called ability. At the same time industrial psychologists have employed "motor aptitude" tests for selecting employees in the belief that these tests are "predictive" of performance levels on the job. Aptitude refers to the potential of persons to perform a specific kind of activity, and an aptitude test is designed to detect underlying abilities within persons and to predict how well they will perform after they have had practice in that activity.

There is a wealth of information that has accumulated over the past 25 years which suggests that the notion of "general motor ability" is a myth and that selecting personnel through the use of a motor aptitude test battery is, at best, ineffective and may even be counterproductive.

A. DEVELOPMENT OF MOTOR ABILITY TESTS

Although it is always hazardous to speculate about the origin of one idea, the notion that there is such a thing as general motor ability was probably triggered by the work done by psychologists in identifying a so-called Intelligence Quotient. In the early part of this century, psychologists who developed intelligence tests contended that the tests measured a general ability to utilize abstract concepts effectively, implying reasoning, imagination, insight, and adaptability as the mental processes involved in intelligent behavior. The claim was that general intelligence was being measured and intellectual ability was believed to be represented by this term. The primary purpose of these tests was to determine scholastic aptitude, and they did predict to some extent academic achievement (Cronback, 1960).

There is no question about the popularity of intelligence tests. During World War I nearly 2 million men were screened for intelligence and assigned to various specialties on the basis of the scores; throughout the 1920s, '30s, and '40s schools used intelligence tests scores to group, career counsel, and even to screen students for college admission. The popularity of the intelligence tests may have been the primary stimulus for those who were working with motor activities—physical educators, coaches, industrial psychologists—to seek a similar assessment instrument for motor ability.

In any case, between 1920 and 1940 several physical educators devised instruments for the measurement of general motor ability. In 1927, David K.

Brace (1927) published a test designed to measure "inherent motor skill." At the University of Iowa, Charles McCloy (1937), one of the most esteemed physical educators of the 1920–1940 era, revised the Brace Test, and attempted to produce a test that would measure "motor educability," meaning the "ease with which an individual learns new motor skills." Other test batteries were developed by Granville Johnson (1932), whose battery of tests was designed to measure "native neuromuscular skill capacity," and by Frederick Cozens (1929) who developed a test that purported to measure "general athletic ability."

The basic idea behind the notion of a general motor ability is that there is an underlying ability which enables certain individuals to be able to perform well in any motor task they attempt and also that they will learn new motor skills to a high level of proficiency quickly. In essence, the suggestion is that there is a motor equivalent of general intelligence.

The various general motor ability tests caused quite a stir throughout the field of physical education for about a decade; physical education classes were grouped on the basis of the scores, prospective athletes were selected for teams from the scores, etc. But then evidence began to accumulate which indicated that, in fact, motor ability tests did not do what it was first claimed they could do. One of the first attacks on these general motor ability tests came from a developer of one of them, David K. Brace. In 1941, in a study designed to ascertain the efficacy of several tests of general motor ability, motor educability, etc., Brace (1941) reported that none of the tests, including his own, was predictive of ability to learn motor skills. He wrote, "Conclusions from the data would appear to indicate that either the so-called learning tests do not measure ability to learn or that the other measures obtained have little relationship to ability to learn motor skills." More damning evidence came about a year later. Gire and Espenschade (1942) correlated the scores on the Brace, Iowa Revision of the Brace, and the Johnson Test with students' ability to learn basketball, volleyball, and baseball skills. Their findings pretty much destroyed the creditability of these instruments. They said, "Thus, it may be concluded that no test of 'motor educability' studied measured accurately the ease with which the subjects in this study learned new skills or relearned old ones in basketball, volleyball, and baseball. . . ."

More recently, the most persistent and consistent opponent of the general motor ability (GMA) notion has been Franklin Henry of the University of California, Berkeley. His own research and the research of his graduate students have shown rather convincingly that there is no such thing as GMA. Two basic strategies have been used by Henry and his students in dismantling this concept. First, they tested groups of athletes and nonathletes on a variety of motor skills (but not sports skills) and found that the athletes performed no better on these tasks than the nonathletes. A second strategy was to administer two or more different motor tasks to the same subjects and assess the relationship between performance on the various tasks by correlational analysis. If the notion of general motor ability is valid, the performers who score well on one task should score high on other tasks—in other words, the correlation between any two motor tasks should be rather high. Several studies designed to assess this relationship found that the correlation coefficients between the performance and/or learning motor tasks were very low. For example, Bachman (1961) had over 300 subjects perform on the stabilometer and a free-standing ladder task which he designed and built. Correlations between both performance and learning the tasks were mostly below 0.20 for age groups from 6 to 26; and Bachman concluded that the "results show little more than zero correlation between performance of the two tasks...[and] motor learning is remarkably task specific. No correlation was found that was significantly different from zero...." A number of other similarly designed investigations have reported similar results (Lotter, 1961; Henry and Smith, 1961; Oxendine, 1967; Marteniuk, 1969a). Several investigators have even studied the relationship between rate and amount of skill acquired by two body parts of the same subject. The basic hypothesis was that if a general motor ability factor existed, some degree of correlation would be observed in the rate and degree to which the skill was acquired by the two body segments. In general, these studies have found that skill was specific to the body segment involved (Singer, 1966; Hanley, Massey, Morehouse, and White, 1971). These studies provide strong support for Henry's (1956) contention that motor task performance and learning depend on numerous independent abilities, not a general unifying motor ability. He suggested that the "all-round" athlete is just a case of an individual with many specific abilities and not the proof of the existence of a general motor ability. Henry (1958) summarized the findings in this way:

...it is no longer possible to justify the concept of unitary abilities such as coordination and agility, since evidence shows that the abilities are specific to the test or activity....The theory of specific motor abilities implies that some individuals are gifted with many specific abilities and others have only a few; it follows that there will inevitably be significant correlations between total test battery scores when tests involving many abilities are lumped together. The general motor factor which thus makes its appearance is a sample, fundamentally, of how many specifics the individual has, and general motor ability does exist in this sense.

Although the evidence is rather clear that the general motor ability hypothesis is unfounded, because of the low correlations between motor tasks, there is an unsettling fact that the correlations are, nevertheless, typically positive, leading to the conclusion that there may be abilities common to some motor tasks. Moreover Eckert (1964) reported moderate correlations between speed of limb movement and strength and Nelson and Fahrney (1965) found moderate to high relationships between tests of strength and movement speed.

B. CLASSIFYING MOTOR ABILITIES

The work of Edwin Fleishman and his colleagues over the past 25 years provides a clarification of the two extreme positions—general motor ability and specificity of motor ability—concerning the abilities underlying performance on a motor task. Fleishman has employed factor analysis to extract factors from a large group of motor tasks. Each factor is believed to represent a basic underlying motor ability, and each motor ability has been named according to the tasks which make up a factor. (For reviews of this work see Fleishman, 1966, or Fleishman, 1972.)

Using over 200 different tasks and administering them to thousands of subjects, Fleishman has been able to account for performance on this wide variety of tasks by a relatively small number of abilities. He has classified these motor abilities into two broad categories, one of which he calls "psychomotor abilities" and the second of which he calls "physical proficiency." The first set of abilities was derived from studies of manipulative skills and limb coordination tasks, while the second came from gross motor tasks.

The psychomotor abilities and their characteristics are:

1. **Control precision.** This ability requires fine, highly controlled muscular adjustments, primarily in situations in which large muscle groups are involved. This ability extends to arm-hand as well as to leg movements.

2. **Multilimb coordination.** This is the ability to coordinate a number of limb movements simultaneously.

3. **Response orientation.** This ability is general to visual discrimination reaction psychomotor tasks involving rapid directional discrimination and orientation of movement patterns.

4. **Reaction time.** This ability is simply the speed with which a person is able to respond to a stimulus when it appears.

5. **Speed of arm movement.** This is the speed with which a person can make gross, discrete arm movements in which accuracy is not the requirement.

6. **Rate control.** This ability involves making continuous anticipatory motor adjustments relative to changes in speed and direction of a continuous moving target or object.

7. **Manual dexterity.** This ability is demonstrated by skillful, well-directed arm-hand movements in manipulating fairly large objects under speeded conditions.

8. **Finger dexterity.** This involves making still-controlled manipulations of tiny objects involving, primarily, the fingers.

9. **Arm-hand steadiness.** This is the ability to make precise arm-hand positioning movements where strength and speed are minimized.

10. **Wrist-finger speed.** This ability is best measured by printed tests requiring rapid tapping of the pencil in relatively large areas; it is of limited generality.

11. **Aiming.** This ability is best measured by printed tests requiring the rapid placement of dots in very small circles under highly speeded conditions (Fleishman, 1972).

The abilities identified as physical proficiency abilities are:

1. **Extent flexibility.** This is the ability to flex or stretch the trunk and back muscles as far as possible in either a forward, lateral, or backward direction.

2. **Dynamic flexibility.** The ability to make repeated, rapid, flexing movements in which the resiliency of the muscles in recovery from stretch or distortion is critical.

3. **Explosive strength.** The ability to expend a maximum of energy in one or a series of explosive acts.

4. **Static strength.** The maximum force which a person can exert, for a brief period.

5. **Dynamic strength.** The ability to exert muscular force repeatedly or continuously over time.

6. **Trunk strength.** A more dynamic strength factor, specific to the abdominal muscles.

7. **Gross body coordination.** This is the ability to coordinate the simultaneous actions of different parts of the body while making gross body movements.

8. **Gross body equilibrium.** This ability involves individuals maintaining their equilibrium despite forces pulling them off balance, while they are blindfolded.

9. **Stamina.** This is the ability to continue maximum effort, requiring prolonged exertion over time (Fleishman, 1972).

The essence to the compilation of this list of motor abilities is not a single general ability but can best be described in terms of a number of broad relatively independent abilities. The same individuals may be high on some abilities and low on others; but the individual who has a great many highly developed basic motor abilities can become proficient at a great variety of specific tasks. The so-called all-round athlete has either acquired or has "built-in" abilities which underlie success in a given skill.

Fleishman (1967) warns that the list of motor abilities that he has extracted is not to be considered a final, complete list. He says, "...we do not present these factors as any kind of final list of perceptual motor categories...." Limitations such as the number and types of tasks which were used as well as the subjective nature of some steps in factor analysis necessitate that the work on this subject be continued.

Fleishman's work has not only helped to clarify the issue of generality versus specificity of motor skill performance and learning, but perhaps one of his most interesting findings is that as the learning of a motor skill proceeds, changes occur in the *particular combinations* of abilities contributing to performance. As noted above, several studies (Bachman, 1961; Oxendine, 1967; Marteniuk, 1969) have found low correlations for motor learning, when the same subjects had to learn two or more motor tasks. Fleishman and his colleagues (Fleishman and Hempel, 1954) demonstrated that the particular combinations of abilities contributing to performance on motor tasks changed as practice on these tasks continued. This finding, combined with their extraction of a number of relatively independent motor abilities, provides a partial explanation for the findings of motor learning specificity—the rate of learning and ultimate proficiency level depend upon the unique ability structure of each person. This suggests, then, the presence of certain potentials for learning a skill.

The pioneer experiment which demonstrated the changing structure of abilities contributing to performance as learning proceeded involved a piloting-type task which required the subjects to manipulate a stick and rudder in response to visual patterns. Scores were obtained at eight different points during the practice and were correlated with performance on a battery of printed and apparatus tests of hypothesized abilities; the results were then subjected to factor analysis. The analysis showed that there was a marked shift in the nature of factors contributing to early and late performance, the changes were progressive and systematic throughout the learning and a factor specific to performance on the task itself increased with practice; indeed, it became the major component of the skill in the late stages of learning (Fig. 18.1) (Fleishman and Hempel, 1954). Using a discrimination reaction time task, a later study also demonstrated a shift in the nature of abilities contributing to performance for early to late learning (Fleishman and Hempel, 1955).

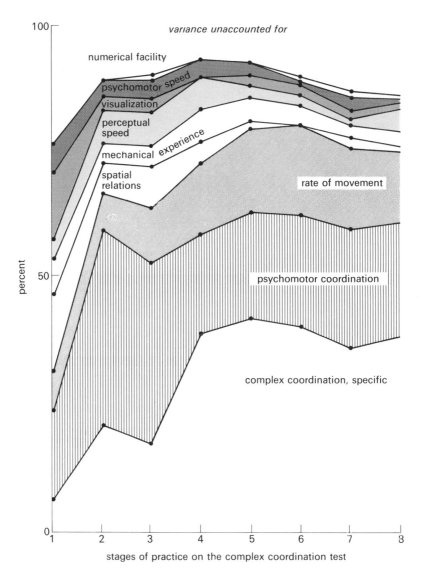

Fig. 18.1 Changes in factor structure as a function of practice. Percentage of variance (shaded area) represented by each factor at various stages of practice. (Based on Fleishman and Hempel, 1954.)

The finding that different abilities contribute to performance at different stages in learning suggests that persons who possess those abilities which contribute to performance in the initial stages of learning will begin at a relatively high level and those who possess abilities which contribute to performance at later stages of learning will achieve high proficiency levels later in learning. The research to test this hypothesis has consistently supported it.

Fleishman and Rich (1963) gave a visual spatial test and a kinesthetic sensitivity test to a large group of subjects, then divided them into groups high and low on visual spatial ability and into groups high and low on kinesthetic sensitivity. Then the subjects learned a two-hand coordination task. The superior visual spatial ability group exhibited early advantage but as practice continued the poorer visual group caught up. Conversely, the superior kinesthetic sensitivity group began at about the same initial level as the poorer group, but as practice continued the former pulled away and performed much better than the poorer group in the later stages of learning (Fig. 18.2). These findings seem to indicate that if visual cues are predominant in early control of the task, individuals who have superior visual spatial ability do better in the early learning stages of the task. On the other hand, if kinesthetic cues are dominant late in the learning of a task, persons with superior kinesthetic perception will outdo others in late stages of learning.

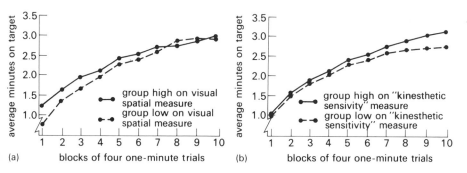

Fig. 18.2 In (a) the superior visual group (high spatial measure) clearly has an early advantage but, as training progresses, the poorer visual group catches up. In (b) the two kinesthetic groups begin at the same level but, in the later stages as kinesthesis becomes more important, the kinesthetically more sensitive group surpasses the less sensitive group. (Based on Fleishman and Rich, 1963.)

Taken together, these studies suggest that the pattern of abilities related to performance changes in a relatively systematic way from one stage of practice to the next, until a point at which the skill is mastered and the pattern of abilities required for performance at the high level of performance is stabilized (Hinrichs, 1970).

One thing that stands out in the studies by Fleishman showing the changing role of abilities as learning continues is that visual spatial ability tends to be a major factor contributing to proficiency in the early phase of learning a variety of motor tasks. In the piloting coordination task (Fleishman and Hempel, 1954), spatial relations were significant only in the first stages of practice; in the discrimination reaction time task (Fleishman and Hempel, 1955), they were the main factor at the beginning of practice but decreased in contribution to performance in the final phase; and in the two-hand coordination task the group with superior spatial orientation showed initial performance supremacy (Fleishman and Rich, 1963). More recently, Stallings (1968) has confirmed the earlier findings; in her study the group scoring high on spatial orientation maintained superiority of performance in the early learning stage, but spatial orientation became progressively less important as practice continued.

Another thing that stands out clearly in these investigations which has some interesting implications for motor skills instructors is the fact that individual differences in initial proficiency have relatively little relation to ultimate proficiency. There are slow learners and fast learners for particular tasks, and early performance is not predictive of final proficiency. Many motor skill instructors have assumed that initial performance is related to ultimate proficiency and the rate at which it will be attained. Some athletic coaches, for example, have selected their teams on the basis of player performance on a few practice tries because they believed that the best performers at that point had the best potential for further improvement. The findings which consistently show that the abilities which underlie this early superiority are not necessarily the abilities which underlie later proficiency level should make coaches pause before they quickly dismiss the poorly skilled. In two studies done in Canada, Percival (1971) divided performers into two groups, an "initial high performer" group and an "initial low performer" group. One study employed a baseball throw for accuracy and another involved shooting a hockey puck at a target. In both studies the "initial low performer" group attained the same level of proficiency, or better, than the "initial high performer" group, after 12 practice sessions.

Although it is little more than a hunch at this time, shifts in abilities underlying performance suggest that instructors might carefully analyze the task which they are teaching for the specific abilities needed to perform it and then either use teaching methods which emphasize those abilities at each level or use instructional methods which emphasize the abilities needed to perform at the high proficiency level. A study by Parker and Fleishman (1961), in which three groups learned a motor task under different instructional conditions, demonstrated that the group receiving guidance with emphasis on the ability components of the task, as they changed over the course of learning, learned faster and reached a higher level of performance than the other groups (See Fig. 17.1, Chapter 17).

Despite the enthusiasm of teachers for ability grouping, there is little research support for this method when measures of physical performance are the standard for judgment. In a comprehensive review of the literature, Nixon and Locke (1973) state, "In general, homogeneous grouping appears to be no better than ordinary methods of assignment to class." When the literature on the specificity of motor skill learning is considered, it is quite understandable why homogeneous grouping is ineffectual, since motor skills classes are typically grouped by scores obtained on some general motor ability test.

INTELLIGENCE AND MOTOR BEHAVIOR

Ever since the ancient Greeks coined the saying, "A sound mind in a sound body," the notion that there is a positive relationship between intelligence and motor ability has existed. At the same time there have been those who have believed that there is an inverse relationship between the two—perhaps the term "dumb jock" characterizes this belief. Actually, there is very little evidence to support either of these two extreme positions.

In one of the first texts on motor behavior, Clarence Ragsdale (1930) reviewed the studies that had been done up to that time and concluded that there was no consistent finding that intelligence and motor behavior are related. Overall, the large body of research which has been done on this topic since that time has yielded essentially the same results. The results of the studies can best be summarized with this statement: There is a low but positive relationship between intelligence and motor ability (Harmon and Oxendine, 1961; Singer, 1968a; Singer and Brunk, 1967).

This conclusion could probably be expected, given the variety of motor ability test batteries which have been used and given the fact that correlational and factor analytic studies have demonstrated that intelligence is not a single, unitary ability. It should be noted, though, that some recent research by Ismail and his colleagues (Ismail and Gruber, 1967) at Purdue University have found significant positive relationships between a few motor task items, especially "coordination" and balance items, and intelligence; factor analysis was used in this work (Ismail, Kane and Kirkendall, 1969).

19

Practice and Motor Behavior

Motor skill acquisition is dependent upon a variety of conditions, and practice is one of the most important of these. Complex motor skills required for riding a bicycle, driving an automobile, shooting a basket, or hitting a baseball must be practiced many times before they can be done effectively and efficiently.

As noted in previous chapters, motor learning involves the establishment of appropriate motor programs which correspond with proper movement execution, and motor programs of the type which are used in games, sports, and dance activities are developed through practice. Moreover, learning proceeds through phases, or stages, each of which requires practice, and practice influences the rapidity with which the phases are passed through and the ultimate level of proficiency.

Practice may take various forms, and in this chapter several of the more important practice factors are examined.

RESEARCH ON PRACTICE

Experimental psychologists conducted extensive research on various practice variables in motor learning during the period between 1900 and 1940, with the decade of the 1930s as the peak for this kind of research. Since then, their excitement about this topic has dwindled. Interestingly, about the same time psychologists' interest in this topic began to diminish, physical educators' interest increased and, since World War II, there has been considerable interest in practice variables in motor skill learning and retention by physical educators.

THE EFFECTS OF PRACTICE

The two most obvious effects of practice on the learning of motor skills is first, increased speed of performance and second, increased accuracy, or reduction of errors. Most improvement in skilled performance is dependent on increasing the speed and accuracy of movements. As was noted in Chapter 10, most motor tasks can be performed the first time if done slowly enough for various sensory mechanisms to guide the performance. However the difference between the skilled and unskilled performer is that the skilled performer can perform with very little sensory guidance, and this has the effect of increasing speed of performance. Accuracy of performance also normally increases with proper practice—basketball players become better shooters and baseball hitters make contact with the ball more frequently when they swing.

There may be more subtle effects of practice on the development of a motor skill. For example, it appears that abilities which are necessary for the learning of a task vary as the individual becomes more proficient. Abilities which contribute to performance in the initial phases of learning are not the same abilities that contribute to performance as proficiency increases. Thus, practice serves the purpose of guiding the learning process through the various "ability" levels toward proficiency.

INSTRUCTION BEFORE PRACTICE

The time given over to instruction to the learners of motor skills may be viewed as part of the practice period, and instructions are commonly thought to be an important factor in the learning experience. Other than some general guidelines, there are few specific prescriptions for instructional techniques which have proven to be effective for enhancing learning rate across many motor tasks.

The notion that the learner must develop a cognitive map of the task to be learned suggests that an important first job of the instructor is to instill in the learner's memory a perfect image or template. This may be done most advantageously by having learners observe skilled performers executing the task before they actually practice physically. Observational learning studies have demonstrated marked facilitation of a variety of tasks directly following visual observation of another's performance (Keele, 1973).

Once the cognitive map is established, the individual may begin to practice the movements. The feedback from the movements can then be compared with the map stored in memory; if there are discrepancies, the motor program can be altered and feedback again can be compared with the map and so on until the appropriate movement pattern is established (Posner and Keele, 1973).

The method of providing demonstration and requiring learners to observe other performers has some drawbacks to which an instructor must be sensitive. Some persons do not have the patience to observe models for extended periods. Moreover, even when models are observed, the learner may not perceive critical aspects of the movement pattern or the tactics employed in execution. Finally, some learners can see others perform, but cannot translate this information into a usable model for their own performance.

An instructional technique that is related to observation of a model but requires somewhat more active participation on the part of the learner is called verbal pretraining. Here learners are required to learn certain aspects of the task, such as the sequence of events, in the hope that they will transfer this learning when they begin to actually practice. An example of verbal pretraining was employed by Adams and Creamer (1962) who had subjects who were to learn to follow an alternating wave form by moving a hand control, simply watch the wave before trying to track it and respond to the changes in direction with vocal responses. Subjects who performed the verbal pretraining subsequently performed the tracking task more accurately than did subjects who did not have the pretraining.

Another form of instruction often employed during the introduction of a motor task is verbally describing the mechanical principles that underlie the correct execution of the movements. Since this topic is discussed in some detail in Chapter 21, it will not be dealt with here.

PRACTICE INTENTIONS

Practice is essential for acquiring complex motor skills. Merely observing and thinking about a motor skill will not suffice for the acquisition of a high level of proficiency in that skill. No one ever learned to shoot a jump shot or serve a tennis ball with any effectiveness by merely watching someone else or by just thinking about these skills. It is only through repetition of the desired movement pattern that skillful response sequences are developed. Practice will not, however, necessarily result in proficiency. Skill improvement will occur only if conscientious attempts to improve are made. Practice must be done with an attempt to improve. The fallacy of the old adage "practice makes perfect" may be seen by observing an adult's handwriting. Although the task (handwriting) is practiced daily, most individuals' handwriting does not improve; in fact, it gets worse in many cases. So practice may actually perpetuate errors.

Little improvement in performance occurs unless there is intent to improve. One explanation for this fact is that if motor learning occurs to some extent as a result of the pairing of feedback resulting from the execution of a movement pattern, if the movement pattern is successful (e.g., the basketball goes into the basket), an emotionally satisfying state results for the individual who is intent upon becoming proficient. When executing the movement again, the learner will attempt to perform correctly so as to receive the satisfaction again. If one performs and does not experience the emotionally satisfying set of stimuli because correct performance is not important to one, the feedback does not become paired with a satisfaction. Thus, there is no particular effort to perform correctly in subsequent practice (Mowrer 1960).

Another explanation of why improvement does not occur if there is no intent to improve might go like this: If one incorporates the feedback from a performance into a verbal-cognitive process of some sort, and this process facilitates forming hypotheses and strategies for making modifications in subsequent performances, if one has no particular interest in improving, one will probably not employ this process to any extent; the result will be little improvement in performance.

A third explanation for no improvement when there is no intent to improve makes use of Consolidation Memory Theory. As you recall, unless the short-term stage is allowed to persist, there will be little long-term memory Information that has entered STM may be enhanced by cognitive rehearsal maintenance of information in STM seems to facilitate transfer to LTM. Persons who are intent upon improving probably do more thinking about the task and their movements between actual practices; they cognitively rehearse, thus strengthening the processes which lead to LTM. A study by Tulving (1966) illustrated that unless there is intention to remember, mere repetition is not sufficient for storage into LTM.

AMOUNT OF PRACTICE

Assuming intention to improve, the more one practices, the higher the level of proficiency. Of course, physical ability limitations place an upper limit on the ultimate proficiency one can attain, but there is no current method for assessing what that ultimate level may be, and there are numerous cases in which improved performance has continued over many years. Crossman (1959) reported improvement in proficiency on a fine motor skill (cigar making) extending over seven years and many thousand trials. (See Fig. 16.11.

Many sports athletes must practice ten or more years to achieve sufficient skill to compete at the national or international level.

Active practice is a form of repeating the process which results in memory; the transfer of information to long-term memory seems to require repetition through rehearsal. The more often a task is repeated, the more likely it is to be embedded in long-term memory. Moreover, active rehearsal acts to organize material in memory, and such organization facilitates memory (Keele, 1973).

The more one practices, the higher the level of skill and the more one retains proficiency when practice is terminated or interrupted. In other words, active rehearsal serves to prevent forgetting and to increase the resistance of stored information to subsequent interfering events.

PRACTICE SCHEDULES

The relationship between practice periods and rest periods has interested psychologists since the earliest learning experiments. In the fields of physical education and coaching, the distribution of practice has been a problem because there is a limited amount of time available and usually there are numerous skills to be taught. Over the past 60 years more motor learning investigations have been concerned with practice schedule phenomena than with any other specific topic of motor learning investigation.

The major questions with regard to practice schedules are: Should learners continuously practice on a skill with only a few brief rest periods, or should they practice for short periods of time with more frequent and prolonged intervals of rest? Which practice schedule is best for speed of skill acquisition? highest levels of skill? retention?

The two basic variables with which practice-schedule studies have been concerned are the time of continuous practice and the interval between practice trials. Practice schedules for skill learning may take the form of either continuous practice with little or no temporal interval between trials, or one of a few practice trials followed by rest intervals of no formal practice. A practice schedule which requires continuous practice with short and/or infrequent rest intervals between trials is called "massed" or "unspaced" practice. When there are rest intervals longer and/or more frequent than this between trials or between a set of a few trials, this is called "distributed" or "spaced" practice. The term massed practice has been defined to be practice periods of several minutes to several hours in duration or by several practice trials to hundreds of trials in each practice period. The infrequent intertrial rest periods have varied from a few seconds to a day or two. Distributed practice has been characterized by shorter practice periods and more frequent rest intervals than massed practice.

The meanings of "massed" and "distributed" have varied from experiment to experiment, so research on distribution of practice in motor tasks has been beset by inadequate and inconsistent definitions. Indeed, Nixon and Locke (1973) have noted that, "Although studies of schedule patterns commonly are labeled as investigations of massed versus distributed practice, they may better be considered contrasts of varying degrees of distribution."

Notwithstanding the definitional problems associated with research on this topic, the advocates of massed practice suggest that performance and learning are most efficient and effective by practicing continuously over an extended period of time with few and short rest periods. Conversely, the supporters of distributed practice have argued that performance and learning are best accomplished by rather brief practice periods with frequent and extended rest intervals. Most investigations which have been designed to test these two contentions have used rather simple motor tasks, such as the rotary pursuit, mirror tracer, and other fine motor skill tasks. These tasks make it possible to control many variables, but some questions arise as to the applicability of the findings to gross motor tasks such as those found in sports and dance. However, several studies using gross motor skills have confirmed the basic findings obtained in studies using fine motor tasks.

A. MASSED AND DISTRIBUTED SCHEDULES AND FINE MOTOR SKILLS

For most fine motor tasks that have been studied, the results show that performance tends to be superior for the distributed group, especially after the first few trials. On the other hand, the results for learning are not so clear-cut, and it appears that there is actually little difference in the two schedules when learning is assessed. Since most of the early investigations did not differentiate between performance and learning, only the performance data were reported and so the superiority of distributed practice for performance was commonly applied to learning, too.

In what has become one of the classic studies, Lorge (1930), using mirror drawing, mirror writing, and a code substitution task, found that subjects who had practiced with a rest period of one minute or one day between trials produced better performances after 20 trials than a continuous practice group did (Fig. 19.1). Nance (1946) reported that distributed paced practice was superior to massed unpaced, distributed unpaced, and massed paced practice. He says that "it is probable the superiority of distributed

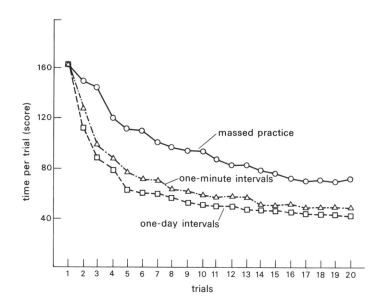

Fig. 19.1 Learning curves under three different schedules of practice on a mirror-tracing task. One-minute rest intervals between trials and one-day intervals were nearly equal, and both were better than massed practice. The lower the score, the better the performance. (Based on I. Lorge, 1930.)

practice is based upon the magnitude of the work-rest ratio and not upon absolute length of trial or rest taken separately."

Rest intervals which have been found to be beneficial vary from a minute to several days, but much depends on the task and the length of the practice period. Basically, the longer and more intense the practice period, the longer the optimal rest period. Kientzle (1946) found that subjects learning to print letters upside down showed better performance improvements when given brief rest periods than did subjects who were given no rest. She found that on this task, rest intervals beyond 45 seconds did not significantly increase performance. These results, and others, suggest that short rest periods are quite effective in producing recovery from any debilitating effects of massed work. Of course, the optimal cycling will depend upon the intensity of the work and the duration of work between trials. Generally, the more intense and longer the work, the longer the duration of the rest period for maximal recovery, but any period of rest is better than no rest, as far as performance is concerned.

In 1960 Dorothy Mohr (1960) reported that a review of the psychological literature turned up 45 studies related to massed and distributed practice. Of these studies, 40 reported results favoring distributed practice, three favored massed practice, and two found no significant differences. These findings were of performance results, and they show the clear advantage of distributed practice for performance.

Studies in which assessment of practice schedules has been made after the massed and distributed groups have had a substantial rest interval between trials (five minutes or more) demonstrate that the actual proficiency of the massed group is very similar to the distributed group. Moreover, massed practice subjects who are shifted to a distributed schedule typically show performance nearly equal to that of the distributed group, implying that the learning of a motor task is a function of the actual practice time and is not wholly dependent upon conditions of practice distribution. Finally, when learning formulae have been employed to assess the effectiveness of practice schedules, little learning difference has been found.

In an often cited study of rotary-pursuit learning, Digman (1959) reported that performance under the massed condition was poorer than under the distributed condition; indeed, within some sessions performance actually deteriorated under the massed condition. However, the performance of the massed group was better at the beginning of each new session than it was at the end of the previous session, and over the course of the experiment the level of performance approached that under the distributed condition (Fig. 19.2).

More recently, Whitley (1970) employed a foot-tracking task to assess performance and learning under massed and distributed schedules. He also reported superior performance for the distributed group which was virtually eliminated when the massed group was switched to the same prac-

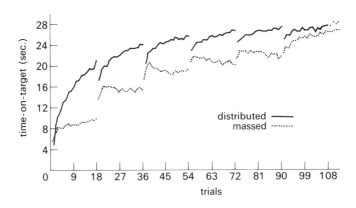

Fig. 19.2   Mean performance for distributed and massed practice groups on the rotary-pursuit apparatus. (Based on Digman, 1959.)

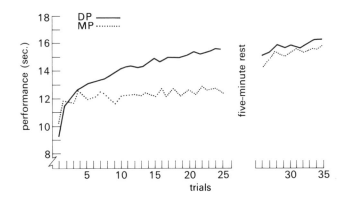

Fig. 19.3   Performance curves for distributed practice (DP) and massed practice (MP) groups on a foot-tracking task. (Based on Whitley, 1970.)

tice schedule as the distributed group after a five-minute rest. He concluded that the practice schedules affected performance, but not learning (Fig. 19.3). Essentially the same results were reported by Carron (1969) who had subjects perform a discrete-trial motor task, called the peg turn. He concluded that "while increasing the amount of massing does have a deleterious effect on performance, it does not reduce the amount of learning."

B. DISTRIBUTED AND MASSED PRACTICE AND GROSS MOTOR TASKS

Studies of the distribution of practice for gross motor skills have generally supported the findings of studies using fine motor tasks for performance, but they have produced equivocal results for learning. Two major factors, other than the type of skills involved, may be responsible for the differences in findings. First, the practice and rest periods tend to be quite different; studies with fine motor tasks often use practice and rest periods for a few seconds to a few minutes, whereas investigations with gross motor tasks often employ practices of several minutes to hours and rest periods from hours to up to several days. A second reason for the differences is that the fine motor tasks used in the studies have typically been continuous tasks, i.e., rotary pursuit, while the gross motor skills have usually been discrete or serial in nature.

   In a study conducted by Young (1954), groups of students practiced archery and badminton on two-day-a-week schedules. She found archery to be learned more efficiently when practiced four days a week, while badminton skills were acquired faster when practiced twice a week. Scott (1954) reported that beginning swimmers who practiced four days per week learned faster than those who practiced two or three days per week, thus suggesting that for learning to swim a relatively massed schedule is best. Niemeyer (1959) found that a practice schedule of 30 minutes of practice three times per week produced faster learning than a practice schedule of 60 minutes twice per week for swimming, badminton, and volleyball. In this study, the "mass schedule group" (60 minutes, twice a week) had 30 minutes more practice per week than the "distributed schedule group."

Singer (1965) used a novel gross motor skill (bouncing a basketball off the floor and attempting to make a basket) under massed and distributed practice schedules and found that acquisition of the skill was significantly better under the distributed practice conditions—24-hour rest between practice periods (Fig. 19.4). Employing both the stabilometer and the Bachman ladder, Stelmach (1969) designed a study with four groups of subjects; each subject in a group performed on one of the two motor tasks under one of the two conditions. Distributed practice consisted of alternating 30-second trials of practice and rest; massed practice was continuous for eight minutes. Performance during the last minute of practice prior to the rest interval was significantly poorer for the massed groups. After a four-minute rest period, when both groups performed on a distributed schedule, no

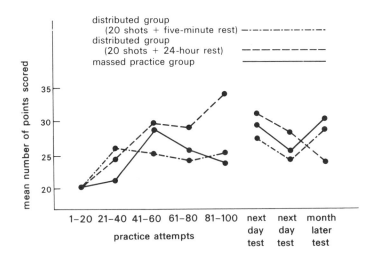

Fig. 19.4   Effects of distributed and massed practice schedules on the acquisition of a novel basketball skill. Measured by the mean number of points scored. (Based on Singer, 1965.)

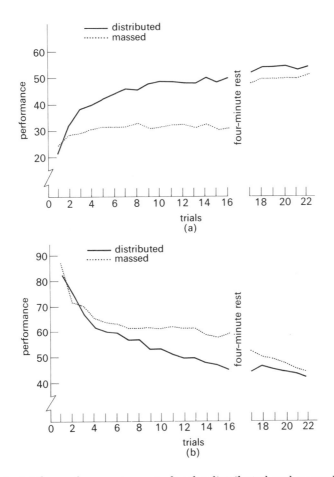

Fig. 19.5 In (a) the performance curves for the distributed and massed groups on the stabilometer. In (b) the performance curves for the distributed and massed groups on the Bachman ladder. (Based on Stelmach, 1969.)

difference was found in the amount of learning (Fig. 19.5). On the other hand, Caplan (1970) reported that massed practice produced less learning on the Bachman ladder than did distributed practice.

C. OPTIMAL REST PERIODS AND CHANGING PRACTICE SCHEDULES

Just how much rest is optimal between practice periods remains a problem. There are limits to the length of the rest period which can be beneficial to learning. After long rest periods of, for example, weeks or months, some forgetting will occur and time for relearning will be necessary when practice is begun again. The optimum distribution of practice obviously lies somewhere between the overcrowding which disrupts practice and the separation which allows a loss of previous gains before practice is resumed.

There is no consensus in the research literature concerning the effectiveness of changing practice schedules as learning progresses. Garry (1963) states that "the practice period should be short when new motor skills are being introduced for the first time...." He goes on to say that "massed practice is desirable when peak performances of a well-established skill is required." On the other hand, Dore and Hilgard, (1938), on the basis of their research, concluded that practice schedules should be massed in the early learning phase and should be changed progressively to distributed in later stages. Harmon and Miller (1950), using a billiards-shooting task, kept constant the units of practice, number of practices, and length of practice periods, while the time intervals between the practice periods were varied for each of the four groups. They concluded that relative massing at the beginning of the learning is preferable to widely spaced practice intervals at the beginning. Oxendine (1965) had subjects practice mirror tracing on three different schedules: massed-to-distributed, distributed-to-massed, and a constant schedule. He found that the group learning by constant units of practice produced more effective overall learning than did groups using either of the changing schedules. But the schedule of gradually lengthening work periods (distributed-to-massed) was superior to the progressively shortened work periods (massed-to-distributed).

D. RETENTION AND PRACTICE SCHEDULES

As noted in Chapter 16, the effects of practice distribution on retention have not been studied to any extent. However, the few studies that have examined this variable suggest that retention of motor skills is superior under distributed practice (Lynn, 1971), although Singer (1965) reported better retention for a skill learned under massed and relatively massed conditions.

E. PRINCIPLES FOR PRACTICE SCHEDULES

It is obvious that the research findings on the distribution of practice do not justify the formulation of any hard and fast "laws." However, drawing on the results of the various investigations reported above, and many others that could not be included, several principles may be proposed.

1. Distributed practice produces superior performance.
2. There is very little difference in learning between distributed and massed schedules, but distributed schedules have a slight advantage.

3. Distributed practice is preferable when the energy demands of the task are high, the task is complex, the length of task performance is great, the task is not meaningful, and motivation of the learner is low.

4. Massed practice is preferable when the skill level of the learner is high and when peak performance on a well-learned skill is needed.

5. Massed practice may be preferable when the skill is highly meaningful, when motivation is high, and when there is considerable transfer from previously learned tasks to the new task.

6. To the extent that intertrial rest can be reduced without decreasing the amount of learning, the efficiency of a practice session can be increased.

7. In coaching, the demands of preparing a team to play contests may necessitate much massing of practice. The coach frequently cannot spread the practice schedule for a given skill over several weeks. Skill learning must be done within a short period of time in order to provide the players with the needed skills to compete against scheduled opponents. When the principles listed above are taken into consideration, the coach need not be overly concerned about whether a massed schedule will adversely affect learning, although its effect upon immediate performance may be detrimental.

F. THEORIES ABOUT DISTRIBUTION OF PRACTICE

Why is performance better under distributed schedules than under massed schedules? The most commonly proposed interpretation of these results is that massed practice produces an inhibitory effect on performance, but has no effect on learning. Diminution in the inhibitory effects during rest periods would account for both reminiscence and for the fact that performance under the two conditions approaches the same level after a rest interval.

The classical statement of inhibitory effects is that of Clark Hull (1943) who postulated two types of inhibition processes: (1) Reaction inhibition (I_R), and (2) Conditioned inhibition $(_SI_R)$. With regard to I_R, Hull said, "Whenever any reaction is evoked in an organism, there is left a condition or state which acts as a primary, negative motivation in that it has an innate capacity to produce a cessation of the activity which produced the state." According to this notion, as a consequence of making any response, there is an increment in a tendency not to repeat it. In addition, the longer the individual practice session, the more reactive inhibition builds up, and the greater is the drive not to respond as the practice continues. Hull states, ". . . the net amount of functioning inhibitory potential resulting from a sequence of reaction evocations is a positively accelerated function of the amount of work (W) involved in the performance of the response in question." The reaction decrements which Hull attributed to I_R bear a resemblance to the decrements commonly attributed to "fatigue," but I_R denotes a decrement in action evocation potentiality, not an exhaustion of the energy available to the performer.

A second characteristic of I_R, according to Hull, is that "each amount of inhibitory potential diminishes progressively with the passage of time according to a simple decay or negative growth function." This extends the notion of inhibition to the dissipation of it over time, in much the same way as fatigue is dissipated by rest.

Applying reactive inhibition to practice schedules, in distributed practice conditions, where the ratio of work to rest is at least somewhat equal, I_R accrues and dissipates in equal amounts; thus, performance is not adversely affected. But in massed practice conditions, I_R builds up as the performer continues to practice, thus depressing performance. Rest intervals allow inhibition to dissipate and, when practice resumes, performance levels are initially much better than just before the rest period.

Hull's second inhibitory process, conditioned inhibition $(_sI_R)$ is viewed as a negative habit which, when the stimuli in the practice situation become conditioned to I_R, produces a reduction in the tendency to respond. In other words, if I_R is allowed to build up, failures to respond will be reinforced by reducing what is seen essentially as a drive not to respond; in this way, $_sI_R$ is developed.

Inhibition theory does not provide a very satisfactory explanation of what may in fact be several distinct phenomena, but unfortunately there is so far no clear superior account to take its place.

The Hullian theory is formulated in behavioral, rather than in neurological, terms. A neurological explanation for differences in performance under massed and distributed schedule makes use of information about alterations in brain activity to simuli, especially repetitive stimuli.

By the use of an electroencephalograph (EEG), it is possible to record the electrical activity of the brain. When a person is in an alert but resting state, the EEG commonly shows the alpha wave pattern. This consists of relatively high amplitude, synchronous waves of between 8–13 Hz. The neurological response to a novel or unexpected stimulus involves the appearance of low-amplitude, fast, desynchronized wave patterns. Normally, these replace the alpha waves and are known as "the alpha block." The alpha block is associated with behavioral arousal, orienting movements, and widespread autonomic charges, i.e., increased heart rate, dilation of the eyes, etc. It is assumed that this arousal response results in an increased ability to detect, classify, and respond appropriately to the incoming stimulus information; in short, the individual is able to perform well in this state. A continuing repetition of stimuli leads to a habituation of the arousal response. Habituation of the arousal response includes changes that may decrease the sensitivity of individuals to a stimulus as well as their readiness to respond.

With regard to practice schedules, the neural response to the initiation of practice is undoubtedly an alpha block and the arousal response. Under distributed practice, the frequent rest periods followed by a new practice period are likely to provide enough novelty and changed conditions to maintain the alpha block and, therefore, high performance. On the other hand, the prolonged repetition under massed conditions is likely to result in habituation, and, therefore, a decrement in performance as practice continues. The notion that the decremental effects of massed practice are due to decreased arousal is capable of explaining a number of results that cannot be accounted for by inhibition theories (Catalano, 1967; Catalano and Whalen, 1967; McIntyre, Mostoway, Stojak, and Humphries, 1972).

PRACTICE UNDER FATIGUED CONDITIONS

The literature on the subject of the effects of fatigue on motor behavior is both vast and depressing; vast because the topic of fatigue has been of interest to human-factor researchers of industrial and military organizations as well as to researchers of sports behavior; depressing because this topic has been beset by methodological and conceptual problems that have rendered much of the findings confusing and contradictory. The conceptual inadequacies of fatigue research stem in large part from the word "fatigue" itself. The word suggests a unitary phenomenon, yet it is obvious that there are a number of separate and diverse dimensions of the word. There is first the subjective awareness of tiredness and second the objective measure of tiredness. It is clear that reports which performers make about their feelings of tiredness bear little relation to objective measures of performance; there may even be a negative correlation. At the same time, objective measures of fatigue are not easily made, and the relationships between the various measures are not altogether satisfactory.

Two of the most evident methodological problems of research on this topic have to do with the time of task performance in relation to the induced fatigue and the amount and extent of induced fatigue. Most investigations have had subjects perform on a motor task immediately after inducing the fatigue state, but several recent investigations have had the subjects perform the motor task while they were simultaneously performing a "fatiguing task." With regard to the amount and extent of induced fatigue, there has been no uniformity. Investigators have used treadmills, bicycle ergometers, and bench step-ups, and fatigue has been indexed by various work loads performed by the subjects, various heart rates, and even subjective feelings expressed by the subjects.

There is a rather substantial body of literature which shows that fatigue induced before performance or interpolated between trials to maintain the fatigue condition throughout practice hinders performance in tasks such as body steadiness, static balance, dynamic balance and mirror tracing (Ross, Hussman, and Andrews, 1954; Johnson, Christian, and Arterbury, 1968; Nunney, 1963; Schmidt, 1969; Pack, Cotten, and Biasiotto, 1974). But performance on tasks such as speed of arm movement and tapping speed seems to be enhanced by prior induced fatigue (Phillips, 1963; Ross et al., 1954), while performance on the rotary pursuit and maze performance are unaffected by induced fatigue (Gutin, 1970). Although these findings appear contradictory, most evidence indicates that physical fatigue is detrimental to performance; how detrimental depends upon such factors as condition of the subjects, the demands of the task, and the actual extent of the fatigue.

The research regarding the effect of fatigue on learning is contradictory. Several investigations have found that learning was unaffected by fatigue (Alderman, 1965; Carron, 1969; Cotten et al., 1972; and Schmidt, 1969). However, some of these earlier studies induced fatigue only before performance of the task to be learned so recovery from fatigue during practice was likely. Studies in which fatigue was severe and was maintained throughout the practice period have shown that learning was adversely affected by fatigue (Caplan, 1970; Carron, 1972; Carron and Ferchuk, 1971; Godwin and Schmidt, 1971; Thomas et al., 1974), suggesting that in order for fatigue to interfere with learning, subjects must remain fatigued throughout the practice period.

The effect of fatigue on learning the Bachman ladder climb was assessed by Pack and his colleagues (1974) who manipulated fatigue by having subjects perform on a treadmill until their assigned heart rate was achieved. Then they practiced the Bachman ladder, returning to the treadmill after each practice trial. The learning score data indicated that subjects whose assigned heart rate fatigue level was 150 to 180 beats per minute showed a decremental effect on learning of the task. It appears, then, that practicing a motor task under conditions of severe fatigue impairs the learning process.

Most research on the effects of fatigue on motor learning has employed the fatiguing conditions before or during the practice—they have been concerned with the proactive effects of fatigue. Common experience and consolidation memory theory would suggest that fatigue induced immediately after a learning experience might disrupt memory consolidation, and thus inhibit learning. Strong exterioceptive stimuli shortly following a training trial interfered with the memory of that trial for mice (Jacobs and Sorenson, 1969) and Hutton and his colleagues (1972) reported preliminary findings from two animal experiments in which fatiguing exercises were introduced after the learning trials. Results suggested partial support for the hypothesis that fatigue introduced after practice on a task depressed learning.

The nervous system is the primary limiting factor for all kinds of work. There is a wealth of neurophysiological data which indicates that exhaustive exercise tends to depress neural mechanisms associated with alert, attentive behavior. Afferent and efferent neurons lose sensitivity and reactivity with long-repeated, rapid stimulation and thus show a fatigue effect—receptors fail to respond to stimuli and motorneurons either fail to transmit impulses or secrete an inadequate supply of transmitter substance at the neuromuscular junction to fire the muscle fiber. In the CNS, fatigue produces an increase in the resting EEG wave pattern, suggesting that the person is less attentive to stimuli and there is a diminished effect of stimulants on arousal responses of cortical and subcortical structures (Pineda and Adkisson, 1961).

MENTAL PRACTICE

It is possible to facilitate the learning of a motor skill by "mentally" practicing the skill between practice trials. Although numerous studies have confirmed this fact, little systematic application of this information has occurred in physical education and athletic coaching. The general belief that "physical" learning is different from "mental" learning and the knowledge that actual practice of the movements of a skill is necessary for skill acquisition have probably perpetuated the notion that the only way to learn motor tasks is to actually perform the task.

A cognitive, or mental, rehearsal of a motor task without any overt motor movements is called mental practice. When tennis players imagine themselves going through the movements of serving a tennis ball, they are involved in mental practice. Basketball players who think through their jump shots while not actually performing are mentally practicing. The word "mental" means that persons are thinking about a particular task and imagining themselves performing it. They are thus producing a pattern of neural impulses in the brain.

Since the classical implication of the word "mental" carries with it the notion of a "nonphysical" phenomenon, perhaps the term "mental practice" is unfortunate. The activity of the nervous system during mental practice is certainly "physical" in the sense that body cells are functioning and electric current is being passed along these nerve cells. The term "covert rehearsal" is occasionally used to describe this form of practice, but since the term mental practice is most commonly used, we will use it in this book.

Mental practice investigations date back more than 30 years and the past 10 years have witnessed a sustained interest in studies on this topic. Richardson (1967a, 1967b), reporting on an extensive review of mental practice studies, says, "An examination of the literature over the past 30 years shows that at least 25 studies have been explicitly concerned with the effectiveness of this procedure."

Typically, experiments on mental practice contain three groups: (1) A physical practice group; (2) A mental practice group; and (3) A group that used a combination of physical and mental practice and/or a group that does not practice at all.

A variety of novel motor skills have been used in these studies, i.e., finger maze, ring-tossing, toy paddle-ball, novel juggling tasks, etc. Likewise, various sports skills have been used, i.e., basket shooting, tennis serving gymnastic stunts, bowling, etc.

A. MENTAL PRACTICE AND MOTOR LEARNING

The literature is too extensive to discuss all of the studies that have been completed on mental practice, but we shall cite several of these studies as representative of the work that has been completed on this topic involving motor tasks.

Vandell et al. (1943) reported the pioneer study on mental practice and motor skill learning. They used junior high school, senior high school, and college students as subjects and had them practice basketball free-throw shooting and dart throwing. These investigators found that the physical and mental practice groups improved, while the no-practice groups did not improve. They concluded that mental practice was almost as effective as actual practice, for the conditions of their experiment. The value of this investigation, however, is limited because there was no statistical analysis and only 12 subjects were used.

Twining (1949) divided college men into three groups and had them practice a ring-tossing task. One group practiced daily for 22 days; a second group tossed rings only on the first and 22nd day, while mentally practicing each day between the first and 22nd day; a third group did not engage in any type of practice between test days. He found that the group that actually practiced tossing each day showed the most improvement. The "mental" practice group showed significant improvement, but not as much as the "physical" practice group. The no-practice group displayed no significant improvement.

Egstrom (1964) also used college men but he divided them into six groups and had them learn a novel paddle-ball task. Each group used a different combination of physical practice and mental practice. He reported that physical practice and combination physical practice–mental practice groups made the greatest improvements. He also found that a group that used mental practice during the first half of the experiment and then changed to physical practice showed improvement in each stage of the experiment. He suggested that mental practice and physical practice might be alternately used in physical education programs.

Stebbins (1968) divided college students into five different treatment conditions: control, mental, physical, mental-physical, and physical-mental. The subjects practiced a simple hand-eye throwing task. He concluded that mental practice alone did not produce any improvement in learning the task; the greatest amount of improvement was made by using a combination of practice conditions.

Many other studies could be identified which show the effects of mental practice on motor learning. Instead, Richardson's conclusions, made after an extensive review of mental practice studies, will suffice to place this topic in perspective. He says:

Despite a variety of methodological inadequacies, the trend of most studies indicates that MP [mental practice] procedures are associated with improved performance on the task. Statistically, significant positive findings were obtained in eleven studies....Seven further studies show a positive trend....Three studies report negative findings....

Results continue to associate various conditions of mental practice with improved learning rate. In a more recent review of the mental practice research, Corbin (1972) summarized the findings this way:

There seems to be little doubt that mental practice can positively affect skilled motor performance, especially when practice conditions are "optimal." It is equally clear, however, that mental practice is not always an aid to performance and that factors such as the practice type, the skill task, and the nature of the performer ultimately reflect the extent of behavior change resulting from MP.

B. WHEN TO PRACTICE MENTALLY

At what time during the interval between physical practices is mental practice most effective? Is it most effective if done immediately after a practice trial, at a point midway between practice trials, or just before a practice trial? This question has not been studied to any extent. In the studies that have been done, investigators have employed different periods in the interval between practice sessions for mental practice with generally consistent positive findings, regardless of when the mental practice was done. So it appears that this form of rehearsal may be done at any time between practices.

Although physical educators and coaches have frequently encouraged learners to mentally rehearse a motor skill just before performing it, studies of subjects mentally rehearsing a skill just prior to performing are not plentiful. Waterland (1956) encouraged her mental practice group to imagine the kinesthetic "feel" of the bowling movements just before delivering each ball down the alley. Under these conditions, the performers produced a smoother action, greater speed of delivery, and made higher scores than the group which practiced without this preperformance mental rehearsal.

C. SKILL LEVEL AND MENTAL PRACTICE

Clarke (1960) found that physical and mental practice were equally effective in basketball free-throw shooting with varsity and junior varsity high school players, but a novice group seemed to profit more from physical practice. This raises an interesting point with regard to the effectiveness of mental practice with groups of different skill levels. More recently, Corbin (1967a, 1967b) investigated this problem and his research suggests that mental practice can be effective only if the subjects have experience with the task and if physical practice precedes their exposure to mental practice. The findings of these studies suggest that skilled performers may benefit more from mental practice than beginners may. However, the research on this topic is too sparse to make any hard and fast rules, particularly inasmuch as a great deal of the overall mental practice research has been done with beginners and learning rate has rather consistently been found to be facilitated.

D. MENTAL PRACTICE TIME

Apparently it is not necessary to devote a great deal of time to mental practice; indeed, it seems that learners can fully concentrate on mental rehearsal for only a few minutes at a time. Although not extensive, the few studies that have attempted to examine this variable suggest that three to five minutes of mental practice at one time produced the best results (Twining, 1949; Shick, 1970).

E. RETENTION AND MENTAL PRACTICE

The effects of mental practice on skill retention have not been studied to any extent. In his extensive review of the literature, Richardson (1967a, 1967b) indicated that only two of the studies he reviewed had examined retention, and he said that the results did not allow any conclusions. Oxendine (1969) reported that the retention of the various practice groups in his study did not exhibit retention differences.

F. TECHNIQUES OF MENTAL PRACTICE

Mental practice may be used immediately preceding, following, or during the performance, and there are two general strategies that may be employed in the rehearsal. First, learners may focus their attention on the task and imagine, or visualize, themselves executing the *correct* movement pattern. This could be likened to a closed-loop film strip, with learners performing over and over, in their minds. A second technique involves rehearsing game tactics between contests or even during lulls in a contest. In this technique, learners think through what they should do if the ball suddenly comes to them, or if their opponent or teammate makes a certain maneuver. One of the oldest coaching dictates in baseball makes use of this technique—"Before each pitch is made, think of what you should do if the ball is hit to you."

G. THEORIES OF MENTAL PRACTICE

Why does mental practice result in improved performance? For this question, as for many questions in motor learning and performance, there is no satisfactory answer at the present time. But several theories have been advanced to account for this phenomenon.

It has been hypothesized that motivation is partly responsible for the effectiveness of mental practice. It has been suggested that mental practice groups become more motivated than nonpractice groups because the former groups become "ego-involved" when asked to "think about" or mentally rehearse a task. In many experiments, the mental practice group meets together regularly, while the nonpractice group is used only at the first and last test periods.

Another theory might be called the "symbolic-perceptual hypothesis." According to this theory, mental practice allows the subject to gain perceptual "insights" into the movement pattern. These new insights result in reduced errors and improved performance. There is some support for this notion in what is called the "general factors" theory of transfer of learning. This will be discussed more fully in Chapter 21 "Transfer of Motor Learning."

Consolidation Memory Theory may be employed to explain how mental practice enhances learning. Information requires rehearsal to ultimately achieve long-term storage. This rehearsal may take the form of overt movements or, apparently, may take the form of covert rehearsal; in other words, covert rehearsal may have some of the same characteristics of activating and maintaining short-term memory processes as overt practice, and in so doing bring about a more robust long-term memory. In essence, this notion hypothesizes that mental practice activates many of the neural components in the brain which are responsible for actually directing the movements. The neural component which is not, of course, fully activated in mental practice is the motor component which actually sends signals to the muscles during execution of the movement. An analogy might be the automobile with its engine running but the gears in neutral; all of the components of the engine are activated except the mechanism which makes the wheels turn. This theory implies that the effect of this neural activity modifies the circuitry so as to bring about more effective performance when the task is performed again.

Many years ago Jacobson (1930) and others discovered that by placing electrodes on muscle groups and recording the electrical activity of the subjects while they imagined themselves performing a task the muscular activity during the mental activity was localized to the muscle group that would be involved in the actual performance of the imagined activity. Jacobson noted that "when the subject imagines that he is steadily bending one of his arms, electrical phenomena simultaneously occur in the biceps region of the arm." More recently, Schramm (1967) assessed the electromyographic responses during mental practice and reported that, during the act of imagining, neuromuscular activity is recorded for those muscles which are concerned with movement.

20

Feedback and
Motor Behavior

It has been repeatedly emphasized that there are numerous factors which affect the efficiency of motor skill learning and performance. Certainly one of the most critical of these factors is feedback, and at various points in this volume we have already described some of the ways in which feedback functions in motor control and skill acquisition.

Feedback is the information which an individual receives as a result of some response. That feedback plays a prominent role in motor behavior is generally agreed upon by most researchers. Indeed, the positive influence of feedback learning and performance is one of the best established findings in motor behavior research literature. Bilodeau and Bilodeau (1961), two of the eminent researchers of this topic, say:

Studies of feedback or knowledge of results (KR) show it to be the strongest, most important variable controlling performance and learning. It has been shown repeatedly, as well as recently, that there is no improvement without KR, progressive improvement with it, and deterioration after its withdrawal.

Furthermore, they state:

No other independent variable offers the wide range of possibilities for getting man to repeat, or change his Rs [responses] immediately or slowly, by small or large amounts.

That feedback improves learning and performance is a principle that holds for children and adults and for groups as well as individuals. The research consistently shows that feedback increases the rate of improvement early in practice on a new task, enhances performance on tasks that are overlearned, and increases the frequency of reports that tasks seem less fatiguing and more interesting with feedback than under conditions in which

411

feedback is withheld. Furthermore, the benefits of feedback apply to a wide variety of tasks.

As noted in previous chapters, motor skill acquisition is essentially the learning of appropriate motor programs which correspond with proper task execution. In establishing a motor program, feedback is compared against a model or standard of the desired output. If there is a mismatch between the feedback and the model, motor program modification is needed. As the feedback comes to match the desired result, then the motor program can be used again with no modification—the correct movement response has been learned.

In previous chapters our emphasis has been on how central and peripheral mechanisms of the nervous system served feedback roles; in this chapter we shall further elaborate on this type of feedback, but we shall give greater attention to the role that instructors play in providing feedback.

THE STUDY OF FEEDBACK

The study of feedback became prominent in the psychological literature in the early 1900s, usually under the conceptual framework of "reinforcement" or "reward and punishment" terminology. The pioneer theorists were specifically dealing with learning theories. Such men as Thorndike, Hull, and Skinner are credited with making major contributions to feedback theory prior to World War II.

During the past 25 years developments in cybernetics, and the theories that it has spawned, have come to have increasing influence on the study of motor behavior, especially feedback. Cybernetics is the science of control and communication processes in both living organisms and machines, and it deals with the theory of such systems as the nerve networks in animals, electronic computing machines, feedback (or servo systems) for the automatic control of machinery and other information processing systems, which includes the human nervous system. Central to cybernetics is the notion of servomechanisms* for the continuous control of a system. Motor behavior scientists have made extensive conceptual and theoretical use of cybernetics as they have sought to understand human motor behavior.

A. RESEARCH AND FEEDBACK

Research on feedback has typically involved determining the effects of providing or withholding various kinds of information about performance during and/or for varying time intervals after performance. Studies with motor

---

*A servomechanism is essentially a machine that is controlled by the consequences of its own behavior.

tasks have used a wide variety of materials with subjects performing under various conditions. But the vast majority have employed discrete rather than continuous tasks and fine motor skills, limited in time and extent of performance. The tasks have required subjects to position levers, draw lines, turn knobs, and aim guns. It may be seen that much of the research on the effects of feedback on motor behavior has been largely limited to simple, discrete motor responses; studies using gross motor task have been conspicuously few, presumably because of the rigid control necessary when feedback is the critical variable.

TERMINOLOGY AND FEEDBACK

The variety of terms that have been employed in the feedback literature is truly bewildering, and as yet there is not complete agreement on the appropriate terminology to describe the various aspects of this topic. Bilodeau and Bilodeau (1961) some years ago wrote, "... there is no agreement on the definition, never mind the function. Indeed, there is not even widespread agreement as to name; knowledge and feedback represent the core words, modified by such words as...." They go on to list over 12 modifiers. The situation is much the same today.

Feedback terminology and the various modifiers has been classified by several schemes (Holding, 1965; Bilodeau, 1969; Del Rey, 1971). Since the selection of terms is arbitrary, we shall adopt the terminology shown on Fig. 20.1. Feedback is the root word, and means the information one receives about behavior and/or the consequences of that behavior.

Feedback may be either intrinsic or augmented. Intrinsic feedback is response-produced feedback that is supplied to the performer as an inherent consequence of the performance. Augmented feedback is the provision of special information which is ordinarily not present in a task; it is extrinsic to the individual and takes the form of either verbal information by an instructor or an external stimulus, such as a feedback circuit from a machine, which supplements the feedback obtained from the senses. The basketball jump shot may be practiced with only intrinsic feedback or the performer may receive augmented feedback to supplement intrinsic feedback. When learners execute a jump shot, they receive feedback regarding their body movements during the shot. They also see the results of their movements—the ball goes into the basket or misses the basket in some direction. This is an example of solely intrinsic feedback; that is, all the feedback is inherent in the task. Now, augmented feedback may be provided by an instructor who may give specific information about why errors in shot direction occurred or who may simply say, "Excellent shot," if the ball goes into the basket.

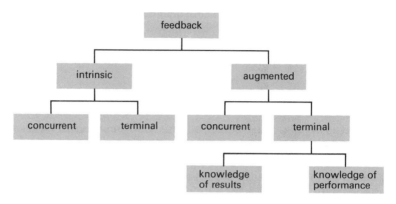

Fig. 20.1   Feedback terminology.

When feedback is being supplied while the performer is moving, it is said to be concurrent. When it is supplied after the performance is completed, it is called terminal feedback. One form of intrinsic concurrent feedback is that which the performers receive from the sensory systems during execution. Concurrent augmented feedback may be provided during a tracking task performance as a constant indication to performers of whether they are on target or off target throughout the performance. Intrinsic terminal feedback is information that individuals receive as a normal consequence of their actions—basketball players see whether the ball goes in the basket, tennis players see whether the serve goes into the appropriate service area. Augmented terminal feedback may be supplied by some mechanical device, such as a light, which may indicate the consequence of the movement, or it may be communicated by an instructor or other observer. This form of feedback may communicate information about the learner's *movement patterns*, in which case it is called knowledge of performance (KP), or about the *results or changes in the environment* that the movements produced; this is called knowledge of results (KR).

Selecting the "appropriate" terminology is certainly arbitrary, but we shall use the scheme listed in Fig. 20.1, except when reporting a specific investigator's research; at that time the researcher's own terminology will be used.

INTRINSIC FEEDBACK

Fortunately, many motor tasks supply intrinsic feedback during and/or immediately after the response is made. Such tasks as kicking a soccer ball or serving a tennis ball provide feedback as a consequence of the actions. When a soccer ball is kicked, the ball either goes into the goal or misses in one direction or another. Proprioceptive feedback supplies data regarding the body movements which are associated with varying degrees of deviation from the target, and visual feedback provides information about directional deviations. The tennis serve either hits the net, goes out of bounds, or lands in bounds. Thus, the learner can feel and see immediately what the consequences of the movements are.

Complex human skillful responses are virtually impossible without proprioceptive feedback. In the disease *tabes dorsalis*, the sensory pathways from the legs to the brain may be completely destroyed, while the motor pathways from the brain to the legs remains intact. Victims of this disease may, therefore, retain motor control of their legs but will lack proprioceptive feedback from them, so they must rely upon vision to tell them what their legs are doing. Thus, they must constantly watch their feet as they shuffle along. This dramatically illustrates the importance of proprioceptive feedback to skillful performance. This is not meant to suggest, however, that all learned movements must be guided by peripheral feedback from the proprioceptors or other sense modalities. As noted in Chapter 10, skilled movements may be initiated by a central motor program and executed without feedback.

Although the precise roles that the various sensory systems play in providing intrinsic feedback for learning have not been ascertained, there is good evidence that they play a prominent role. Learners commonly receive visual and auditory information about the success of their responses but they also receive feedback about amount of force applied, locations of limbs, body postures, and pressure exerted via the somatosensory receptors. Although neurophysiological evidence is unclear about how and to what extent these receptors provide feedback, there is good evidence that they are a rich source of information to the learner.

Adams (1971) suggests that intrinsic feedback via the sensory systems is important for developing the perceptual trace which in turn is responsible for making corrections and structuring appropriate motor responses. It also appears that early motor learning is primarily under visual control, with control gradually shifting to kinesthesis as learning progresses (Rock and Harris, 1967; Fleishman and Rich, 1963). Fitts (1964) writes:

Visual control probably is very important while an individual is learning a new perceptual-motor task. As performance becomes habitual, however, it is likely that proprioceptive feedback or "feel" becomes the more important.

AUGMENTED FEEDBACK

Some motor tasks either do not provide feedback as a consequence of the behavior or provide feedback which is fragmentary and incomplete. In order for learning to continue, an instructor or training aid may serve to provide learners with feedback regarding the consequences of their behavior. Various aids—videotape, films, and "gimmicks"—have been used as training aids to augment information to learners.

In general, both concurrent and terminal augmented feedback has been found to enhance learning and performance. Even if the task itself supplies feedback about the subject's performance, supplemental information frequently enhances learning. Reynolds and Adams (1953) found that on a target-pursuit task during which subjects could see whether or not they were on the target, additional information in the form of a clicker, which sounded when the subjects were on the target, clearly enhanced learning and performance on the task. The clicker was especially helpful later in practice, when the subjects were able to remain on the target for long periods of time. Smode (1958), using a tracking task in which subjects learned to keep centered a randomly varying needle by rotating a dial, found that performance

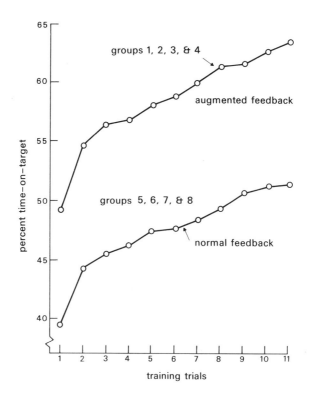

Fig. 20.2 Learning curves for motor tasks with and without augmented feedback. (Based on Smode, 1958.)

was greatly enhanced with augmented feedback (Fig. 20.2). Fitts and
Leonard (1957) found that augmented feedback in the form of a continuous
series of clicks at the rate of two per second enhanced performance in a
speeded perceptual task. Robb (1968) investigated the course of learning an
arm movement pattern under varied conditions of feedback. She found that
the group which received the greatest variety of feedback produced the
most effective learning pattern.

Augmented feedback about movement errors is usually presented to the
learners in experiments via verbal, visual, or kinesthetic means. There is
clear evidence that verbal and visual augmented feedback is effective at enhancing learning with a wide variety of motor tasks, but the role of kinesthetic augmented feedback is not clear. Lincoln (1956) and Connolly and
Jones (1970) provide limited support for the notion that verbal, visual, and
kinesthetic augmented feedback are equally effective in informing subjects
about their performance. The former reported the verbal and kinesthetic
error information was equally effective in a crank-turning task, and the
latter found error scores for visual and kinesthetic feedback on a matching
task did not produce significant differences in performance. More recently
Chew (1974) reported that verbal, visual, and kinesthetic error information
were equally effective at producing learning of a linear, self-paced positioning task. Other investigators have suggested that kinesthetic cues are less
effective in early learning than visual cues and therefore augmented visual
feedback is more appropriate (Fleishman and Rich, 1963; Rock and Harris,
1967).

The studies above convey the impression that augmented feedback always enhances motor learning and performance but, in fact, this is not the
case. There is some evidence that when sufficient feedback is inherent in
the task, the use of additional feedback does not further affect the acquisition or performance of the motor task (Bilodeau, 1969; Haywood and Glad,
1974).

Most studies of knowledge of results (KR) have dealt with some type of
accuracy on a fine motor, discrete task; few studies on this topic have been
conducted using gross motor skills. But those that have been done generally
corroborate those done with simpler tasks. Howell (1956) studied the effect
of providing feedback to subjects by showing them force-time graphs on
their sprint start after each practice trial. Another group of subjects did not
receive this information. The first group successfully learned the desired
force-time pattern and improved their speed and momentum; the second
group made very little improvement. Malina (1969) studied the effects of different KR practice conditions on the speed and accuracy of overhand throwing performance. He reported marked differences in the patterns of throwing performance under the various feedback conditions; groups receiving
speed and speed-and-accuracy KR were superior to a no-KR group on throw-

ing velocity, and accuracy and speed-and-accuracy feedback groups were superior to the no-KR group on throwing accuracy.

As with fine motor tasks, there have been reports that augmented feedback does not enhance motor learning for certain gross motor tasks. Bell (1968) had subjects practice the badminton long serve under four different conditions. She reported that no differences were found between groups which could be attributed to the different KR conditions. She concluded:

Where sufficient knowledge of results is inherent in the task, the direction of practice through the use of additional knowledge of results does not further affect the acquisition or retention of gross motor skill at the beginning levels of performance.

Fitts has suggested that augmented feedback may be particularly useful during advanced stages of learning in which learners are nearing their hypothetical limit of ability to discriminate available feedback. Augmented feedback is especially useful at this time "because of the more precise information it provides to the learner."

A. AUGMENTED FEEDBACK FOR OPEN AND CLOSED SKILLS

In Chapter 16 it was noted that motor skills may be classified as either "open" or "closed," depending upon the extent to which a performer must conform to a prescribed standard sequence of movement during execution and the extent to which effective performance depends upon environmental events. In closed skills the goal is to acquire a stereotyped movement pattern; the performer attempts to execute a precisely defined movement pattern, and the environment is an unchanging factor, as in shot putting, diving, etc. On the other hand, open skills demand the absence of stereotyped movements; there is a variety of responses, each response is a match to a particular set of requirements in the environment. Here the movement pattern must be constructed uniquely for each execution because what is required is a different response to each situation. In an open skill, no single movement pattern will accomplish the goal in all situations. There is not a single instep kick in soccer but rather numerous responses all called the instep kick; each one is different depending upon the speed to be imparted, location of where the ball is meant to go, etc., yet all are called instep kicks.

The instructor may augment information available to the learner for either performance or results. It has been suggested that for closed skills, in which one consistent pattern is the goal, knowledge of performance (KP) is the most powerful and appropriate form of augmented information, while knowledge of results (KR) is the most appropriate for the learning of open skills, where a variety of motor patterns is the goal (Gentile, 1972). KP provides information about the performer's movement patterns, about the spatial and temporal employment of the body's parts. KR provides information about the consequences of the performer's movement, the results or changes in the environment that the performer's movement produced. Recent studies have supported the contention that KP is more effective with closed skills and KR more effective with open skills (Del Rey, 1971; Hampton, 1970).

FREQUENCY AND WITHDRAWAL OF FEEDBACK

How often should augmented feedback be given? Should it be administered after every performance, or intermittently? That is, is the total number of feedbacks in a set of performances (absolute frequency) more important than the proportion of performances on which feedback is given (relative frequency)? Bilodeau and Bilodeau (1958a) compared the learning rates of four groups that received feedback after every trial, after every third, fourth, or tenth trial while performing a linear positioning task while blindfolded. Performance improved only on the trials immediately following the presentation of knowledge of results (KR). Moreover, when they plotted the error scores for only the responses that followed KR, the responses were almost identical for the four groups—in short, there was no learning during trials without KR. The implication here is that it is the absolute frequency, the actual number of KRs provided, that determines rates of learning and that relative frequency is unimportant for learning. That is, whatever the distribution of KR, non-KR trials neither hinder nor facilitate the learning produced by KR trials. Taylor and Noble (1962) had subjects learn to respond to the Selective Mathometer, using 100, 75, 50, and 25 percent KR. They reported that 100 percent-KR groups displayed the most efficient skill acquisition. They also found that in early withdrawal of KR trials, that this group was slightly more susceptive to cessation of performance (this they called extinction).

A. WITHDRAWAL OF FEEDBACK

The research is rather consistent in the finding that when KR is provided during training and then withdrawn, performance deteriorates in succeeding trials. The extent to which this happens differs, however, and the problem is to ascertain whether certain methods of administering KR during learning leads to better maintained performance than do others in which KR is withdrawn. A rather dramatic example of the consequences of removing KR is the now classic study of Elwell and Grindley (1938). They used an apparatus in which subjects employed two levers to direct a spot of light on a target, and in the initial stage of the experiment the light clearly indicated where on the target they had landed. In the second phase of the study, KR was removed by switching off the light, so the subjects were unable to see where on the target they had landed. There was an immediate drop in performance (Fig. 20.3). Moreover, the subjects were annoyed by the change in conditions, they became bored and careless, and even began arriving late for practice sessions. Seashore *et al.* (1949) reported a marked diminution in ranging scores by trainees on the Pedestal Sight Manipulation Test* when the red filter arrangement, which indicated hits on the target, was stopped. Bilodeau, Bilodeau, and Schumsky (1959), using a lever-displacing task, found no improvement without KR (KR was the amount and direction of the reported error), progressive improvement with KR, and deterioration of performance after the withdrawal of KR.

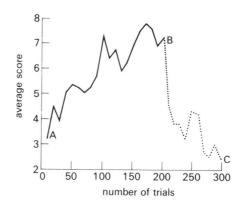

Fig. 20.3 The reduction in performance with withdrawal of knowledge of results. AB is the average curve of performance while subjects received knowledge of results. BC is the average curve after knowledge of results was withdrawn. (Based on Elwell and Grindley, 1938.)

The closed-loop theory of motor learning proposed by Adams (1971) postulates that withdrawal of KR after a task has been well learned should not result in a performance decrement, and this has been supported in studies using simple, self-paced positioning tasks and brief ballistic tasks. According to Adams, KR is used to detect errors and correct responses during the early phases of learning, and this process results in the development of a perceptual trace, which is a response recognition mechanism, made up of

---

*The Pedestal Sight Manipulation Test requires that subjects keep a dot on a moving target by manipulating the sight with their hands.

how the response looked, felt, and sounded. If KR is withdrawn after limited practice in which the perceptual trace has not been well developed, a performance decrement occurs. But, since the perceptual trace is strengthened with learning, gradually a strong perceptual trace develops and forms a composite representation, or image, of the feedback qualities of the correct response and thus operates as a reference mechanism for evaluation of current responses. At this point, response-produced feedback can be compared to the perceptual trace, enabling the learner to associate response-produced feedback with response outcome, and thus accurate movement may be maintained without KR. Some support for this notion has been reported for simple, self-paced positioning tasks and ballistic tasks (Schmidt and White, 1972; and Newell, 1974). In these studies KR was withdrawn at different points along a series of practice trials. The results supported the prediction of Adam's theory which proposed that criterion performance is maintained during KR withdrawal because a strong response recognition has been developed which serves as a reference for evaluation of response-produced feedback.

B. ACCURACY OF FEEDBACK

In general, the efficiency of motor learning is directly related to the precision of feedback; that is, the more precise feedback is relative to performance on a motor task, the more efficient acquisition of skill will be (Smoll, 1972; McGuigan, 1959; Trowbridge and Cason, 1932). However, some investigators have found little advantage in increasing precision of feedback beyond a certain level with lever position, rudder control, and knob rotation tasks, suggesting that there may be some optimal level of precision beyond which the learner cannot process and translate the information into meaningful performance improvements.

The "optimal-level hypothesis" proposes that increased precision, up to a point, improves performance, but further increases do not enhance, and may even have detrimental effects on, performance (Gill, 1975; Rogers, 1974). In studying the effects of varying KR precision levels on a linear positioning task, Gill (1975) reported that KR precision level (error scores in either centimeters or millimeters) did not affect actual performance but extremely precise KR had detrimental effects on performance evaluation and the labeling process of estimating performance by the subjects.

Although there may be an optimal precision level at which additional precision is no more beneficial to the learner, this particular level would have to be obtained for each task. So it seems that the motor skill instructor should employ as much precision as seems reasonable. If this is done, there is little evidence that learning will be greatly deterred.

DELAY OF FEEDBACK

Just as feedback schedules are important factors in motor behavior, so is the time lapse between performance and feedback. Since the consequences of delaying concurrent feedback and terminal feedback are so dramatically different, it is essential to treat these two feedback conditions separately.

A. CONCURRENT FEEDBACK

Some tasks lend themselves to concurrent feedback utilization and others impose limits on the feasibility of concurrent feedback, because of the speed and frequency with which movements must be made (such as the golf swing). In motor tasks in which intrinsic concurrent feedback can be used in task performance, any delay, even a delay as short as a fraction of a second, seriously hampers, or even makes impossible, appropriate execution. The effects of this kind of feedback lag is dramatically illustrated in delayed feedback of speech. In this condition, average persons stutter, slur their words, or omit whole syllables, and speak as if in a state of intoxication. Similar effects have been reported for various types of motor acts.

Chase and his colleagues (1961a, 1961b, 1961c) conducted several experiments in which sensory feedback was delayed and/or decreased. In one study they compared the effects of a 244-millisecond delay in auditory feedback for repetitions of a simple speech sound and the repetitive motor act of key tapping. They reported that both response classes produced more errors and disruption in timing because of the delay. The amplitude of motor responses and the intensity of spoken sounds were disturbed.

K.U. Smith and his colleagues (Smith and Smith, 1962; Smith 1962) have demonstrated the disastrous effects of delaying concurrent visual feedback on motor activities. Employing complex television camera-videotape arrangements, Smith has modified the visual feedback so that performers see themselves doing things shortly after they are actually done. Time delays as brief as 1/5 of a second produce an entire breakdown of performance. Smith writes:

> ...various studies of delayed sensory feedback, both visual and auditory, have produced strikingly similar results. Delays of even a small fraction of a second cause serious disturbances of behavior organization, often accompanied by emotional effects.... All evidence indicates that there is little, if any, effective adaptation to conditions of delayed feedback.

B. TERMINAL FEEDBACK

As noted above, terminal augmented feedback is that information which is provided to the learner after a trial or performance, and this commonly akes the form of KR. When considering the application of KR, there are several time intervals involved in the interresponse interval; that is, the time between Response 1 and Response 2 (Fig. 20.4). First is the KR-delay interval, which is the period following the end of the response until KR is presented to the learner. Second, the time interval that follows the presentation of KR until the learner must make the next response is called the post-KR-delay interval. Finally, the third interval is the total amount of time from the end of one response to the next response and it is called the interresponse interval; it incorporates the first two intervals.

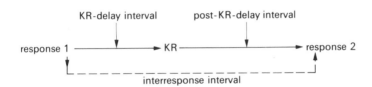

Fig. 20.4   Various time intervals between responses.

In addition to the question of the effects of just sheer delay of KR on motor learning, there is also the issue of introducing into either the KR-delay interval and/or the post-KR period some intervening (usually called interpolated) task for the learner to perform. The question at issue here is whether the interpolated task performed during one or both of the KR-delay intervals influences learning.

1. The KR-delay interval

The KR-delay interval is the interval that has most often been studied over the years, but the results of this research have led to some confusion about the consequences of this type of feedback delay on human learning. There are two main reasons for this confusion: First, results of studies with lower animals have been generalized to humans and, second, there has been a mixing of results for studies in which there was no interpolated task required of the learner and results of studies in which the KR-delay interval was filled with an interpolated task.

Many years ago, studies with animals clearly established the fact that delay of feedback produced learning decrements (Hamilton, 1929; Roberts, 1930) but the classic study by Lorge and Thorndike (1935) called into question the application of animal results for humans, for humans, since that delaying KR did not deter learning. The subjects performed a ball-tossing task at a target which they could not see. The results showed that delays of KR up to six seconds did not affect improvements.

The Lorge and Thorndike study triggered an ongoing controversy which is still active today. In terms of sheer numbers of studies supporting one side or the other, the research is overwhelmingly in support of Lorge and Thorndike's original finding—that is, that the mere delay of KR does not adversely affect human motor learning (Alexander, 1951; Bilodeau and Bilodeau 1958b; McGuigan, 1959; Larre, 1961). Perhaps the Bilodeau and Bilodeau (1958b) study provides the most convincing evidence that delay of feedback during the KR-delay interval does not deter learning. Five studies were undertaken, each one providing KR delay, one up to one week! The studies failed to show that KR-delay had any effect on the learning of the skills. Bilodeau and Bilodeau (1961), in a review of delay of KR studies, say that "to delay or to give immediate KR can be quite immaterial for learning to make relatively simple Rs [responses] when the periods between Rs are relatively free of specially interpolated Rs."

The evidence is not completely unequivocal, however; support for KR delay effect has been presented by several investigators (Greenspoon and Foreman, 1956; Dyal, 1964, 1966). But the evidence strongly supports the conclusion that KR delay alone does not affect the learning of simple motor tasks, providing the KR-delay interval does not require interpolated activity by the learner.

Studies concerned with the effect of interpolated activity on the KR delay period are not numerous, and the findings do not lead to a definite conclusion. Research on this subject has used two basic interpolated activities. In the first KR is given a number of trials after the response to which it actually refers (e.g., a one-trial delay is: Response 1, Response 2, KR for Response 1, Response 3, KR for Response 2 . . .); in the second, the interpolated activity is some type of verbal or motor task performed during the KR delay interval.

Lorge and Thorndike (1935) and Bilodeau (1956) reported that when KR was given following the response to which it referred it produced decrements in learning. The Lorge and Thorndike subjects tossed balls at a target they could not see and received KR after an interval filled by another throw which referred back to the previous throw. Bilodeau (1956) studied the effect of delay of knowledge of results in an experiment in which additional responses had to be made during the delay. For example, in a two-trial delay condition, knowledge of results of the first trial was given only after the third trial had been completed, knowledge of results of the second trial were given after the fourth trial was completed, etc. She reported that with one-two-, three-, or five-trial delays, rate of learning and level of accuracy achieved within 30 KR trials decreased with the number of trials by which KR was delayed. This basic finding was replicated more recently by others (Lavery, 1964; Lavery and Suddon, 1962). On the other hand, Larre (1961) reported no differences due to amount of interpolated activity, when KR was delayed for a given number of trials or responses, and others have reported that verbal or motor tasks used as interpolated activities do not adversely affect motor skill acquisition, when employed during the KR-delay period (Boulter, 1964).

At the present, it is difficult to reconcile the differences in findings for the KR-delay interval. From a theoretical viewpoint, the Consolidation Memory Theory would suggest that the unfilled KR interval would not adversely affect, and may enhance, learning because the short-term trace of the response could be well maintained. Thus, from what has been said about short-term memory, we should expect lapse of time as such to have either no effect or an enhancing effect, but it would seem that intervening activities and shifts of attention might be disruptive to learning. Adams's (1971) closed-loop theory would suggest the KR-delay should not affect either the perceptual trace or the motor trace, the two traces assumed to be strengthened during learning. More theoretical and empirical study will be necessary to fully settle the issue of the effects of KR-delay periods on motor learning.

From an instructional standpoint, there is no compelling evidence for delaying feedback. The principle that information about the correctness of performance should be administered quickly has been used successfully in teaching a wide variety of verbal and motor tasks. So it appears that KR should be provided as soon as possible after a response is completed but also that, if a delay must occur, the instructor need not be overly concerned because the delay will not have disastrous results.

2. Post-KR interval

The period between the administration of KR and the next response has not had the research interest that the KR-delay interval has experienced, but, in general, the research that has been done suggests that unfilled post-KR intervals have little effect on motor learning. In one of the earliest studies of this topic, Brown (1949) reported that post-KR length is related to the acquisition of motor skills, but contradictory findings have been reported by several investigators since then (Bilodeau and Bilodeau, 1958a; Boucher, 1974; Magill 1973, 1975). These more recent studies indicate that the length of the post-KR period does not affect motor learning.

It has been proposed that there is an optimal post-KR period, that up to a certain length performance should improve providing that the period is long enough to process the KR, but beyond that point performance should decline. Adams (1971) states that "increasing the post-KR interval up to a point will improve performance." Although this notion is intuitively and theoretically appealing, there is little empirical evidence to support it.

Research of the effects of post-KR intervals that are filled with interpolated verbal or motor activities has produced equivocal results, and at
present no firm conclusions may be made. Several investigators have reported that post-KR activity adversely affects performance (McGuigan et al.,
1964; Boswell and Bilodeau, 1964) but others have found interpolated tasks
to have no affect on performance (Blick and Bilodeau, 1963; Magill, 1973)
when the task was motoric. Boucher (1974) reported that the use of pron-
unciation of difficult multisyllabic words adversely affected performance
early in practice but not later in practice, but Magill (1973; 1975) reported
results indicating no effect on performance when the verbal activity was
counting backward.

In the post-KR interval, the learner is assumed to process the information by developing new strategies and hypotheses about the nature of the
task and how to accomplish it, resulting in the selection of new motor programs to correct errors. In relation to consolidation memory theory an unfilled period should facilitate consolidation providing that the period is not
too brief for neural processing, while an interval with interpolated activity
should disrupt short-term neural processing, but there is some evidence that
motor short-term memory processing may be somewhat different from
verbal short-term processing, since several investigators have found kines-
thetic-distance forgetting to be unrelated to interpolated activity (Posner
and Konick, 1966; Williams et al., 1969).

Adam's (1971) motor learning theory gives important consideration to
the post-KR period because presumably it is during this period that the
learner is evaluating and forming new response strategies for the next
response, especially in the early phase of learning. Thus, the strengthening
of both perceptual and motor traces are dependent on this period. Adams
suggests that too brief an interval will not allow for enough processing but if
the intervals are too long, performance will decline. As noted above, this
proposition needs further empirical support.

There is little need for the motor skills instructor to be overly concerned
about the post-KR interval, providing its duration is neither less than a second or two nor extremely long, i.e., days or weeks. Post-KR between these extremes can be useful to the learner.

3. The interresponse interval

The interresponse interval (IRI) has typically not been held constant in the
studies of KR delay and post-KR delay. This lack of constancy has been suggested as the main reason for the equivocal results. But the validity of this
assertion is still unsettled. Bilodeau and Bilodeau (1958b), on the basis of the
results of two of their studies, suggested that the IRI is the critical variable,

with learning being enhanced with shorter intervals. However, recent research by Magill (1975) and Shea (1975) failed to support this conclusion; Magill reported that different lengths of interresponse yielded no differences in effects on motor learning the locations of three specified positions on serial order with a manual lever, and Shea reported similar results using a discrete positioning task.

The issue of the effects of IRI is, of course, related to the issue of retention of motor skills. Both consolidation memory theory and Adams's (1971) motor learning theory consider that the strength of a motor program for response execution is dependent upon the IRI. For Adams, the perceptual trace is weakened through forgetting during the IRI, causing a performance decrement, and decay of neural connections which constitute long-term memory has the same consequence from a consolidation memory theory standpoint.

It appears that the motor skills instructor need not be overly concerned about adversely affecting motor learning, provided that the IRIs are not too short, which might produce the performance decrements described for massed practice, or too long, which might produce memory loss.

FUNCTIONS OF FEEDBACK

Learning is a modification of behavior brought about by experience and is measured by changes in performances in the direction of some criterion. In order for learners to modify their behavior to achieve the criterion, or goal, they must know whether or not their responses are bringing them closer to the criterion; they need information about their responses. While this fact is rather obvious, there are several subtle factors that are not so obvious concerning the influence of feedback on learning and performance.

Brown (1949) and Ammons (1956) were the first to identify and discuss the three functions which feedback may provide: information, motivation, and reinforcement. It may inform individuals about what they should or should not do, or be doing; it may motivate individuals; and/or it may reward individuals for correct performance and/or punish them for incorrect performance.

Although feedback may certainly serve these three functions, it is practically impossible to establish exactly how and why feedback is working, that is, whether the main effects are informational, motivational, or reinforcing. The nature of the interaction of these variables is not clearly known and few investigators have thrown any significant light on the problem.

A. INFORMATION FUNCTION

Several writers have discussed the informational aspects of feedback. Plausible explanations for this function are plentiful. Feedback is foremost a source of information which results in corrections that eventually lead the learner to correct response. Feedback provides cues or information to learners concerning the type, extent, and direction of their errors. Learners can use such information to correct their errors or to improve their methods of performing the task.

Currently, the leading spokesman for the information function of feedback is Adams (1971). He does not insist that feedback is not used as reinforcement or motivation, but according to him, these are not the primary functions served in human learning.

B. MOTIVATION FUNCTION

Many types of feedback can serve both informational and motivational functions and the manner in which feedback functions to motivate learners is quite complicated. Any type of feedback that serves a cueing function may indirectly affect motivation but the converse is not necessarily true. There are some types of feedback that could not be used to correct errors or to improve one's method of performing the task. Examples of ways of providing feedback which does not give the learner information about a better *method* of performing are total time-on-target scores on a pursuit task, total score on some task after several trials, total score after several throws on a target-throwing task, etc. (Locke, 1967). Any effects on performances from these types of feedback may be attributed to motivational factors, since presumably only the learner's level of effort is affected.

Smode (1958) hypothesized that a higher feedback-of-information schedule would produce superior performances than a lower information-feedback schedule, due to motivational effects. He found that high information feedback facilitated performance and that interest level increased as a function of increased information feedback. He concluded that "the effect of the higher information feedback was mediated by an increase in motivation."

Gibbs and Brown (1955) attempted to isolate and measure the purely motivational factor of knowledge of results. Their subjects worked at an extremely uninteresting and repetitive task (copying pages from difficult scientific reports, encyclopedias, and historical reviews). In the experiment, knowledge of results was casual and incidental. In half the trials subjects could see a counter which tallied each page as it was copied; in half the trials the counter was covered. The subjects were given no incentives or rewards for the work completed; nevertheless, the findings showed that when the subjects could see the counter, their output was significantly higher than it was when the counter was covered. On the other hand, Chapanis (1964) could not replicate Gibbs and Brown's findings with subjects performing a repetitive, monotonous task (punching random digits into a teletype tape). He did offer, however, several suggestions to account for the discrepancy between the results of the two experiments.

Undoubtedly, knowledge of results functions as an incentive and aids performance, even after a task has been well learned. It has been found that if two well-trained groups perform a task, with one group receiving KR and the other group not receiving KR, the group receiving KR will consistently give the better performance.

The way in which feedback exerts its motivational effects is not yet fully understood. One suggestion is that certain types of feedback affect the goal or aim the performers set for themselves; that is, it may motivate the learners to try harder and persist longer at the task. Locke and his colleagues have found that the setting of "hard" goals does facilitate performance (Locke, 1967; Locke, Cartledge, and Koeppel, 1968).

An increase in arousal state, which is one aspect of motivation, may also mediate the effects of feedback on learning and performance. Arousal states have been found to be related to performance and learning; up to a point there are increased learning and performance. It appears that at least part of the differences of learning and performance between individuals can be accounted for in terms of the level of arousal. Why this is so is not clear, but a moderate level of arousal presumably strengthens the consolidation process for long-term memory, and perhaps strengthens the memories already there.

C. REINFORCEMENT FUNCTION

Whether feedback serves informational or reinforcement functions has been debated for some time. Annett (1969) has this to say about the controversy, "There have been numerous attempts to solve the problem of distinguishing between informational and reinforcement effects—none entirely satisfactory." The reinforcement function of feedback is in the instrumental learning tradition in which a class of reinforcing stimuli is presumed to strengthen, or "cement," a relatively stable habit state for the learner. Reinforcement has been defined as an event following a response which increases the probability that the response will be made again when the same stimulus situation occurs. Thorndike (1911) formulated a reinforcement theory called the "Law of Effect." He said:

Of several responses made to the same situation, those which are accompanied or closely followed by satisfaction to the animal will be more likely to recur; those which are accompanied or closely followed by discomfort to the animal will, other things being equal, have their connections with that sit-uation weakened, so that, when it recurs, they will be less likely to occur. The greater the satisfaction or discomfort, the greater the strengthening or weakening of the bond.

The "reinforcement" view of feedback, then, is that feedback is rewarding or punishing, and that a rewarding result preserves the behavior which pre-ceded it by some mechanism.

There are at the present time what might be called several theories of reinforcement rather than just a single reinforcement theory, but there is a great deal of commonality to them. Hull (1943) proposed that the basic na-ture of reinforcement is that it serves as a reduction of a biological need. His theory has been called a "need-reduction" theory. Miller and Dollard (1941) formulated a "stimulus reduction" theory. They postulated that any intense stimulus is drive producing and that reduction in the strength of an intense stimulus is reinforcing. Skinner (1938), one of the most famous learning theorists, takes the position that the nature of reinforcement needs no explanation. He does not ask why something is reinforcing, he tries only to determine whether it has reinforcing properties.

Obviously, reinforcement may be intrinsic or augmented. The satisfac-tion of seeing the basketball go into the basket, the feel of the baseball against the bat, and the feel of a solid tackle all provide intrinsic feedback to the learner. When a movement pattern is executed two stimulus events occur in close temporal proximity. First we feel what our bodies have just done, and second we see the results of our performance, producing either satisfaction or dissatisfaction with the performance. Since the two stimuli are paired in rapid succession, we have the basic reinforcement paradigm in that the feedback of a pattern of stimuli becomes conditioned to an emo-tional reaction of satisfaction or dissatisfaction, according to the Law of Effect. Augmented feedback as reinforcement may come in the form of re-wards or punishment. Rewards may be verbal praise or some material gift. Punishment may take the form of verbal reproof or physical chastisement. Some writers refer to rewards as positive reinforcement and punishment as negative reinforcement.

Experiments comparing rewards and punishment generally show re-wards to be more effective for learning and performance, but punishment has been one of the more widely used feedback techniques. Studies by numerous investigators show that, with humans, negative reinforcement fre-quently has unpredictable and varied consequences, and is generally not nearly as effective as reward. Of course, in some cases punishment is effec-tive. A person touching a burning match is not likely to repeat that behavior. A badminton player hitting a clear shot too short and having it smashed back is likely to stop this behavior and attempt to hit the clear shot deep to his opponent's baseline.

It has been suggested that in instructional situations punishment says "stop doing what you did" but it does not indicate what should have been done. It may merely suppress the behavior without reducing the strength of the drive which gave rise to it. For undesirable behavior to be eliminated, appropriate alternative behavior must be taught and rewarded. One additional weakness of punishment in teacher-learner situations is that interpersonal conflicts between the two participants may arise, causing emotional stress and reduction in learning and performance efficiency.

1. Shaping behavior and reinforcement

Many times in the early phases of learning the ultimate goal, or criterion, may be a long way from present performance levels. If the goal is the only criterion to obtain reinforcement, the behavior leading to it may be impossible for the present and no reinforcement occurs. What is required is a systematic change of reinforcement contingencies to gradually "shape" the behavior toward the ultimate goal. In the shaping procedure subgoals are established which are rewarded as the behavior occurs. At the same time instructions are provided as to what to do.

2. Schedules of reinforcement

The basketball player does not make a basket with each shot. The baseball batter does not hit the ball with every swing. Reinforcement in dynamic motor tasks does not occur 100 percent of the time. Does it make any difference how frequently reinforcement is given to the learner? A very similar topic was discussed earlier in this chapter under the heading, "Frequency of Feedback."

Generally, but depending upon the task, schedules of partial reinforcement* with both animals and humans produce slower learning, but learning continues long after reinforcement stops. Also, a task learned under partial reinforcement is more resistant to extinction.† In a comprehensive review of the literature on partial reinforcement, Jenkins and Stanley (1950) state:

All other things equal, resistance to extinction after partial reinforcement is greater than that after continuous reinforcement when behavior strength is measured in terms of single responses.

---

*The two basic partial reinforcement schedules employed in the laboratory are interval and ratio schedules. In the first, the subject is given reinforcement after specific intervals of time, the time intervals may be fixed (constant) or varied. In the second type of schedule, the ratio schedule, subjects are given reinforcement after making a certain number of responses; here, too, the ratio may be fixed or variable.

†Extinction is the gradual diminution in magnitude or rate of a response upon withdrawal of the reinforcement.

MANIPULATION OF FEEDBACK

It should be obvious from information presented in this and the previous chapter that practice and repetition without feedback are very ineffectual. It seems that one of the critical tasks of an instructor of human movement is to be a "movement diagnostician and a manipulator of feedback." That is, it is first essential to be able to diagnose which are the correct and which are the incorrect movements learners are making while they are performing a motor task; then it is necessary to provide feedback to learners in such a way as to enhance the correct responses and to eliminate the incorrect responses. The better instructors are at accomplishing these tasks, the more effective they are as teachers, since efficient and effective learning and performance are the outcomes.

A. MOST APPROPRIATE FORMS OF FEEDBACK

The value of providing augmented feedback for enhancing motor learning and performance has been well established by extensive research, but the most desirable type of augmented feedback for motor tasks remains to be identified. Aside from the work on KR and KP for open and closed skills, there is virtually no other research to provide guidelines. What is the most appropriate form of feedback is an important question since there may be a great deal of variance in the consequences of different types of augmented feedback. For example, is information feedback more beneficial than reinforcing feedback?

Recently, Haywood and Glad (1974), assessing the effectiveness of informative KR and positive, reinforcing KR, reported that neither was more beneficial than intrinsic feedback which was available to the learner. The results of rewards and punishment on skilled motor performance were investigated by Broughton and Nelson (1967). They selected subjects to perform three motor tasks (grip strength, starting and running six feet, and a 60-second all-out ride on a bicycle ergometer) while the experimenters used positive verbal reinforcement, neutral reinforcement, or negative verbal reinforcement with the subjects. The pattern of performance on all three tests showed that the positive reinforcement produced the best responses, with the grip strength and the starting and running test results significantly better.

21

Transfer of
Motor Learning

When some particular behavior has been learned by an individual, the capability established by that learning may affect to some extent the subsequent behavior of the individual. The effects of the original learning are said to "transfer" to subsequent activities. Transfer of learning refers to the effects of past learning upon the acquisition of a new task. For example, the effect that learning to play tennis has on learning to play badminton would be considered a transfer of learning.

Transfer of learning plays an important role in a wide variety of human behaviors. Language, customs, attitudes, and motor skill acquisition are a few of the human activities in which transfer of learning is important. Our society assumes that school experiences will have transfer value for out-of-school activities. A basic belief in teaching motor tasks is that movement patterns learned for one task will transfer to other tasks; the learning of one task is expected to facilitate the learning of similar tasks. Many teachers of motor skills take positive transfer of learning for granted. They assume that movements for task execution of one type transfer to tasks of another type. For example, general "coordination" or "agility" exercises are frequently used by physical educators and athletic coaches with the expectation that movement patterns learned in this context will transfer to improved performance on specific sports skills.

In view of the fact that teachers of motor activities desire and expect their programs to promote positive transfer of learning, it is essential that instructors in these programs understand the conditions that govern transfer of learning. Directors of motor skill learning can inhibit or enhance the acquisition of skills by their students, depending on their knowledge and use of transfer of learning principles. Instructors who know and understand the principles of transfer that have emerged from countless studies will probably manage the learning environment in such a way as to produce maximum positive transfer and, therefore, efficient and effective motor learning. This chapter examines the various transfer factors which affect motor learning.

THE STUDY OF TRANSFER OF LEARNING

Transfer of learning has been one of the most popular topics for psychological research in the past 70 years. Since so much of our lives revolves around formal learning—in the school and in occupations—and since much of what is taught is based on the notion that what is learned in one setting can be transferred to another setting, it is probably not surprising that this topic has been so extensively studied.

A. RESEARCH ON TRANSFER OF LEARNING

A good deal of the early study of transfer was related to the then prevailing doctrine of "formal discipline" which was a part of "faculty" psychology. This position emphasized that the "mind" possessed special abilities, or "faculties," such as memory, logical thinking, judgment, and attention, which could be trained separately or conjointly. That is to say, memory could be improved by practicing memorizing—any kind of memorizing; or learning Latin could enhance the learning of English. Thus, the objective for the study of certain subjects was to "discipline" the mind, enabling it to cope with virtually any demand that might subsequently be made on it. Latin and mathematics were studied because it was assumed that their study strengthened memory and logical thinking ability. Such ideas served as the focal point for transfer of learning experiments in the first two decades of this century.

Most early investigations on transfer were concerned with whether transfer actually occurred—the effects of experience with one task upon another. Studies to investigate the effects of learning one subject, Latin for example, on the learning of a second subject were common. However, psychologists have increasingly become concerned with determining the variables which influence transfer between tasks and not merely with ascertaining whether transfer occurs.

Experimentation on transfer of motor tasks has been conducted primarily in research laboratories and has been limited primarily to fine motor tasks. Most of the studies investigating motor skill transfer have used the same fine motor tasks that have been used for practice and feedback studies, i.e., rotary pursuit, tracking apparatus, mirror tracing, etc. Relatively few studies involving transfer effects on gross motor skills have been undertaken.

B. TRANSFER TERMINOLOGY

Transfer of learning may be positive, negative, or absent. The influence of prior learning may be such that the learning of one task facilitates the learning of a second task; this is called positive transfer. Positive transfer of learning means that individuals are able to learn a second task more readily than they could prior to learning the original task. When the learning of one task impairs or inhibits learning a second task, this is called negative transfer. Thus, negative transfer means that individuals are able to learn something less readily than they could prior to the original learning. If the learning of one task has no measurable influence on learning a second task, zero transfer is said to have occurred.

There may be both positive and negative transfer in components of a complex motor task, and the net transfer will be a function of the relative amounts of positive and negative transfer from the components to the entire task. Mixed transfer effects might occur by learning to play baseball after having learned to play softball. Basic movement patterns developed for positioning to receive and throw the ball and other components of the task of playing the game would probably show positive transfer, but batting the ball and actually fielding and throwing the ball may show negative transfer initially because of the differences in the size of the ball and the distances of the pitcher and the bases.

C. TRANSFER EXPERIMENTAL DESIGNS

There are many experimental designs which have been used to study and measure transfer, and it is beyond the scope of this book to discuss all of these various designs. The two basic designs are called "proactive" and "retroactive" designs. They may be illustrated as follows:

1. Proactive design

Experimental group:	Learns task 1	Learns task 2
Control group:	Rests	Learns task 2

In this situation, the experimental group learns task 1, while the control group is given no special training, so it is said to rest. Then both groups learn task 2. This type of design is called a proactive transfer design—meaning transfer effects that are the result of previous experience. Thus, if learning task 1 facilitates the learning of task 2, proactive facilitation, or positive transfer is said to have occurred. But if learning task 1 inhibits learning task 2, proactive interference, or negative transfer, is said to have occurred. If both groups learn task 2 at equal rates, this represents zero transfer.

2. Retroactive design

Experimental group:	Learn task 1	Learn task 2	Test task 1
Control group:	Learn task 1	Rest	Test task 1

In this design, both groups learn task 1, then the experimental group learns task 2 but the control group does not. Both groups are then tested on task 1. This type of design is called a retroactive transfer design because task 2 may have a retroactive effect on task 1. If learning task 2 enhances the performance on task 1, there is retroactive facilitation, or positive transfer. If performance on task 1 is inhibited, retroactive interference, or negative transfer has occurred.

3. Transfer measures

A number of transfer formulae have been developed to ascertain the amount and direction of transfer which occurs in a given experiment. The amount of transfer of learning is often expressed as a percentage of transfer. One percentage of transfer formula is as follows:

$$\text{Percentage of Transfer} = \frac{E - C}{E + C} \times 100,$$

where E represents the mean performance of the experimental group on the transfer task and C represents the mean performance of the control group on the transfer task. The maximum amount of positive transfer that can be obtained is 100 percent transfer and the maximum amount of negative transfer is -100 percent.

This formula is appropriate if the measure of performance is such that the larger the value of the measure, the better the performance. For example, if the measure of performance is the number of correct responses, then the formula is appropriate because the number of correct responses becomes larger with better performance.

This transfer formula may be illustrated as follows: If we employ a group that practices a left-hand task for a given amount of time and then is tested on a right-hand task and a control group that is tested on the right-hand task, without practicing the left-hand task, we can obtain a percentage of transfer score. Assume that the experimental group (E) averages a score of 25 on the right-hand task while the control group (C) averages 15, applying the formula we obtain:

$$\frac{25 - 15}{25 + 15} \times 100 = \frac{10}{40} \times 100 = 25 \text{ percent transfer.}$$

The E group shows 25 percent transfer, which means that there was 25 percent positive transfer from the left-hand task to the right-hand task.

This formula must be modified by reversing the positions of the experimental and control groups scores in the formula if the measure of performance is such that the smaller the value of the measure, the better the performance, the formula must be modified to read:

$$\text{Percentage of Transfer} = \frac{C - E}{E \times C} \times 100.$$

This formula is appropriate with such measures as errors, trials to reach some criterion, or time. As errors, trials, or time are reduced in value, performance improves.

A less popular method of measuring transfer is the "savings method." With this technique, the number of trials which the experimental group uses to reach an equivalent level of proficiency with the control group on a motor task are counted. If the experimental group requires fewer trials than the control group, it is said that learning the task which the control group did not learn (such as task 1 in the proactive design above) produced a "savings." Thus, if a control group has reached a certain level of performance after 20 trials on task 2, and the experimental group, after having learned task 1, reaches this level of performance on task 2 after ten trials, this means that ten trials on task 2 were "saved" by learning task 1.

The measurement of transfer of learning is plagued by the problem that the various formulae which may be used do not yield the same results, so the importance of knowing which transfer formula was used in a given study becomes obvious, especially if one wishes to compare the magnitude and direction of transfer obtained in different studies. Moreover, there are several variables which might affect the transfer results, such as conditions under which the subjects were tested, mental practice engaged in by the subjects, etc.

TRANSFER AND SIMILAR ELEMENTS

The evidence that has accumulated over the past 80 years suggests rather clearly that, in general, when similar responses to identical stimuli are required, positive transfer occurs; on the other hand, learning different or incompatible responses to identical stimuli usually results in initial negative transfer. Thus, learning to track and catch a baseball probably facilitates learning to catch a softball. But, surely a baseball player required to run the bases clockwise upon hitting the ball would encounter initial confusion and difficulty. When different responses are required for different stimuli, there is usually little or no transfer. Thus, learning to swim probably does not affect learning to play golf in any way.

The amount of transfer, then, is generally affected by the similarity of the task initially learned to the second task in which the occurrence of transfer is observed. A general principle of transfer is: As responses become increasingly dissimilar for a similar stimulus, the transfer effects shift from positive to negative. Positive transfer occurs when the successive responses learned to identical or similar stimuli are associatively related, and negative transfer results when new, unrelated responses are learned to old stimuli (Fig. 21.1).

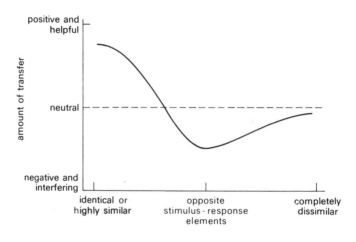

Fig. 21.1 Effects of task similarity on transfer. When tasks 1 and 2 are identical or highly similar, performance on task 2 is facilitated. When the tasks have opposite stimulus-response elements, performance on task 2 is hindered. When the tasks are completely dissimilar, performance on task 2 is unaffected. (Based on Robinson, 1927.)

This principle of task similarity is an outgrowth of Thorndike's (1903) "identical elements" theory of transfer. This was one of the first theories of transfer and was formulated as an effective response to the theory of "formal discipline." Thorndike said, "A change in one function alters any other only insofar as the two functions have as factors identical elements." His identical-elements theory proposed that transfer of learning occurs to the extent that identical components exist in the two specific tasks, and therefore if general training is effective in producing improvement in learning efficiency in a variety of tasks, it is because the components, or elements, of specific tasks are practiced in the process of general learning.

It is difficult to ascertain whether "identical elements" refers to the simplest components of which a whole is composed, or to the general "set" toward the task. However, by general practice, "identical elements" may be as specific as muscular contractions common to the two tasks or as general as methods of gaining "insight" or understanding into the commonality of the two tasks. Similarity has been defined by scales of similarity based upon the judgments of subjects, in terms of variation of a physical dimension such as size or intensity, and in terms of transfer itself.

When a person is required to make new responses to the same or similar stimuli, the general rule is that the responses learned for the first task will interfere with the new responses needed to learn the second task. However, this issue is somewhat complicated, and both positive and negative transfer can occur in this situation. For motor tasks, interference is usually minimal and disappears rapidly.

A. TRANSFER AND SIMILARITY FOR MOTOR LEARNING

As was noted in Chapter 18, there is strong support in the motor skills literature for the specificity of motor learning principle (Henry, 1970), which is that motor skills are not based on a few general factors but are based upon factors which are specific to the task in question. This particular position has been supported for many tasks. Although Fleishman and his colleagues have isolated basic underlying motor abilities using factor analysis, the factors usually account for a relatively small proportion of the actual performance of a task.

Motor skill transfer studies have been concerned with transfer of learning from one task to another, such as from tennis to badminton, as well as from one variation of a task to another variation of the same task. The first is often called task-to-task transfer and the second is referred to as intratask transfer.

1. Task-to-task transfer

Studies of motor skill transfer from one task to another are not numerous but they do consistently support the notion that there is little transfer from one task to another. Motor task studies in which the stimulus and response variables are quite different between tasks confirm the notion that little transfer can be expected. Nelson (1957a) investigated the transfer effect of swimming upon the learning and performance of two gross motor skills (volleyball tap for accuracy and high-hurdle skill). He attempted to answer the question of whether swimming during learning of other gross motor skills results in negative transfer, as had been hypothesized. He found no transfer effect from swimming to the other skills. Lindeburg (1949) measured the transfer effect of table tennis and "quickening exercises" upon reaction time and pegshifting. He found no transfer of learning from the table tennis and "quickening exercises" on reaction time or pegshifting. He concluded that quickening exercises which involve many rapid skillful movements do not improve general coordination. He states that "the results agree with the theory that transfer is highly specific and occurs only when the practiced movements are identical."

There has been some popularity among physical educators in recent years for courses in "movement fundamentals" or "basic skills." The assumption behind offering these courses is that the movements learned in these courses will transfer to enhanced learning of specific sports. There is little evidence for this assumption, but from that which does exist it would appear that such transfer is negligible. For example, Coleman (1967) found no significant differences in bowling performance between groups that experienced a "movement education" course prior to a bowling course, and a group that enrolled only in bowling. In another study, Burdenshaw and her colleagues (1970) assessed the effectiveness of a basic skills course as a prerequisite for learning badminton skills. One group experienced a basic skills course before enrolling in the badminton course. This group performed no differently from a group that enrolled initially in the badminton course.

The findings of these studies are in agreement with research on specificity versus generality which was discussed in some detail in Chapter 18. Rather than reintroduce these findings here, we encourage the reader to review these studies at this time.

In summarizing data on task-to-task transfer with motor tasks it appears that there is typically little transfer of any kind. There is almost never negative transfer and any positive transfer tests to be minimal, thus, the motor skills instructor need not worry about bringing about negative transfer among students, as long as the students do not have to learn contradictory responses.

2. Intratask transfer

There are a number of studies concerned with intratask transfer, that is, transfer from one variation of a task to another variation of the same task. One way of varying a task is to speed up or slow down the rate of practicing the task. Studies of this type have examined the effect of emphasizing speed or accuracy on performance of the task at normal speed. Other studies have been concerned with the transfer effect of practicing parts of the task on performance or learning the whole task. Finally, a few studies have varied the task in a way to make the task easier or more difficult and have assessed the transfer affect when the task is performed normally.

a. Speed versus Accuracy

In 1928 Agnes Poppelreuter (1928) published a study in Germany in which she stated that speed should be retarded until a reasonable level of accuracy was attained. This sparked a controversy in physical education and psychology which still exists today. The controversy has been centered around the appropriate time and place in motor learning to emphasize speed and accuracy, since in motor skill instruction the teacher may impose a set for action, the instruction being for either speed or accuracy or both in combination.

Early studies on this topic by Fulton (1942) and Solley (1952) concluded that early emphasis on speed was more beneficial where speed was necessary in the final performance. However, where both speed and accuracy are important an early emphasis upon both seems to be more effective. Lordhal and Archer (1958) and Namikas and Archer (1960) two years later, examined the effects of transferring from one speed of rotation on the rotary pursuit to a second speed of rotation. Three groups practiced at either 40, 60, or 80 rpm and then all three groups transferred to the 60 rpm speed for testing. In the first study positive transfer ranged from 47 to 54 percent while in the latter it ranged from 42 to 64 percent, but in both cases transferring to the same speed gave the best results. More recently, Jensen (1975) reported similar results, even when the practice speed on the rotary pursuit was gradually built over three practice periods to the transfer speed of 60 rpm. Practicing over three days, one group practiced with a 20-20-40 rpm schedule, a second had a 30-30-45 schedule, a third practiced with a 30-40-50 schedule, and a fourth group practiced with 60-60-60 schedule. The transfer testing speed for all groups was 60 rpm.

Using sports skills, Woods (1967) assessed the effect of varied instructional emphasis on speed and accuracy on the acquisition of a forehand tennis stroke. The most desirable results were obtained by equal instructional emphasis on speed and accuracy simultaneously. An accuracy emphasis followed by a maximum velocity emphasis proved least beneficial. Hornak (1971) found that a teaching sequence of speed, accuracy, and then a combination of the two was a better method of teaching the soccer instep kick, when considering both accuracy and speed scores. Other investigators have found that sports skills that require both speed and accuracy are most efficiently learned by equal emphasis during practice (Jordan, 1966; McCoy, 1968).

The substantial research on this topic is nicely summarized by Nixon and Locke (1973). They say:

Nowhere in the literature is research in more perfect and happy agreement. Instructions for either speed or accuracy produce the intended effects. Tasks that demand equal emphasis profit from equal emphasis throughout the learning process. . . .Certainly the natural proclivity of the teacher to stress accuracy in early trials is contraindicated.

The implications for motor skill learning are quite clear. If a task is to be performed at a given speed, it should be practiced at that speed, even though inaccurate performance results, to facilitate the learning of the task. This method of practice results in faster and more accurate learning than does emphasizing slow but accurate movements and gradually increasing speed. Practicing a task at a slower or faster speed than will actually be used in performance invites momentary negative transfer. Good basketball players, for example, get their jump shot off in less than two seconds. When learning to shoot, players may take longer than two seconds as they attempt to develop an effective movement pattern. Then during a game, since they must perform the shot quickly to prevent it from being blocked, they speed up the movement, which alters the habit they learned in practice; the result is a poor performance. During practice drills, therefore, performers should be executing their skills at "game speed" in order to gain optimal transfer from practice habits to game habits. Thus, the teaching method of requiring beginners to practice a task at a slower tempo than is actually needed for effective execution of the task must be viewed with suspicion. However, the learner should probably not be forced to overstress speed in the early learning stages because this may disrupt performance and impede learning.

b. Level of Difficulty and Transfer

Some transfer studies have examined the effect of modifying a task to make it easier or more difficult and having subjects practice under this modified condition before practicing the task under normal conditions. The question under consideration here is whether it is harmful or beneficial to practice an easy or difficult modification of a task when attempting to learn that task. Investigations of this type have usually made the task "easier" or more "difficult" by decreasing or increasing the size of targets to be followed or hit, changing the speed of the target, or increasing or decreasing the distance of the target from the performer (e.g., pistol shooting, archery).

Regardless of whether the modification is in target size, target distance, speed of target, or whatever, the findings are equivocal; some studies show a superiority of practice with an "easy" modification, others show a superiority with a "difficult" modification, but in general, practice on the actual task to be learned in a normal manner appears to be as valuable as practicing modifications of the task. For example, in one of the few studies where a sports skill was used, Singer (1966) used archery accuracy as the skill to be learned by the subjects. An easy-to-difficult group practiced archery 10 yards from the target; a difficult-to-easy group began at 40 yards from the target; and a control group started at 25 yards from the target. All groups were then tested 25 yards from the target. Singer reported no significant differences in transfer effects from easy-to-difficult compared with transfer from difficult-to-easy conditions. And ultimate success, measured by the Columbia Junior Round, was not influenced by the distance at which initial practice occurred.

In another study involving gross motor skills, Scannell (1968) studied transfer of accuracy training, using a dart throw and a softball throw, when the difficulty was controlled by varying target size during practice. He found no significant difference in the effects of practice with targets equal to, smaller than, or larger than the test target. Thus, this study showed that easy-to-difficult or difficult-to-easy conditions did not make any difference on performance of the test skills. Scannell suggested that "attempts to enforce, in practice, degrees of precision greater than those required in the test situation, while not deterring the subject's progress, will not enhance the progress."

Several writers have suggested that the task as well as other factors may make one condition more favorable than the other. Some tasks may transfer better with an easy-to-difficult arrangement, while the reverse may be true for other tasks. It seems that optimal conditions must be established for each task. Holding (1962) echoes this viewpoint and, in summarizing over 25 articles on this topic, he concluded that "difficulty is not a useful category for the prediction of transfer efficiency, and...the solution lies in examining the skills involved."

c. Whole-Part Transfer

Another transfer variable that is related to practice method is concerned with whether a motor task involving several component movements should be practiced in its entirety with each practice trial or whether it should be divided into component parts and these parts practiced separately, putting together the parts and performing the entire task only after the parts have been mastered. Or should some combination of these two methods be employed? These questions have been studied by many researchers, but because of the many variables and widely varying tasks, the results of the studies are vague, and in some cases conflicting. Nevertheless, this problem is important for those who direct motor learning.

A task to be learned which is capable of being divided into parts may be practiced in two basically different ways: First, it may be practiced as a whole, i.e., it may be practiced from beginning to end at each trial until it is learned, or until a certain level of proficiency is attained. Second, it may be separated into two or more parts, and then each part, or component, of the task may be practiced as a separate unit and then connected with other units to form the whole movement pattern. This second method, called the part method, may be further divided into variations of the part method: (1) a pure part method would find each part, or component, of the task separately learned, and then all the parts repeated in sequence to produce the whole task. (2) A progressive part method would involve practicing the first two components of a skill, combining these to form a whole, next practicing a third component and then chaining it to the first two, adding a fourth component, and so forth. This continues by progressive addition of components until the whole task has been learned. (3) A third part method is called a repetitive part method. It is accomplished by practicing and mastering the first component, then doing the same for components 1 and 2 together, then components 1, 2, and 3 together. This continues until all the parts are mastered.

Much of the early research into the relative effectiveness of whole versus part learning was done with verbal material. We shall not review these studies; instead, we shall focus on studies involving motor tasks. The findings on motor task studies have fairly consistently (considering the inconsistency in this area) replicated the findings of studies which used verbal materials.

The experimental evidence shows that in an integrated motor task the performance of a single component by itself is different from the performance of the same component when it is embedded in the entire task (Beeby, 1930). Shay (1934) taught a gymnastic skill on the horizontal bar to one group using a progressive part method, and he taught the same skill using the whole method to a second group. He reported that the whole method produced superior results. Niemeyer (1959) reported a study where swimming, volleyball, and badminton were taught to two classes by the whole method and to two classes by the part method. His findings shows that students in the whole method group learned to swim sooner, farther, and faster than those taught by the part method. Badminton learning was not significantly affected by the different methods; and the part method was significantly better than the whole method for students in volleyball classes. Lewellen (1951) also found that the whole method was superior to the Red Cross progressive part method in learning swimming skills and developing distance skill. Lersten (1968) had subjects practice on a task which resembled a rho (ρ). Some subjects practiced only the circular component, others practiced only the linear component, a third group practiced only the total task. He found that there was very little transfer of motor skill and it occurred to a significant degree only in the circular component (6.7 percent).

Several writers in this field have endorsed a combination method as the most effective solution to the problem. Although this notion sounds attractive, there is little research to support it. Knapp and Dixon (1952) hypothesized that a combination of the whole and part methods would produce more efficient learning. They used two groups of matched pairs to learn the skill of juggling. Subjects who used the whole method of practice tended to attain the criterion (100 consecutive catches) most rapidly. Their hypothesis that a combination of the whole and part methods results in more efficient learning was rejected.

The findings above suggest that if there is a great deal of integration and interaction among components it may be inefficient to practice on the components first. A general rule for whole versus part learning might be whole practice increases in effectiveness as the integration of the component parts of the skill increases in importance.

Although all motor tasks involve motor patterning, they vary in the degree of integration. Some skills are thus actually composed of several relatively independent activities. When the total task involves separate, independent movements, it seems that dividing the task into parts for practice facilitates learning the whole task. Gagne and Foster (1949) measured transfer of learning on a motor skill with varying amounts of practice on a component part. The task was to learn to throw the appropriate toggle switches on a board as rapidly as possible when certain lights went on. One experimental group received 10 trials on a component of the task before being transferred to the whole task; a second experimental group received

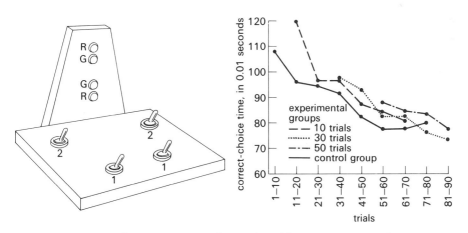

Fig. 21.2   Gagne and Foster measured transfer of learning to a complex motor skill with varying amounts of practice on a component part. The task was to learn to throw the appropriate toggle switches as rapidly as possible when certain lights went on. For the component task, only one upper (red or green) and one lower (green or red) light of the same color were used, and one switch on the left and one on the right. For the complex task, all four lights and all four switches were used. (Based on Gagne and Foster, 1949.)

30 trials; and the third received 50 trials. A control group practiced only the whole task. The learning curves for all groups on the task indicate that the more practice the learners had on the component practice, the greater the transfer to the whole task (Fig. 21.2). The control group's starting average for the whole task was 108; the starting averages for the 1p-, 30-, and 50-trial practice groups were 110, 98, and 89, respectively. However, the control group, which spent all its time on the whole task, learned more quickly than did any of the other groups. Thus, although practice on a component part helped in the learning of a whole skill, the most efficient method of practice was working on the whole task from the beginning.

There are some tasks in which component practice apparently facilitates learning. Adams and Hufford (1962) reported that learning a series of separate movements which were a part of a larger task of flying an airplane showed a great deal of transfer to the performance of the whole task.

Fitts and Posner (1967) suggest the following principle might be applied to the whole-part problem:

If the components of the skill are independent of each other . . ., then it is better to practice each component separately. . . . When, however, the task involves synchrony between the components . . ., much of the learning is concerned with the overall integration of the components and thus is best learned as a whole. A practical exception to this may arise if the components are too complex to allow the beginner to practice the task as a whole. The best plan here is to program practice so as to develop some proficiency in the separate components, choosing component processes that are as nearly independent of each other as possible and alternating between part and whole.

Many other writers have formulated generalizations which apply to the whole-part problem. One of the most frequently mentioned is the whole method seems preferable when the motor task to be learned consists of serial movements which form a chained sequence. For example, tasks which lend themselves to the whole method are tasks in which timing and speed are critical in order not to destroy the total movement pattern, and tasks in which the proper timing and coordination of the whole task might be destroyed if isolated parts of the total task were practiced. Skills such as the tennis serve and the basketball jump shot are composed of almost inseparable links—one link blends into and provides the cue for the next link in sequential manner. The real value of the whole method is that it enables the learner to realize the interrelationships of the component parts of a task to the entire task.

Another frequently identified generalization is if the task is complex and/or is composed of various components each of which can be identified as a complete unit, then the part method of practice may be superior to the whole method. For example, the offensive motor tasks of basketball, i.e., shooting, dribbling, and passing, offer a complex task with several subtasks. Many team sports fall into this category. Individuals may profitably practice the subtasks separately; then, as skill improves, they may learn to use these tasks in combination and in relation to teammates, opponents, and in reference to the rules of the sport. So for complex tasks the whole method might be employed for connecting the components together, after the components are learned by the part method. Furthermore, even when the part method is used, it must be used with reference to a concept of the whole task. Learners must know what the entire task consists of (a general idea of the whole) if they are going to learn the whole task. Thus, it is only after learners achieve a general idea of the whole complex task that they isolate the subtasks and practice them.

Several methodological implications are evident from the foregoing. Instructors of motor learning should first provide an explanation and demonstration of the total task to be learned. They should not break up this total task into parts unless it is obviously too large or too complex for learners to practice in its entirety. The most important characteristic of a motor task is its wholeness. If the task is complex and lends itself to division into subtasks, it may be practiced in isolation, but only in relation to the whole task.

TRANSFER AND GENERAL FACTORS

Clearly, a narrow definition of the term "identical elements" proposed by Thorndike, or even "similar elements," does not fully describe the conditions under which transfer occurs. Up to this point our emphasis has been on specific transfer but we must differentiate between specific and "general" transfer. When we learn a task, we acquire not only the specific movements of the task but also many other aspects of it that make for enhanced performance. These may include such varied things as learning how to fixate attention on certain stimuli, how to organize the task demands into meaningful parts, how to use certain devices to form associations, etc. These general skills, strategies, and other habits acquired for a task may in turn influence learning of quite different tasks. When this influence occurs it is called "general" transfer, and several studies have shown the potential for general transfer when learning motor tasks.

Judd (1908) was the first to take exception to the extent and nature of Thorndike's theory. He reported that boys who had been given instruction on the principles of light refraction were more accurate at hitting a target submerged in water than were boys who had not received this instruction.

He proposed that the learner can use principles and laws as well as general strategy to transfer learning from one task to another. Obviously, this theory allows for a great deal more transfer than Thorndike's identical elements theory, and has therefore been called a "general factors" theory.

A related concept that has arisen in the transfer literature of the past 30 years is "learning-to-learn." Harlow (1949) triggered the current interest in this topic when he reported that monkeys improved the speed with which they could solve problems by increased experience with problem-solving situations. Similar results have been reported subsequently with humans. In tests of verbal material, persons tend to improve their ability to master lists of nonsense words by experience with lists of such words. Learners are said to have learned how to learn; that is, they perceptually organize general features common to the two tasks and use the successful "strategy" of one task to solve the problems of mastering a different task.

A. TRANSFER OF PRINCIPLES

Beginning with Judd's paper, numerous studies have examined the transfer effect of presenting information about principles underlying motor tasks. Judd (1908) extended and reported a study that was started by Scholckow which demonstrated transfer of principles. As noted in the previous section, the specific principles were those of refraction of light. In this study, subjects threw darts at a target submerged in water. When the target was four inches under water, the group that had been given knowledge of the principles of refraction adapted quickly to the situation and produced superior performances over the group which lacked knowledge of refraction principles.

Hendrickson and Schroeder (1941), in an attempt to make a general replication of Judd's study of target accuracy and transfer of knowledge principles on a target submerged in water, had subjects shoot an air gun at a submerged target. Experimental groups were given an explanation of the theory of refraction prior to shooting. With targets at a water depth of six inches, experimental groups learned more rapidly than a control group, and essentially the same results occurred when the target was raised to two inches below the water surface.

In a study in which sports skills were used, Mohr and Barrett (1962), using women students from intermediate swimming classes, taught an experimental group the mechanical principles involved in four swimming strokes while a control group did not get mechanical-principles instruction. Other teaching conditions were the same for the two groups. They found that the experimental group made significantly greater improvement in the strokes after eight weeks of instruction. They concluded that "exposing students to an understanding and application of mechanical principles will effect greater improvement than instruction without reference to those principles."

Montgomery (1961) found that a knowledge of mechanical principles about force and projection had a significant effect upon performance in two gross motor tasks—the standing broad jump and softball throw. Papcsy (1968) reported that eighth grade boys learned a handball skill at a faster rate after having been taught the mechanical principles involved. They also performed better on a bunting skill. Interestingly, the greatest advantage was displayed by the subjects of lower intelligence. Finally, Werner (1972) showed that teaching four science concepts (levers, Newton's First Law of Motion, Newton's Third Law of Motion, and work) to fourth, fifth, and sixth grade students enhanced their performance on a variety of gross motor tasks.

Although the studies cited above may give the impression that every study has demonstrated a facilitation of learning when mechanical principles are employed, this is not the case. Several investigators have reported no advantage to the mechanical principle instruction group (Coville, 1957). However, the fact that instruction in mechanical principles has been found to enhance the learning of a number of motor tasks and that it is typically fairly easy to incorporate this type of information into verbal instructions suggests that instructors might use this technique to some advantage.

B. OTHER GENERAL FACTORS PHENOMENA

Learning for optimal transfer effects might include experiences which permit the learner to form generalizations applicable to the new situation while at the same time helping the learner to distinguish basic components in each task so as to recognize the differences in the tasks. A verbal explanation often attempts to utilize transfer from one skill to another. References such as "the serve in tennis is just like the overhand throw in baseball" attempt to cause learners to transfer their baseball throwing pattern to the tennis serve. Broer (1958) gave an experimental group instruction emphasizing problem solving and mechanical principles of learning volleyball, basketball, and softball basic skills. Also, the experimental group was given one-third, two-thirds, and the same amount of specific instructions on volleyball, basketball, and softball, respectively, as the control group. The experimental group surpassed the control group on all skills tests for the various sports given at the completion of each unit.

A few studies show positive transfer between small pattern motor practice and large pattern learning. For example, Gagne and Foster (1949) investigated the extent to which positive transfer of learning a motor skill occurred following varying amounts of practice on a paper-and-pencil representation of the task. They reported considerable effectiveness of preliminary training on the pictured representation. Cratty (1962) studied the transfer effect of prior practice on three small-patterned mazes on large-patterned maze learning proficiency. He concluded that prior practice on a similar small-patterned maze resulted in initial positive transfer of traversal time on the large-patterned maze and that prior reverse pattern practice caused initial negative transfer.

In a unique study, Vincent (1968) classified two criterion motor tasks (a hop and jump task and a static balance task) by their perceptual components and their motor components. Experimental group subjects then practiced to a high level of competence in the perceptual components of the criterion tasks through the use of practice tasks which were similar to the criterion tasks in perceptual makeup, but not similar in motor demands. He hypothesized that subjects who practiced tasks with perceptual components similar to the criterion motor tasks would exhibit higher proficiency on the criterion tasks than a control group who practiced unrelated exercises. His results confirmed the hypothesis; the experimental groups were significantly superior to the control group on both criterion motor tasks. Vincent suggested that the transfer resulted from the similarity in perceptual components of the practice and criterion tasks, and that perceptual abilities are subject to improvement through practice.

Mental practice was discussed in an earlier chapter, but the general finding of several studies on mental practice and transfer effects has been that mental practice exhibits substantial positive transfer to the learning of motor tasks. Positive transfer of learning has been reported by several scholars on mental or imaginary practice of various motor tasks.

C. SUMMARY OF GENERAL FACTORS

It may be seen from the discussion above that the "identical elements" theory of transfer of training is incomplete. Although it is not possible to identify the stimulus and response characteristics of most tasks, it is fairly obvious that a good deal of transfer cannot be accounted for by an identical-elements theory. The more contemporary view is that transfer effects are best explained as the result of a combination of elements, both specific and general. Some psychologists, on the basis of their research, have advanced what has been called a "two-factor theory of transfer of learning." Two-factor theories propose that individuals not only transfer identical stimulus response elements from task to task but they also transfer general elements, such as principles of problem solving, learning to learn, and "insight."

ADDITIONAL FACTORS AND TRANSFER

There are many additional factors which are known to affect transfer. Factors such as interlimb transfer, degree of initial learning, variation in task difficulty, variety of previous experiences, and effects of learning two tasks simultaneously have been studied, and the results of these studies have implications for motor learning and performance.

A. BILATERAL TRANSFER

When persons practice a motor skill, such as throwing a ball, with their right hands, there is usually (but not always) some positive transfer to their left hands, even though they have not practiced with the left hands. Transfer from a limb on one side of the body to a limb on the opposite side is called bilateral transfer. Several studies have demonstrated the presence of bilateral transfer of skill, and this transfer occurs from hand-to-foot as well as hand-to-hand. Greatest transfer, however, is in the symmetrical muscle group on the opposite side of the body.

Perhaps the earliest report of bilateral transfer with a gross motor task was a study by Swift (1903). He studied the transfer of learning on a juggling skill where the subjects attempted to keep two balls going with one hand, receiving and throwing one while the other was in the air. He found unmistakable evidence that "practice with one hand trains the other." In another of the early experiments on bilateral transfer, Munn (1932) had subjects learn a hand-eye coordination task, catching a wooden ball in which a hole had been drilled with a wooden handle which would just fit into the hole. Both ball and handle were attached to a string. Subjects were given 50 trials with the left hand, then 50 trials with the right hand, followed by 500 trials with the right hand. A subsequent 50 trials with the left hand showed an average amount of transfer due to practice with the right hand of 32.59 percent. Munn explained the difference on the basis of "insight" into the total situation which the learners developed by experience with the task. That is to say, the subject formulates implicit and explicit methods for the task and, since the basic task is the same regardless of which hand is used, the formulation is useful in both situations. Munn's explanation would probably fit into the "general factor" or "two-factor" theory of transfer.

A year after Munn reported his study, Cook (1933) published an article on what he called "cross-education." This study dealt with bilateral transfer on mirror tracing a star-shaped maze. He reported that "cross-education" (bilateral transfer) occurred between all four limbs of the body on the maze task.

Although not a controlled study, one of the most remarkable case studies of apparent bilateral transfer is reported by Jokl (1958). Karoly Takacs, a Hungarian pistol shooting champion, lost his preferred arm. One year later he won the world pistol shooting championship, using his other arm.

Explanations to account for bilateral transfer have been many and varied. In a comprehensive summary of this topic, Ammons (1958) listed over ten reasons commonly given for this phenomenon. Visual cues, familiarity with the general principles of the task, and increased confidence due to experience of original practice are three of the prominent reasons which Ammons lists.

There are many bilateral transfer conditions about which little or no research has been done. For example, does more transfer occur from the dominant to the nondominant hand? Or is the reverse true? Or is the transfer effect due more to the proficiency of the limbs? The answers to these questions must be tentative because of the limited research.

Since so many sports skills involve the use of one or more limbs, we might ask, what are the implications of bilateral transfer to teaching sports skills? In sports where a ball must be thrown, caught, or kicked, it is obvious that most of the practice must be done with the limbs that will carry out these tasks most frequently. That is, football quarterbacks whose right hands are dominant can more efficiently improve their passing accuracy by practicing with their right hands. However, in situations in which fatigue or injury to the dominant limb exists, practice with the other limb may facilitate performance with the dominant limb. Sports which require ambidextrous use of the limbs, such as soccer and handball, may be taught with an understanding that extensive practice with one limb does not necessarily mean no change for the other limb; indeed, it may facilitate rate of improvement when that limb is made to practice.

B. INITIAL LEARNING

In situations where transfer is known to occur, the transfer effect increases with increasing practice on the original task. This finding has been reported by numerous investigators. For example, Duncan (1953), in a study involving lever-moving into radically placed slots, concluded that positive transfer was a function of both first task learning and task similarities.

A critical deterrent to securing positive transfer, when it is expected or known to occur, is incomplete initial practice on the original task. There is an important implication here for motor skill teaching. Superficial practice on the original task is not likely to produce the intended positive transfer. A primary weakness of many school programs is that numerous motor skills are presented with provision for only superficial practice on each one. About the time the motor skills for one sport are beginning to be learned by the students, the teacher moves on to a new "unit" which requires the learning of a new set of motor skills. The learner is never given sufficient time to master a set of motor tasks; the result is that any positive transfer that might occur from task to task is prevented due to the teaching techniques employed. The overall consequence is that most students obtain virtually no mastery of any game or sports skills from their physical education classes.

C. VARIETY OF PREVIOUS TASKS

While there is a great deal of evidence that positive transfer is related to similarity of tasks and the initial learning of a previous task, it is also true that complex motor skills, such as those employed in sports, are dependent upon and built upon a variety of learned skills. Thus, the statements above should not be interpreted to mean that variety of motor experiences is unimportant. Even when the transfer from one task to another is very small, the experience of a wide variety of tasks appears to be important for learning motor skills. It is a common observation of physical educators and coaches that students who have been deprived of a rich background of movement experiences have greater difficulty in learning sports skills. Teaching basketball to a student who does not have a movement background in running, catching, and throwing is quite difficult.

D. SIMULTANEOUS LEARNING OF SIMILAR TASKS

Is it best to learn two similar motor tasks simultaneously or at different times? The limited research indicates that tasks which involved similar movement patterns should not be learned at the same time. Nelson (1957b), in one of the most comprehensive studies of transfer and gross motor skills, studied three basic phenomena:

1. The extent of transfer between two tasks which involve similar movement patterns when the tasks are learned simultaneously.

2. The extent of transfer between two tasks which involve similar movement patterns when the tasks are learned at different times.

3. The extent of transfer when the instructional method emphasized transfer.

He found a favorable effect of learning a tennis skill on learning a badminton skill, a basketball skill on learning a volleyball skill, and a track starting skill on a football starting skill, but the differences were not significant. He concluded that sports skills that involve similar elements and patterns of movements should not be learned at the same time.

GENERAL PRINCIPLES OF TRANSFER OF LEARNING

The enormous amount of research that has gone into the study of transfer has produced a variety of general principles which enable us to predict when transfer between tasks will be likely to occur. Stolurow (1966) formulated a taxonomic system of studies of transfer and listed over 200 principles based on a review of more than 1500 articles. There are a number of these transfer principles which can serve as guides for motor skill acquisition and instruction. Some of these principles are:

1. Transfer of learning is greatest when two tasks are highly similar.
2. When a second task requires the learner to make different, incompatible responses to identical or similar stimuli which appeared in the original task, initial negative transfer will likely result.
3. When a second task is quite dissimilar to the original task, little or no transfer usually results.
4. When successive tasks of the same type are given, the tasks will tend to be learned more and more quickly.
5. Positive transfer increases with increasing initial mastery of the original task.
6. Practice with one limb usually results in positive transfer to all the other limbs.
7. The research on task difficulty and transfer is contradictory; optimal conditions must be established for each task.
8. An understanding of the general nature and basic principles which are important to task performance produces positive transfer.
9. When two tasks involve similar movement patterns, they should not be learned at the same time, for maximum positive transfer.
10. Practice of nonspecific "coordination" or "quickening" tasks will not produce positive transfer to specific sports skills.

22

Motivation: An Overview

Human behavior of almost any type is affected by motivation; in hitting a baseball or running a 100-yard dash, performers must be motivated if they expect to achieve effective and efficient performance. If they are not, they may "go through the motions" but the result is likely to be a poor performance. It is as though no "power" had been supplied to the machine. It is entirely possible, then, for performers to possess a high level of skill and yet perform poorly; indeed, performance is rarely commensurate with skill level.

Performance typically fluctuates from one occasion to another. Although there is a variety of factors which might account for this variation (i.e., fatigue, disease, etc.), certainly one of the most important factors is motivation. Bringing individuals' performance to the maximum of their capabilities requires that they be motivated. To emphasize the importance of motivation, Gagne and Fleishman (1959) say, "There is much evidence to make us think that motivation does not simply add to skill in producing performance, but rather multiplies with it." They suggest the following equation to symbolize this relationship:

$$\text{Performance} = \text{Skill} \times \text{Motivation}.$$

This notation should not be taken as some exact formulation but rather as a very general suggestion which emphasizes how skill level and motivation interact for performance. There are many every-day examples in sports where this equation seems to apply, such as when an individual or team of mediocre ability beats superior individuals or teams when the one with the lesser ability has the greater motivation.

The evidence is clear that behavior is enhanced when an individual is motivated, so persons involved in teaching or coaching motor skills need to be acquainted with the literature on this topic in order to use this knowledge in improving the learning and performance of the individuals under their direction. Those instructors who have the ability to motivate others, recognizing the differences between individuals and situations, will be the most effective in their instructional and leadership roles. There is no more important topic to the person who is attempting to gain a comprehensive understanding of human movement.

Motivation is such an important topic, and its dimensions are so varied and complex, four chapters have been devoted to it in this volume. Even so, only selected aspects of the subject will be discussed, and no claim is made for a comprehensive and in-depth coverage of motivation here. The amount of literature on this subject is awesome, and there is a wide variety of theoretical approaches that could lead us far astray from our main focus—motor behavior. Traditionally, textbook treatments of motivation are concerned with biological drives and instincts, but these play a small role in sports, games, and dance learning and performances. The criterion used as to what information to include in this book was the extent to which it seemed important for basic understanding of motivation and application to motor behavior.

In this chapter basic conceptual and theoretical dimensions of the subject are briefly examined. The following chapter describes the structure and function of the autonomic nervous system (ANS); the reason for including content on the ANS at this point in the text will become evident later in this chapter. The remaining two chapters focus on the two most significant functions of motivation: the arousal and directive functions.

THE STUDY OF MOTIVATION

The topic of motivation is an area within the field of psychology which has captured the interest of numerous scholars. Psychologists with widely differing orientations have studied motivation. On the one hand, physiologically oriented psychologists have been primarily interested in how bodily processes are related to motivation. Their approach has focused on neural and biochemical correlates of an organism's responses. Other psychologists have focused their attentions on attempting to find lawful stimulus-response relationships, or behavioral principles, rather than being concerned with physiological mechanisms in motivation. They have studied conditions such as reinforcement, punishment, deprivation, and how they govern behavior.

In recent years, there has been a growing cooperation between these two extreme camps; each side now recognizes that neither of the extreme positions promises a complete solution to understanding this complex phenomenon. There is an understanding that both physiological mechanisms and environmental contingencies interact to produce complex patterns of motivated behavior.

DEFINITION AND FUNCTION OF MOTIVATION

Like so many other concepts used in the study of human behavior, there is no precise and uniformally accepted definition of motivation. There are even some psychologists who feel that it is not a useful word or, better, that the concept is unneccessary. This, of course, is an extreme position and, since the word is so firmly embedded in the popular vocabulary, it is unlikely that it could be abolished by some researcher's dictate. Moreover, most psychologists feel it is a useful concept, notwithstanding the definitional problem.

For our purposes, motivation will be defined as the internal mechanisms and external stimuli which arouse and direct behavior. It may be seen, then, that motivation involves two basic functions: One is an arousal, or energizing, function which is involved in the mobilization of the bodily resources for vigorous and intense response. The second is a directive function which guides behavior to specific ends. This involves why individuals select a particular behavior at a particular time and why they choose certain goals and not others. Of course these two functions are not mutually exclusive. Certainly, behavior at any one time is the result of the integration of both aspects of motivation. This general orientation to motivation is seen in Hebb's (1972) definition when he says that motivation is a "tendency of the whole animal to produce organized activity, normally varying from the low level of deep sleep to a high level in the waking, alert, excited animal, and varying also in the kind of behavior that results or the kind of stimulation to which the organism is responsive."

MOTIVATION TERMINOLOGY

Some of the terminology which is used in the literature on motivation is unique to the topic, or at least unique in the meanings assigned to various words. Some authorities use several concepts synonymously, while others emphasize the differences between these same words. We have already defined motivation; we shall now define some of the other terms that are frequently used in the literature on this topic. The definitions presented here are believed to represent the most widely accepted definitions for these words:

Need.   A need is a deficiency or lack of an essential element. More generally, it is any lack or deficiency which is inimical to the individual's welfare.

Drives.   Closely related to needs are drives. Drive has been used in a variety of ways and has several different definitions. In general, a drive is a tendency to behave in a particular manner to fulfill, or satisfy, a need. The behavior associated with drives is directed toward eliminating deprivation or moving away from noxious stimuli. Drives seem to compel us to act in a particular way because of tension or arousal instigated by a need.

Motive.   The concept refers to a state of the individual which arouses and directs behavior toward a goal. The word motive is usually considered a specific condition contributing to performance and to the general behavioral level. The words "motive" and "drive" are frequently used interchangeably in the literature because both refer to goal-directed behavior and both are triggered by a need.

Goal.   The word goal refers to objects or situations which an individual is seeking.

Incentives.   Incentives are objects, conditions, or stimuli external to the individual. They may be divided into positive incentives, which the individual tends to approach, and negative incentives, which the individual tends to avoid. In humans, since symbolic processes are so well developed, incentive objects, situations, or states, both positive and negative, can be imagined. In this case, the incentive is internal rather than external. Incentives have two basic functions. One is to evoke a state of arousal in the individual so that he or she will approach or withdraw from the incentive. The second is to instigate directive actions toward it or withdrawal from it.

Reinforcement.   This word refers to some condition which strengthens behavior which has preceded it. A negative reinforcement is an aversive stimulus used to decrease the probability of a response.

TYPES OF NEEDS

Since there is a universal agreement that motivational conditions may affect an individual's rate of learning and performance, a central issue in motivation study is the identification of the conditions which arouse and direct behavior, and an obvious candidate for resolving this issue is needs. The needs which are present in an individual at any one time are many and varied; moreover, they cannot be observed directly, but, like learning, must be inferred from behavior. A major task has been delineating needs.

In the interest of bringing some order to the enormous array of human needs, psychologists have classified them into two general categories. The first is called biological, or physiological, needs. These are triggered by basic biological demands for things such as food, water, oxygen, sex, and elimination. The second category contains what are known as social needs, such as the need for achievement, social status, self-esteem, etc. The needs fluctuate and at any one time some will dominate over others, and the individual's behavior will be controlled by the dominant ones.

Although there is no precise agreement on the number of biological needs, there is agreement that they are unlearned and they are essential to the survival of the individual and the species. There are also wide differences in the number of social needs which psychologists identify, but it is agreed that they are learned. Social needs seem to exist among numerous species of animals that live together. Each individual serves as a stimulus source for other individuals. As a result of this mutual interaction, social needs come to be learned. The human being is certainly the most complex social animal, and all persons must learn a prodigious set of social needs and responses peculiar to their societies and cultures in order to function effectively. Although many social needs are unique to a particular society, there are many that are common to the various people of the world.

MOTIVATION THEORIES

One of the most difficult tasks for the student of human behavior is to describe why a certain behavior occurs. We ask, what was the motivation for that behavior. Psychologists have been wrestling with the problem of motivation for many years, and various theories of motivation have been formulated, but factual knowledge is incomplete and most of the theories have glaring weaknesses. Nevertheless, a brief examination of the more important theoretical notions helps one obtain a "flavor" of the work on this subject as well as an understanding of the approaches, advances, and setbacks which have accompanied its study.

A. PHILOSOPHIC THEORIES

Attempts to explain the "why" of human behavior permeates much of the philosophic and scientific literature throughout history. Philosophic viewpoints about free will, as a basic view of motivation, enjoyed many centuries of acceptance in Western culture. Interwoven with this concept of free will were attempts to explain behavior by use of the concept of "soul." With the rise of science, mechanistic views of motivation emerged and the concepts of "free will" and "soul" were not very useful to the scientist in explaining why a person behaves in a certain way. Instead, it was proposed that mechanical principles governed human behavior. For example, Descartes postulated fluid spirits passing through the nerves as driving agents that moved the body.

B. EARLY SCIENTIFIC THEORIES

The first solid beginning of scientific theory about motivation came from Charles Darwin's (1859) theory of evolution. For Darwin, complex behavior was to be traced to "instincts" which emerge through natural selection. Darwin's "survival of the fittest" notion viewed life as a continual struggle for existence, and the organisms which made the best adaptation to the environment survived while the nonadaptive perished. Thus, motivation was primarily adaptive and competitive. Since the idea of instincts was central to Darwin's theory of behavior, a great deal of motivated behavior was viewed as instinctual.

C. INSTINCT THEORIES

In the later years of the 19th century the concept of instincts gained favor and by the beginning of the 20th century it came into the mainstream of psychological theorizing. Instinct was adopted enthusiastically by respected scholars such as William James (1890), Sigmund Freud (1938), and William McDougall (1912) as an essential concept in explaining motivation. These various theorists identified a variety of instincts and each gave emphasis to particular ones. McDougall identified such instincts as curiosity, repulsion, sex, hunger, gregariousness, acquisitiveness, etc. Freud emphasized two basic instincts: the life instinct and the death instinct; the first is exemplified in the sex drive and the second in the aggressive drive.

D. DRIVE THEORISTS

The instinct doctrine was quite popular in the first two decades of this century, but by the 1920s numerous attacks upon it had weakened its structure and credibility. As the popularity of instinct theories of motivation dwindled, a successor, called "drive theory," rose to take the limelight. The concept of "drive" was introduced in 1918 by Robert S. Woodworth (1918) to describe the tendency which propels an organism to action as opposed to the habits which guide behavior in one direction or another. The main drives that came to be identified with this proposition were hunger, thirst, sex, and pain. In the 1930s, Walter B. Cannon (1932) introduced the concept of "homeostasis" which integrated the concept of drive with physiological mechanisms.

1. Homeostasis

Homeostasis may be explained in this way: In order for an individual to survive, many physiological and chemical functions must maintain some sort of equilibrium. Temperature, blood pressure, oxygen, carbon dioxide compositions, sugar content, and water balance must all be maintained within certain limits. When there is a disequilibrium of any of these, and other mechanisms, there is said to be a need to correct this imbalance, and compensatory actions are mobilized to counteract the disturbance and restore equilibrium.

Increasing heart and respiration rates are reactions to exercise, and are responses to oxygen need. Homeostasis is the internal regulatory process that is responsible for maintaining this internal equilibrium. Behavior produced from basic physiological needs ensures the survival of the animal or species by maintaining this internal equilibrium, which is called the "homeostatic state." Thus, whenever the cells or tissues of the body are deficient in a necessary chemical substance, homeostatic mechanisms are mobilized by the central nervous system to correct this deficiency. The term "tissue need" is often used to describe such a deficiency. The body also has "expulsion needs," which arise out of an accumulation of metabolic waste materials which must be expelled from the body. The word "drive" in this context refers to a state of tension and activity that is aroused by one of these needs. Hunger is one example of a biological drive based on a tissue need for food.

The functioning of biological drives is essential to the maintenance of homeostasis. Homeostatic mechanisms have often been compared to thermostats. Whenever there is a deficiency or surplus of some substance in the body, the thermostat that is particularly sensitive to that function is activated and initiates regulatory measures.

2. The comprehensive drive theory of Clark Hull

"Drive theory" was greatly advanced by a comprehensive theoretical formulation devised by Clark Hull (1943) in the 1940s and reformulated by him in the early 1950s (1952). His theory was developed around the notion that all behavior is motivated by homeostatic drives, or secondary drives based on them. Needs were believed to stimulate specific sensory receptors and elicit afferent impulses toward central controlling mechanisms; these mechanisms, Hull proposed, acted like a kind of automatic switchboard, directing the impulses to the muscles or glands the action of which was necessary to reduce the particular need. Satiation or drive reduction, according to this theory, depends exclusively upon the cessation of drive stimulation.

If the responses reduced the drive stimulus, these responses acquired reinforcement properties so that on future occasions, if the same drive stimulus recurred, the same responses would tend to be used again. In essence, the Hull's drive-reduction model first assumes that the behavior of an organism is influenced by the operation of internal drives or tension-like states that seek reduction or relief. This drive-reduction point of view became one of the most influential theories relating learning and motivation during the 1940s and 1950s.

E. CONTEMPORARY ADVANCES IN MOTIVATION THEORY

Drive theory has been the center of numerous investigations during the past 25 years. Although these investigations have yielded much evidence in support of the theory, formidable attacks have been leveled at it, and these attacks have exposed a number of weaknesses in it. One group of critics has argued that four or five biological needs do not seem to account for all human needs, and that many behaviors are unrelated to the basic biological needs. They point out that the range of human behavior is too variable to be grouped into a few simple needs. Drive theorists have countered this criticism by postulating "secondary needs" as underlying the primary needs. They have also added to the number of primary needs, by adding such things as an exploratory need, a manipulative need, etc.

Another criticism of drive theory is based on evidence that is incompatible with a homeostatic conception of drive involving stimulus reduction or tension reduction. A number of observations of various species, including humans, show that they exhibit behavior that actually *increases* stimulation, rather than reducing it. Animals exhibit curiosity and exploratory behavior even when they are not hungry or thirsty. Monkeys will manipulate objects, such as puzzles, and learn how to disassemble them with no obvious reinforcement except that which is provided by the objects or the achievements themselves (Harlow, 1950). Butler (1953) reported that monkeys under his care learned to press on a panel on the side of their cage which, when pushed, opened and allowed them to view the laboratory and the activity going on in it; presumably this provided the animals more stimulation than merely sitting alone in their cages.

A type of stimulation quite different from external stimulation has been found to be an effective reinforcer. In this case, the stimulus is delivered to certain areas within the brain by means of a brief electrical current. Olds and Milner (1954) reported that rats with permanently implanted electrodes in specific sites in the brain could be made to learn tasks while the only re-inforcement for performance was electrical stimulation to the brain. This demonstrated that reward mechanisms were not dependent upon drive reduction, and it revived one of the oldest motivation theories, hedonism.* In the same year, Delgado and his colleagues (1954) reported that electrical sti-mulation of certain brain sites produced aversive effects in cats. This sti-mulation could be used to motivate the learning of behaviors to terminate the stimulation. The identification of both "pleasure" and "aversive" areas of the brain has stimulated a good deal of research concerning a hedonistic approach to motivation during the past 20 years.

Taken as a whole, it is evident that the view of motivation based solely on a drive- or stimulus-reduction theory becomes hard to defend. A great deal of evidence is incompatible with the stimulus-reduction notion of drive theory.

1. Arousal theory

A motivational theory that has come to have increasing attention in the past two decades is called activation or arousal theory (both names have been used) (Duffy, 1962). Theorists of this persuasion have been concerned with two basic issues. First there has been concern about examining the notion that persons are motivated to seek levels of stimulation that are optimal for general function. The underlying notion here is that for a given person there is a level of arousal that is normal or appropriate for that person, and behavior is motivated towards achieving and maintaining that normal state of arousal, and that individual will engage in behavior to decrease his or her arousal level when it is too high and increase it when it is too low (Korman, 1974). The second major interest of the activation theorists has been on the effects of arousal on behavior. The concern here is on the ways in which the fluctuating of arousal states affect behavior. More will be said about this in Chapter 24.

Although arousal theory is an interesting perspective for predicting behavior under different conditions, there are, however, several theoret-ical, methodological, and measurement questions that are still to be resolved with it. It does, nevertheless, overcome several weaknesses of the Hullian approach which predicts that behavior ceases once the reduction of the stimulus is achieved.

---

*Hedonism is the notion that the individual acts in such a way as to seek pleasure and avoid pain. This notion had its root in Greek antiquity, where it was argued that the desire to achieve the "greatest pleasure" was universal in mankind.

2. Expectancy-value theory and consistency theories

Two other motivational theories which have generated much interest and research support in the past 20 years are the expectancy-value theory and an
interrelated set of formulations collectively called consistency theory. The
basic position of the former is that behavior is a function of both the characteristics of persons at the time (i.e., their needs and demands) and the
characteristics of the particular environment as it is perceived by individuals; in other words, "behavior is a function of the expectancy of value
attainment at that time and in that particular environment and the actual
degree of value (or incentive) that is available" (Korman, 1974). The underlying notion here is that individuals will behave in ways that will maximize
their outcomes, in light of the value of the outcomes they see available to
them, the kinds of outcomes they desire, their rational expectancy of achieving the outcomes in that particular situation (Korman, 1974).

Consistency theory postulates that balance or consistency among cognitions is the end or goal of behavior. When there is a discrepancy or inconsistency in cognitions, changes take place to restore the equilibrium. The
essence of this theory is that individuals are motivated to maintain a consistent relationship between their beliefs, likes, dislikes, etc., and their behavior. Behavior is aroused when inconsistency is developed and becomes
directed toward reducing it (Heider, 1958; Osgood and Tannenbaum, 1955;
Festinger, 1957).

These models of human motivation have provided significant advances
in our understanding of behavior. But they, like other theories of motivation,
suffer from various weaknesses. For example, the constructs of expectancy
and consistency appear to be far more complex than they were originally
thought to be, and much refinement will be necessary in order to uncover
their antecedents and experimental determinants before they are brought
under the necessary experimental control to provide adequate theories of
motivation.

3. Maslow's theory of self-actualization

A contemporary motivation theory that is not tied to the notion of reducing
biological drives or seeking pleasure or reducing discomfort is known as
self-actualizing theory or humanistic theory. This model of human motivation emphasizes the individual's yearning to explore, to create, to be loved,
or to feel self-respect, and its acknowledged originator is Abraham Maslow
(1954). Basically, the theory proposes that human strivings and the direc-
tionality of behavior are organized around a "hierarchy of needs," with the
lowest level being the physiological needs for such things as food, water, etc.
The next higher level is the safety needs; these are followed in the hierarchy

lowest   *physiological needs*—satisfying hunger, thirst

          safety needs—security, stability

          belongingness and love needs—affection, identification

          self-esteem needs—prestige, self-respect

highest   self-actualization needs

Fig. 22.1   Maslow's hierarchy of needs. (Based on Maslow, 1954.)

by belongingness and love needs, self-esteem needs, and finally, at the highest level, self-actualization needs (Fig. 22.1). According to Maslow, motivation follows a developmental pattern from lower needs to higher needs, and the prepotency of the higher needs increases as needs immediately below them are satisfied.

For Maslow, the fundamental motive is the motivation to express human potentialities in their most complete and effective form; this is the need for self-actualization. Self-actualization is defined by Maslow (1954):

It refers to man's desire for self-fulfillment, namely, to the tendency for him to become actualized in what he is potentially. This tendency might be phrased as the desire to become more and more what one idiosyncratically is, to become everything that one is capable of becoming.

This theory proposes that humans are capable of a meaningful, viable, potential-fulfilling existence, and that they have the ability to implement a meaningful, self-actualized existence, but social conditions tend to prevent them from achieving this state.

At this time, there is very little systematic research support for the theory, and the work that has been done on the postulated hierarchy of needs is equivocal (Alderfer, 1969; Lawler and Suttle, 1972; Trexler and Schuh, 1971). Factor analyses of the instruments which have been developed for assessing the Maslow hierarchy have reported conflicting findings; Beer (1966) found the items did cluster together in the manner predicted by the theory, but Payne (1970) reported that they did not.

MEASURING MOTIVATION

Many investigators who study motivation use lower animals exclusively or primarily, and by far the bulk of studies on motivation have been done with animals. There are, of course, a number of obvious advantages to using animals: It is fairly inexpensive to maintain an animal colony in a laboratory; it is easy to control animals' prior experience (but not that of humans), which is important in motivation studies; rapid reproduction keeps a ready supply of new subjects available; and various kinds of surgical manipulations can be performed, such as implanting electrodes in the brain, which would be illegal to do with human brains.

Psychologists who use animals as subjects have used a variety of methods to assess motivation. They have deprived the animals of food or water, they have applied electric shocks of various strengths, they have made lesions in specific parts of the brain, and they have implanted electrodes in specific parts of the brain. The purpose of all of these manipulations is to assess their effects on the behavior of the animals.

There is no universally accepted method of assessing human motivation, and this lack of adequate assessment methods has restricted the development of systematic information about this topic. Because of the wide differences in theoretical constructs, there has been considerable variety in the methods of measuring motivation, and each method has met with severe criticism by its detractors. The strict experimental psychologists claim that clinical methods of measuring human motivation are nothing more than codified subjective impressions of little reliability and doubtful worth. The clinical psychologists, on the other hand, claim that the experimentalists tend to avoid direct confrontations with human motivation and try to apply extrapolations from lower animals which may or may not be valid.

A. SELF-RATING METHOD

The simplest and one of the oldest methods of assessing human motivation is the self-report inventory. This method employs a standardized interview schedule or a written questionnaire. Subjects are asked by the interviewer or via a printed questionnaire how they "feel" about a given topic, or they might be asked to respond to questions about likes, dislikes, wants, aspirations, anxieties, and habits.

There are numerous instruments of this kind, but they all have limited value because the relevance of the motivational constructs they measure may be great in one environmental context, but not in the next; in addition, they frequently do not contain clear, unambiguous questions, and responses are easily faked by respondents. These are only a few of the problems that are common to most of them.

Projective instruments

Projective instruments are a special form of self-report in that the test materials consist of ambiguous figures or pictures to which the subject must respond. The ambiguous materials may be inkblots, incomplete sentences, or scenes. The subject is asked to write or tell stories about the stimulus items. These stories are then analyzed and coded as to the motives, needs, wishes, and so forth, which are assumed to have been projected by the respondent onto the characters in the test items and which manifest themselves in what is said or written about the items.

Projective tests assume that persons' perception of the world is greatly influenced by personal needs and therefore that respondents will tend to project their own needs and desires into the stimuli. Instead of describing what they see, subjects are presumed to describe their own motives without always realizing what they are doing. It is believed that unconscious motives will be revealed by the responses the subjects make. It is further assumed that a psychologist or psychiatrist is able to identify and interpret these hidden motives from the subjects' responses.

B. OBSERVATION METHOD

A second method of measuring human motivation is to have an observer assess motivation from observation of behavior. This has been a favorite method of clinical psychologists who believe that this method is particularly fruitful for uncovering unconscious motives. The student of human behavior can probably discern glaring weaknesses in this method. Judgments by observers, even highly trained observers, vary considerably in their reliability. Since behavior is so multidetermined, it is difficult to ascertain with any certainty why the behavior occurred. Also, the "halo" effect cannot be ignored; that is, observers may project their own motives into their judgments of behavior. A common experience in everyday life illustrates this point: As two individuals attempt to describe the behavior of a third person, especially if they have strongly different viewpoints about that person, they invariably describe conflicting observations about the behavior of the third person. Finally, this technique, as well as the self-rating method, suffers from a very serious weakness: neither technique has been subjected, to any extent, to the experimental method.

Motivation under induced conditions

A related method of assessing motivation is by observing behavior under various motivationally induced conditions. The subject is given a task and permitted to perform it under varying motivational conditions. From observation of the resultant behavior, different conditions may be evaluated as to their motivation properties. Motivational conditions that have been used are deprivations, material rewards, verbal praise, individual competition, team competition, electric shock, verbal reproof, etc. One of the main effects of motivation on behavior is its influence on selection of goals, so in some cases conditions are arranged to permit the subject to select goals—such as achievement or affiliation. Some persons may respond to incentives emphasizing achievement, whereas others respond to affiliation incentives. The presence of a motive, then, is inferred from the behavior a person exhibits and the incentives which are effective. The frequency, intensity, and persistence of responses exhibited by an individual are other ways in which motivation may be inferred from behavior.

C. AUTONOMIC NERVOUS SYSTEM RESPONSE METHOD

A third method of measuring motivation involves measuring the activity and reactivity of the organs and tissues innervated by the autonomic nervous system (ANS), a system which is known to mediate motivated behavior. As you recall, one of the components of motivation is a state of arousal, and during arousal there are changes in heart and breathing rates, blood pressure, muscle tension, electrical activity of the brain, and so on. These changes are neural correlates of what is meant by an arousal or activated state, and there is evidence that behavioral patterns do vary with arousal level.

Grossman (1967) lists the various physiological responses that are commonly measured because they seem to be affected by motivation-producing stimuli:

1. Pilomoter responses (movements of the hair)—this is the most frequently used index of emotionality in laboratory animals.
2. Skin electrical resistance.
3. Cardiac activity—heartbeat
4. Blood pressure
5. Respiration rate
6. Muscular tension
7. Skin temperature
8. Gastrointestinal activity
9. Electrical activity of the brain
10. Biochemical measures
    a) Norepinephrine—epinephrine
    b) Steroids

In order to understand how these physiological responses occur, it is necessary to have an understanding of how the ANS functions. Knowledge of ANS activity also provides a foundation for understanding the arousal and directive functions of motivation. Therefore, the following chapter deals with this specialized part of the nervous system.

Before concluding this chapter, it needs to be pointed out that although the assessment of ANS activity can be carried out rather precisely, there are only moderate correlations between different measures of physiological arousal; thus, whatever each of these measures is assessing, i.e., heart rate, brain wave activity, muscular tension, each is measuring something separate from the others, in addition to the commonality which exists.

23

The Autonomic Nervous System

In the first few chapters of this book the structure and functions of the somatic nervous system were discussed; thus, the parts of the central nervous system (CNS) and the peripheral nervous system (PNS) which convey impulses from the sensory receptors, organize them in the brain, and deliver impulses to the skeletal muscles were described in those chapters. There are, however, essential nervous system functions which occur in conjunction with the somatic nervous system activities but which are carried out by another component of the nervous system, the autonomic nervous system (ANS). The ANS consists of neurons located in both the CNS and PNS which control the response of smooth muscles and glands. This chapter describes the structure and functions of this component of the nervous system.

THE AUTONOMIC NERVOUS SYSTEM

All of the various body organs and tissues must be regulated and, when necessary for action, mobilized before effective and efficient behavior can take place. This regulation is not under voluntary control in the full sense of the word voluntary. That is, you do not normally regulate your heart rate, breathing, pupil dilation or constriction, or perspiration. These are only a few examples of involuntary control. The activity of many other organs and tissues is modified without voluntary regulation. The part of the nervous system most directly involved in the bodily adjustments described above is the autonomic nervous system (ANS), which consists of a network of efferent neurons in the brainstem and spinal cord that transmit impulses to their destinations in the PNS. These motor impulses innervate smooth muscles of the visceral organs, such as the heart, stomach, blood vessels, and glands.

This system is itself activated primarily by neural centers located in the brainstem, hypothalamus, and parts of the cerebral cortex.

It is, then, the ANS which functions to control and regulate the internal environment of the body. It utilizes reflex controls over effectors to achieve homeostatic balance or to mobilize the body's resources for action. Homeostasis, meaning self-regulation, is primarily a function of the ANS. For example, temperature regulation is one homeostatic function. As environmental temperature rises, sweat glands are activated which promote body cooling, and peripheral vasodilation of the arterioles and capillaries of the skin allows blood to be brought to the surface for cooling. In cold temperatures, the skin arterioles constrict to keep blood away from the surface; skeletal muscles increase their tone, and shivering may occur to produce more heat from the muscles.

Internal physiological adjustments to emergencies are primarily controlled by the ANS. Preparations to strengthen the body to meet physically demanding situations include acceleration of the heartbeat, increase in blood pressure, release of glucose from the liver and conversion of glycogen

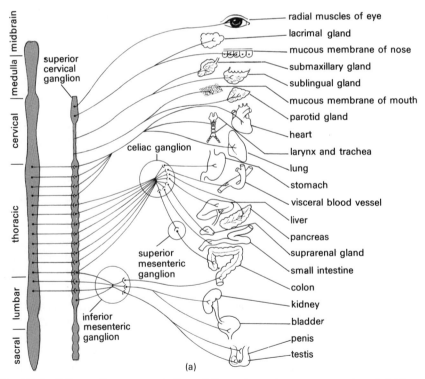

Fig. 23.1 Schematic representation of the autonomic nervous system. (a) The sympathetic nervous system (thoracolumbar).

to glucose in muscles, secretion of epinephrine and norepinephrine by the adrenal glands. These are only a few of the adjustments which help to strengthen and prepare the body for action. It would be impossible to perform effectively or efficiently in games and sports skills without an ANS.

The activity of the ANS is also primarily responsible for bodily changes accompanying emotional states. Since the ANS is so important in mobilizing the body for action on the basis of sensory stimuli and aiding the body to return to a more normal state when a high degree of mobilization is necessary, it has been called the "center for emotions" by some psychologists. In fact, one psychologist says, "emotion is the activity and reactivity of the tissues and organs innervated by the autonomic nervous system."

AUTONOMIC DIVISIONS

The ANS is a motor system which supplies structures of the body which are typically not under voluntary control, such as the smooth and cardiac mus-

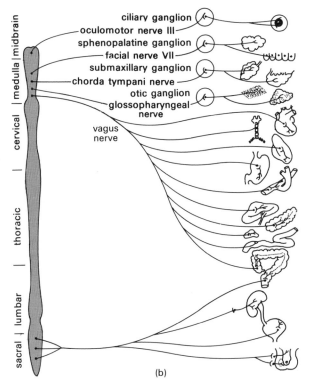

Fig. 23.1 (cont.)   (b) The parasympathetic system (craniosacral). (Based on DeCoursey, 1968.)

cles and the glands. It is divided into two major divisions: The sympathetic, or thoracolumbar, division and the parasympathetic, or craniosacral, division (Fig. 23.1). There are several reasons for this division. First, the nerve fibers have anatomic distributions which are distinct from each other. Second, the two divisions secrete different types of transmitter substances at their nerve endings. Third, the effects produced on the internal organs and tissues by the two divisions are generally opposite to each other. In general, the sympathetic division stimulates somatic activity and inhibits vegetative functions; that is, it prepares the body for action; while the parasympathetic division promotes vegetative functions, meaning it helps the body maintain a homeostatic, or normal, internal environment.

Both the autonomic efferent axons and the somatic efferent axons originate with cell bodies located in the spinal cord and brainstem but, unlike somatic efferent fibers, the autonomic fibers do not go directly to efferent organs. Instead they make synaptic connections with peripheral ganglia containing neurons the axons of which actually innervate the effector organs. The cell body of the first autonomic neuron is located in the lateral intermediate (intermediolateral) gray column of the spinal cord or in nuclei in the brainstem, and the cell body of the second neuron is located in a ganglion outside the CNS. Since the axon of the first neuron synapses with dendrites and cell bodies in a ganglion, it is called preganglionic. The second neuron projects its fibers from the ganglion to muscles or glands and it is, therefore, called postganglionic.

A. THE SYMPATHETIC DIVISION

In the sympathetic, or thoracolumbar, division, there is a long nerve trunk on each side of the vertebral column that extends from the base of the skull to the coccyx. Each is known as a sympathetic trunk, or "ganglion chain." These two chains of ganglia outside the vertebral column look like a pair of beads; the beads are a succession of approximately 22 enlargements produced by masses of nerve-cell bodies, called ganglia. The ganglia chains receive preganglionic fibers from the spinal cord from the first thoracic vertebral level down to the third lumbar level. Although there are no sympathetic efferent fiber connections from the spinal cord in the cervical or sacral regions, that does not mean that these levels do not receive sympathetic fibers. The sympathetic chains extend up to form cervical ganglia which supply various mechanisms of the neck and head and the chains extend down into the sacral level to provide sympathetic innervation to the organs of the lower trunk and body, bladder, genitals, colon, and legs.

In addition to these ganglia chains, the sympathetic division has "collateral" ganglia. The largest of these collateral ganglia are the celiac, superior mesenteric, and inferior mesenteric. The heart, lungs, liver, intestines, stomach, blood vessels, adrenal medulla, and glands are the most important structures which are innervated by the sympathetic ganglia.

The sympathetic division is characterized by short preganglionic fibers, about one centimeter long, and long postganglionic fibers, except when the preganglionic fiber extends through the ganglion chain to a collateral ganglion, in which case there is a short postganglionic fiber to the organ supplied.

Nerve fibers to the sympathetic chain connect the chain with each spinal nerve just as it emerges from the intervertebral foramina. The preganglionic fibers then leave the spinal nerve and travel through small whitish nerves called white rami (preganglionic fibers of the ANS are also called white rami communicantes) into the sympathetic chain. These fibers appear white because they are myelinated. The preganglionic neurons may synapse with postganglionic neurons within the ganglion that they first enter, or they may pass through one or several ganglia and synapse within other ganglia at lower or higher levels, or they may project uninterrupted

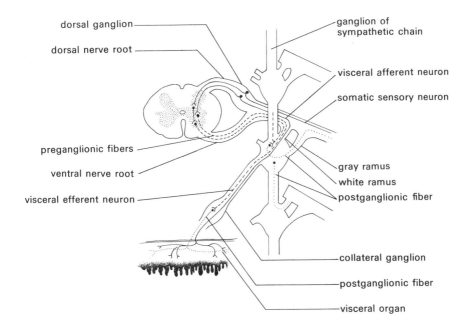

Fig. 23.2 Relationship between preganglionic and postganglionic transmission in the sympathetic system. (Based on DeCoursey, 1968.)

through the ganglion chain to synapse in one of the collateral ganglia (Fig. 23.2). Each preganglionic axon typically synapses via its collaterals with a number of ganglion cells. This arrangement is important because it provides for rapid and widespread responses which are characteristic of the sympathetic division.

Axons from nerve cell bodies located in the sympathetic ganglion chain are called postganglionic fibers, and they leave the chain in bundles called gray rami (or gray rami communicantes). These fibers appear gray because they are unmyelinated. They are distributed in two major ways: some return to spinal nerves and proceed to involuntary peripheral muscles, blood vessels, and smooth muscles in the skin, or to sweat glands. The others go directly to visceral-organ blood vessels and various visceral organs in the neck, head, abdomen, and pelvis.

B. THE PARASYMPATHETIC DIVISION

The parasympathetic, or craniosacral, division of the ANS consists of two segments: the cranial and the sacral. The cell bodies of the preganglionic neurons of this division are located within the midbrain, brainstem, and sacral regions of the spinal cord; hence the name craniosacral.

Unlike the sympathetic ganglia, parasympathetic ganglia are not located in a well-defined ganglion chain. Instead, the axons leaving the cord as preganglionic fibers usually pass all the way to the wall of the organ to be stimulated, at which point they synapse with postganglionic neurons. Thus, the postganglionic fibers are actually located near or within the organ the nerve is serving; the unmyelinated postganglionic fibers are, therefore, very short. Two other differences in the two divisions are that each preganglionic axon of the parasympathetic division has synaptic connections with very few cells whereas preganglionic sympathetic axons typically innervate numerous cells, and the postganglionic fibers innervate fewer organs than do the postganglionic fibers of the sympathetic division. For example, there are no parasympathetic fibers reaching the sweat glands or smooth skin muscle.

In the parasympathetic division, most of the preganglionic fibers originate in the tenth cranial nerve (vagus nerve). Indeed, about 85 percent of all parasympathetic fibers pass through the vagus nerve. This nerve sends parasympathetic fibers to the heart, lungs, and most of the organs of the abdomen. Some parasympathetic fibers begin in the other cranial nerves to supply the head, to innervate voluntary and involuntary muscles of the eyeball, face, and salivary glands. Additionally, there are a few parasympathetic fibers arising from sacral segments of the cord. These fibers reach the bladder and other pelvic viscera.

C. OVERALL FUNCTIONS OF THE AUTONOMIC DIVISIONS

The parasympathetic division is considered an antagonist of the sympathetic division, when a structure is innervated by both divisions. When the sympathetic division is an accelerator, such as with the heart, then the parasympathetic division is the inhibitor; that is, it slows down the heart to a normal level, but usually not below normal unless it is stimulated by drugs or pressure on a nerve. The parasympathetic division tends to act selectively on structures and is concerned mostly with maintaining regular, normal bodily functioning. The sympathetic, on the other hand, tends to react as a whole, particularly in sudden emergencies or dramatic environmental changes. As a result, the heartbeat increases, blood pressure rises, overall

organ	effect of sympathetic stimulation	effect of parasympathetic stimulation
eye: pupil	dilation	constriction
ciliary muscle	no effect	contraction
gastrointestinal glands	constriction	stimulation and copious secretion of many enzymes
sweat glands	sweating (cholinergic)	no effect
heart muscle and coronaries	increased activity (vasodilation)	decreased activity (vasoconstriction)
systemic blood vessels		
abdominal	vasodilation	no effect
muscle	vasodilation	no effect
skin	vasoconstriction or vasodilation	no effect
lungs: bronchi	dilation	constriction
blood vessels	mild constriction	no effect
gut: lumen	decreased peristalsis and tone	increased peristalsis and tone
sphincters	increased tone	decreased tone
liver	release of glucose	no effect
kidney	decreased output	no effect
basal metabolism	increased	no effect
adrenal cortical secretion	increased	no effect

Fig. 23.3 Effects of the autonomic nervous system on selected organs of the body.

rate of metabolism increases, blood sugar, or glucose, increases, and mental altertness is enhanced. Thus, the sympathetic division prepares the body for action and aids a person to react to emergency situations (Fig. 23.3).

AUTONOMIC TRANSMITTERS

One of the major differences between the sympathetic and parasympathetic divisions is that they secrete different chemical substances at the post-ganglionic terminals where they innervate tissue and organs. But first it should be noted that both divisions secrete the same transmitter at the pre-ganglionic terminals; at the preganglionic fiber terminals in all sympathetic and parasympathetic fibers the chemical transmitter that is secreted is acetylcholine.

A. THE SYMPATHETIC DIVISION

It is in the postganglionic fiber that there is a difference in chemical trans-mitter. Most of the postganglionic fibers of the sympathetic division secrete norepinephrine (also called noradrenalin) and traces of epinephrine (also called adrenalin), commonly referred to collectively as catecholamines. Postsynaptic sympathetic neurons that secrete catecholamines are called adrenergic neurons.

Norepinephrine is the transmitter agent released at the synapse by most postganglionic sympathetic fibers. This substance is synthesized by the nerve cell and stored in the axon terminal within vesicular structures and is released in response to neural stimulation. Although it is possible that adrenergic neurons may release minute quantities of epinephrine, current evidence indicates that norepinephrine is the neurotransmitter. Small amounts of norepinephrine from the postganglionic terminals may diffuse into the general circulation but it is not likely that this occurs to any extent.

Norepinephrine and epinephrine are removed at the sympathetic end-ings by reabsorption into the sympathetic nerves and by destruction by o-methyl transferase, an enzyme. Catecholamines are also secreted by the adrenal medulla gland and they circulate in the blood. In the blood, they are not destroyed or removed until they diffuse into tissues; then they remain active sometimes for many minutes.

Experiments with animals have found that norepinephrine is essential for active behavior, and any depletion of this neurochemical results in inability to produce normal amounts of movement. Drugs which cause deple-tion of norepinephrine centrally produce sedation or depression, while drugs which increase or potentiate brain norepinephrine are associated with behavioral stimulation or excitement and generally have an anti-depressant effect on humans (Schildkraut and Kety, 1967). Conditions that cause stress are known to deplete norepinephrine in the brain for periods up to 24 hours. Since neurochemical systems adapt to repeated demands on their resources, depletion of norepinephrine becomes less severe if demands are continually placed on the system. Thus, repeated exposure to any stressful experience will eliminate the behavioral deficit. Moreover, it is possible to counteract the effect of stress with drugs, such as parayline, thus protecting norepinephrine against depletion (Poortmans, 1969).

Not all of the sympathetic postganglionic terminals are adrenergic. For example, the sweat glands and the adrenal medulla do not follow the sympathetic transmitter pattern of adrenergic secretions. Postganglionic fibers to the sweat glands transmit their impulses by the release of acetylcholine, and impulses passing down the splanchnic nerve release acetylcholine which discharges the catecholamines from the adrenal medulla.

B. THE PARASYMPATHETIC DIVISION

The postganglionic terminals of the parasympathetic division secrete acetylcholine. They are, therefore, cholinergic at both the preganglionic terminals and at the postganglionic ends; thus, these postganglionic neurons are called cholinergic. The enzyme cholinesterase destroys acetylcholine at the parasympathetic nerve endings just as it does at the somatic axon endings, but this destruction does not occur as rapidly. In fact, at the parasympathetic endings, the acetylcholine will sometimes last for several seconds, allowing it a long-action period.

To review, the transmission flow in the ANS is generally as follows: impulses travel over preganglionic fibers and synapse with ganglion cells, releasing acetylcholine. Impulses are then carried over postganglionic fibers and certain chemical substances are secreted at these fiber terminals. These chemicals serve as transmitters, and, when released, initiate activity in tissues and organs, or they may alter the existing activity.

AUTONOMIC CONTROL LEVELS

Just as with control of skeletal motor activity, the ANS may be examined as a series of levels of control which differ in function from one level to the next. The highest level is the cerebral cortex; next is the hypothalamus, then the brainstem and spinal cord; the lowest level is the ganglionic level.

A. THE CEREBRAL CORTEX

Very little is known about the role of the cerebral cortex in control of the ANS. But the cerebral cortex does appear to be involved in ANS responses to emotional states. It is known that portions of cortex in the prefrontal and temporal lobes can enhance or depress the degree of excitation of the lower level centers. Fear, anger, or apprehension can alter various organs which are mediated by ANS fibers; indeed, there is no visceral activity that cannot be modified, even completely disorganized, by emotional states. For example, fear or anger may completely upset the digestive processes while at the same time it is causing heart rate to increase, sweat glands to secrete, and blood pressure to increase. Sports performers are well acquainted with these phenomena which often occur just before contests. They are called "butterflies" in the sports world.

B. THE HYPOTHALAMUS

The hypothalamus consists of a series of nuclei which lie on the floor of the diencephalon behind the optic chiasm and between it and the pons (Fig. 23.4). Located here are many of the centers for initiating the complex reaction mechanisms which maintain a homeostatic, or physiological, balance in our internal environment and which help to organize the outward expression of emotions. Because of these mechanisms, the hypothalamus has been called by some authors the highest level of autonomic control of bodily mechanisms. We refer to it here as the second highest level.

The hypothalamus receives afferent transmission input from many pathways, and many of the functions of this organ are carried out in conjunction with connections to lower centers such as the brainstem. Afferent transmission relaying in the thalamus projects signals to the hypothalamus. Of course, there is input from the cerebral cortex, especially the frontal lobes. These, and many other afferent fibers, provide a complex network of input, but little is known about their diffuse connections and effects except that they interconnect all of the hypothalamic nuclei. Efferent fibers from the hypothalamus scatter widely. The majority of fibers descend to the brainstem and connect with the motor and visceral areas throughout the brainstem. Others supply parts of the pituitary gland.

This structure also functions as an important link between the CNS and the endocrine system. Located near the pituitary gland, the hypothalamus has cells which discharge neurohormones which act upon various parts of the pituitary gland in such a way as to cause it to form and release chemical mediators, which then activate various glands throughout the body. Thus the hypothalamus influences endocrine activities such as metabolism, growth, electrolytic balance, and many others. It is obvious, then, that the

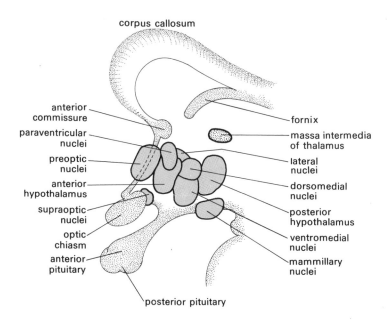

corpus callosum

anterior commissure

paraventricular nuclei

preoptic nuclei

anterior hypothalamus

supraoptic nuclei

optic chiasm

anterior pituitary

fornix

massa intermedia of thalamus

lateral nuclei

dorsomedial nuclei

posterior hypothalamus

ventromedial nuclei

mammillary nuclei

posterior pituitary

Fig. 23.4 The hypothalamus, showing the main nuclei of this structure. (Based on Woodburne, 1967.)

hypothalamus plays a critical role in the overall behavior of individuals. It may be said to act as a coordinating center for the ANS.

The exact role of the hypothalamus is certainly not completely understood, but the mechanisms which are at least partially under its control are water balance of the body, appetite, blood pressure, temperature regulation, sexual behavior, and emotional expressions.

1. Water balance

Cells of the supraoptic nucleus of the hypothalamus are sensitive to changes in the osmotic pressure of the blood, and this changes with its water content. The activities which are critical to maintaining water balance involve the responses of these hypothalamic cells to changes in osmotic pressure. Osmotic pressure changes trigger neurosecretory cells to discharge neurohormones which act on the pituitary gland; this then results in the release of an antidiuretic hormone (ADH) into the blood from the posterior pituitary gland. ADH, when released into the blood due to lack of water, travels to the kidneys and promotes reabsorption of body fluids rather than their excretion as urine; it also promotes the activity of water intake.

2. Appetite and hunger

Appetite and hunger are controlled by the hypothalamus and, normally, the adjustment of food intake to energy requirements is very sensitive and appears to depend on calorie content or blood temperature. Two theories have been proposed to explain the regulation of appetite: first, a drop in the blood or body temperature stimulates the lateral hypothalamic nucleus and initiates eating or the search for food; second, the cells of the lateral nucleus are sensitive to changes in the blood sugar content. During periods of hypoglycemia (low blood sugar) the cells stimulate eating or search for food.

3. Blood pressure

One of the most important areas for the regulation of blood pressure and blood volume is the hypothalamus. Stimulation of specific parts of the hypothalamus causes an increase in blood pressure and blood volume.

4. Temperature regulation

Hypothalamic centers maintain a constant regulation of body temperature. Responses to a warm environment seem to be initiated by mechanisms in the anterior of the hypothalamus, which have the effect of cooling the body. These mechanisms cause vasodilation in the skin, sweating, and panting in furry animals. On the other hand, the posterior hypothalamus normally acts to cause changes needed to regulate body temperature against cold. These changes are vasoconstriction in the skin, shivering, epinephrine secretion, and piloerection. These two parts of the hypothalamus act in coordination in a manner like a thermostat.

5. Sexual behavior

Sexual behavior involves more than control by the hypothalamus. However, experiments have found that when the anterior hypothalamus is stimulated, it produces male-mounting behavior in rats. This particular function of the hypothalamus has not been studied to the same extent as other functions.

6. Emotion

While the cerebral cortex is an important center for emotional control because an understanding of the significance of sensory data takes place there, the hypothalamus is particularly important in the phase of emotional reactivity which depends upon autonomic responses. The most widely accepted theory of emotion is the so-called Papez-MacLean theory (Papez, 1937; MacLean, 1949). According to this theory, a group of subcortical structures located in the medial and ventral parts of the forebrain, between the diencephalon and cerebral cortex, such as the hippocampus, fornix, cingulate gyrus, and the mammillary bodies of the hypothalamus, and collectively called the limbic system, is responsible for emotional expression, organization, and experience. The theory is a general description of what experimenters have established, which is that the limbic system is the central system in emotion. Of particular importance to the Papez-MacLean theory is the hypothalamus, which is the principal center in which the various components of emotional reaction are organized into definite patterns. The hypothalamus is, then, the focal, organizing structure in emotional behavior.

The hypothalamus and limbic structures seem to be as much involved in "pleasant" emotions as they are in rage and fear emotions. It has been found that rats and other animals with electrodes permanently implanted in a specific part of the lateral hypothalamus or in the limbic system will press a lever to deliver an electric shock to themselves; in fact, they will deliver as many as 3000 shocks per hour. These animals will learn mazes, cross electrified grids, and forego food just for the opportunity to stimulate portions of their hypothalamus or limbic system. Olds (1956) has called these areas of the brain "pleasure centers." Electrical stimulation in other parts of the brain results in the animals refusal to repeat the stimulation after the first response; indeed, they will act to shut off the electricity if it is initiated by the investigator.

C. THE BRAINSTEM AND SPINAL CORD

The level of ANS control below the hypothalamus is the brainstem and spinal cord. The brainstem contains ANS centers which are concerned with functions such as reflex respiration, circulation, heart rate, salivation, intestinal activities, and various other functions (Fig. 23.5).

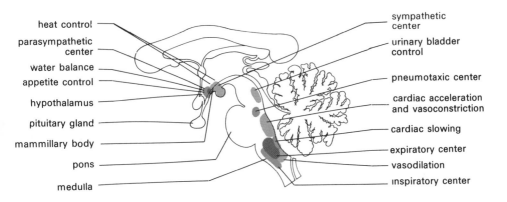

Fig. 23.5   Main autonomic nervous centers in the hypothalamus and brainstem. (Based on Guyton, 1964.)

Brainstem neurons receive input from the cerebral cortex, hypothalamus, and collaterals from ascending sensory fibers and reflex pathways. They project fibers to the nuclei of several cranial nerves and also to neurons descending to the spinal cord, especially those going to thoracic regions, the first three segments of the lumbar cord, and the second and third sacral levels.

Although these ANS centers are reflexive in nature, they are functionally restricted. For example, the respiratory centers do not actually control the vasomotor centers, although they may affect them. But the hypothalamus, projecting to both, may regulate or activate them simultaneously—for example, when respiration and blood pressure increase during emotional states. Of course, these centers do function on a reflex level, as in the regulation of blood pressure, but they are frequently integrated with somatic activities. In respiration, for instance, skeletal muscles are involved.

Some idea of how brainstem centers function in autonomic control can be obtained by studying decerebrate animals. A decerebrate animal, you will recall, is one in which all the nerve-fiber tracts above the midbrain have been severed. Descending impulses from the cerebral cortex and hypothalamus are thus interrupted. A decerebrate dog will continue to breathe by itself and its blood pressure will be maintained reflexively at about normal. But it cannot eat or regulate body temperature or adjust to any dramatic environmental changes. Reflex salivation may occur after taste of a food in decerebrate animals. If a light is flashed in the eyes of a decerebrate animal, the pupils of both eyes narrow and restrict the amount of light which can enter. This is known as the light reflex.

ANS control in the spinal cord is concerned with the more specific functions in more specific parts of the body. Spinal-cord ANS neurons arise in the intermediolateral portion of the gray matter of the cord and they receive input from all other levels of autonomic control. The axons of these neurons are known as preganglionic fibers. We have discussed the preganglionic fibers in a previous section of this chapter.

D. GANGLIONIC LEVEL

The lowest level of ANS control is the ganglionic level. This level consists of the various autonomic ganglia, such as the sympathetic ganglion chain. Preganglionic fibers from the brainstem and spinal cord project into the ganglia where they synapse with ganglion neurons located there. The axons of these ganglionic neurons form the postganglionic fibers of the ANS. These have already been discussed earlier in this chapter.

AUTONOMIC EFFECTS

We are now ready to identify and discuss some of the autonomic effects on various tissues and organs of the body. (Refer to Fig. 23.3.) Because of their importance in ANS functioning, the adrenal medullae will be discussed first and in more detail than other structures which are innervated by autonomic fibers.

A. ADRENAL MEDULLAE

The adrenal glands rest on the superior surfaces of the kidneys. Each gland consists of an outer region (the cortex) and an inner region (the medulla). These two regions are different in origin, cellular makeup, types of hormones which they secrete, and function, so each adrenal gland is actually two glands in one. The functioning of the adrenal medullae is of great importance in ANS responses.

Preganglionic fibers of the sympathetic division enter each adrenal medulla and make contact with modified ganglion cells of this structure. Acetylcholine, which is secreted by the preganglionic terminals that come in contact with the medullary cells, is the normal stimulus for the discharge of medullary hormones. These medullary cells are regarded as modified postganglionic neurons, and their functional activity appears to be controlled by preganglionic fiber activity.

The cells of the adrenal medulla produce epinephrine and norepinephrine, collectively called catecholamines. These hormones flow throughout the body to cause sympathetic effects everywhere. The adult human adrenal medullary glands secrete about ten times more epinephrine than norepinephrine. Thus, epinephrine is the primary neurohormone (hormones which are discharged into the blood stream to act on distant tissues and organs) secreted by the adrenal medulla. Substantial amounts of norepinephrine are, nevertheless, produced in the medulla. You will recall from an earlier section that the postganglionic nerves of the sympathetic division secrete only traces of epinephrine, and norepinephrine is the primary transmitter substance of the sympathetic postganglionic-fiber terminals.

Whether epinephrine and norepinephrine are secreted by the same adrenal cells or whether there are different cells for the production of each hormone is unknown at present. Evidence is accumulating that there are two cell types, each responsible for the secretion of one hormone. Thus, it may be that epinephrine and norepinephrine arise from different adrenal medullary components and are released separately.

The catecholamines are similar in some of their biological actions but there are differences in the nature and degree of their effects. Epinephrine has a more pronounced effect on cardiac activity than does norepinephrine increasing the frequency, force, and amplitude of contraction. Epinephrine increases the blood flow through skeletal muscles, liver, and brain; norepinephrine has no effect or decreases flow. The peripheral vascular effect of epinephrine is to cause vasodilation; norepinephrine produces vasoconstriction. Epinephrine has a much greater effect on metabolism than norepinephrine does, increasing the metabolic rate by as much as 100 percent above normal. Epinephrine injected into human subjects causes restlessness, anxiety, and a feeling of fatigue; norepinephrine does not produce these symptoms. This list of differential effects of the catecholamines is illustrative, and is not meant to be definitive.

The behavioral manifestations of the differential effects of epinephrine and norepinephrine have been studied by several investigators. Drawing on the evidence that the adrenals secrete both of these hormones, they have studied the comparative effects of these two hormones on behavior. Studies on animal and human subjects indicate that active aggressive behavior is associated with high secretion of norepinephrine, while passive anxiety and depression are associated with high secretion of epinephrine.

It has been found that overtly aggressive animals, such as the lion, have a relatively high amount of norepinephrine, while animals which depend on passive or flight behavior, such as the rabbit and some domestic animals, have a relatively high amount of epinephrine. With human subjects, those whose primary behavior pattern was to express their anger outwardly in aggressive actions were found to have a high rate of secretion of norepinephrine, while subjects whose anger or fear was manifested in passive anxiety and depression secreted high amounts of epinephrine (Funkenstein, 1955).

The neurophysiological mechanism for this differential secretion of adrenal medulla hormones seems to be located in the hypothalamus. Stimulation of certain portions of the hypothalamus evokes the adrenals to secrete epinephrine; stimulation of other areas evokes norepinephrine secretion. Thus, it appears that different emotional states may activate different portions of the hypothalamus, causing the secretion of one or the other of the adrenal medullary hormones.

The adrenal medulla is under constant stimulation and it is generally agreed that there is a basal level of secretion of its hormones. This basal rate is altered tremendously during emergencies. Stress stimuli such as severe temperature changes, trauma, hemorrhage, threatening situations, and hypoglycemia greatly accelerate adrenal medulla activity.

Although the effect of vigorous physical activity on catecholamine secretion has been clouded by experimenter methodology, there is a rather consistent finding of an elevation of catecholamine response to exercise in both trained and untrained subjects (Poortmans, 1969). However, Hartley and his colleagues (1972) reported that after an extensive conditioning program norepinephrine values almost doubled during the first 40 minutes of exercise but the augmentation in norepinephrine during exercise was only half the increase seen before the conditioning program; and epinephrine response was unchanged by a physical conditioning program.

B. THE EYE

The ANS controls two functions of the eye: pupillary opening and lens focusing. The sympathetic division dilates the pupil of the eye by contracting the radial fibers of the iris. Parasympathetic stimulation produces constriction of the pupil by contracting the circular muscle of the iris. This parasympathetic regulation is reflexive and occurs in response to the light entering the eye. The sympathetic response occurs primarily during periods of excitement.

Lens adjustment for focusing is regulated by the parasympathetic division. Parasympathetic stimulation causes contraction of the ciliary muscle. This releases tension on the ligaments, which normally hold the lens in a flattened state, and causes the lens to become more convex. This permits the eye to focus on close objects.

C. SALIVATION AND DIGESTION

Salivary glands in the mouth, glands for secretion of digestive juices, and fundic glands of the stomach are almost totally regulated by the parasympathetic division. The sympathetic system has little effect on these tissues and organs, except mass firing of the sympathetics causes vasoconstriction of the blood vessels supplying these tissues and organs.

D. SWEAT GLANDS

Sympathetic fibers stimulate the sweat glands. Large quantities of sweat are secreted when sympathetic nerves are stimulated, whereas no effect is produced by parasympathetic stimulation. Postganglionic sympathetic fibers to sweat glands are cholinergic (secrete acetylcholine) in contrast to most sympathetic fibers, which are adrenergic. Also, sweat glands are activated by hypothalamic centers which control parasympathetic activity

rather than the sympathetics. So, although the postganglionic fibers inner
vating the sweat glands are sympathetic, sweating may be considered a
parasympathetic function.

E. THE HEART AND CORONARY ARTERIES

The heart's activity is increased by sympathetic stimulation. The rate and
force of heartbeat are increased. Also, coronary arteries are dilated to
supply increased nutrition to cells throughout the body. Constriction of the
coronary arteries and a decrease in the heart rate to a normal steady state
result from parasympathetic stimulation. Thus, parasympathetic activity on
the heart and coronary vessels is basically opposite to sympathetic stimula
tion, decreasing the overall activity of the heart and vasoconstricting coro
nary vessels.

F. BLOOD VESSELS

Except for the skeletal muscle vessels and the coronaries, most blood vessel
are constricted by the sympathetic division. This control of the blood vessels
is one of the most important functions of the sympathetic division. The
sympathetics act to vasodilate blood vessels in the skeletal muscles during
exercise or hard work, permitting increased blood flow. While sympathetic
activity is causing vasodilation in the skeletal muscles, it is causing vasocon
striction in other parts of the body, except in the heart and brain, which
shunts the blood away from the visceral organs and causes an enormous
shift of blood flow to the working muscles. The parasympathetic division has
little effect on blood vessels, but it dilates them when it does act on them.

G. THE LUNGS

The ANS has very little effect on the lungs, but the bronchi are dilated by the
sympathetic division. Conversely, mild constriction on the bronchi is caused
by parasympathetic stimulation. All effects of ANS activity in the lungs are
slight because of the meager supply of ANS fibers.

H. GASTROINTESTINAL TRACT

Approximately 85 percent of all the parasympathetic fibers are found in the
gastrointestinal tract, and the parasympathetics increase peristalsis and
decrease the tone of the intestinal sphincters, thus permitting rapid propul
sion of materials along the tract. Sympathetic action inhibits peristalsis and
constricts the sphincters. This slows digestion and propulsion of material in
the tract.

I. RELEASE OF GLUCOSE

The sympathetic division activity produces a rapid breakdown of glycogen into glucose in the liver and the liberation of glucose into the blood. This sympathetic effect resembles glucagon in hastening the breakdown of glycogen to glucose, but whereas glucagon mobilizes only the glycogen stores in the liver, epinephrine causes the breakdown of the glycogen in muscle cells, too. Muscle glycogen is for the use of the muscles only and, by stimulating its breakdown, epinephrine allows for the drawing on a private energy supply by the muscles. This provides a quick supply of nutrition to the tissue cells.

J. THE KIDNEYS

Sympathetic activity brings about vasoconstriction of the renal blood vessels and inhibits the production of urine. The bladder is also prevented from emptying. This has the effect of retaining fluid in the circulatory system, which increases the blood volume and venous return to the heart. This causes increased cardiac output and keeps blood pressure up to a desired level.

K. METABOLISM

Sympathetic stimulation has the general effect of increasing the metabolism of the body, since the catecholamines increase the rates of chemical reactions in all cells. The metabolic rate of all cells of the body is enhanced by these hormones. This increased rate of metabolism is important, of course, in sustaining the body during exercise or intensive work.

L. ADRENAL CORTEX

In a complex and indirect way, sympathetic stimulation causes the secretion of hormones in the adrenal cortex. The mechanism by which this occurs is as follows: The hypothalamus has humoral connections with the anterior pituitary gland via a rich blood interchange. This blood transport system between the hypothalamus and anterior pituitary is called the hypothalamic-pituitary portal system. Sympathetic stimulation causes neurosecretory cells (cells which discharge neurohormones into the circulatory system to act as hormones upon distant tissues and organs) in the hypothalamus to secrete hormones which enter the blood supply going to the anterior pituitary. The hormones carried by this portal system cause the anterior pituitary to secrete several hormones, one of which is the adrenocorticotropic hormone, abbreviated as ACTH. ACTH travels in the blood to the adrenal cortex, where it causes the secretion of adrenocortical hormones (Figs. 23.6

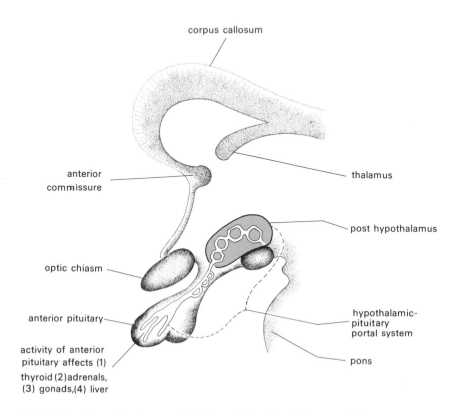

corpus callosum

anterior
commissure

thalamus

post hypothalamus

optic chiasm

anterior pituitary

hypothalamic-
pituitary
portal system

activity of anterior
pituitary affects (1)
thyroid (2) adrenals,
(3) gonads,(4) liver

pons

Fig. 23.6   General schema of the hypothalamic-pituitary portal system.
(Based on Woodburne, 1967.)

and 23.7), especially hydrocortisone which circulates in the blood and
metabolizes to produce at least 11 different steroids. Several of these are
collectively called hydroxycorticoids and another group constitutes the 17-
ketosteroids. Elevated levels of hydrocortisone are found in the blood
plasma of acutely disturbed or anxious persons, and the levels are increased by stress.

These hormones are needed in large quantities during periods of stress.
They are concerned with a wide variety of metabolic mechanisms, and they
aid in the repair of tissue cells which may be damaged during stress to the
body. Since these hormones are so important in the adjustment and adaptation to stress, it may be seen that the entire mechanism described above provides a means by which stress can affect a multitude of bodily activities.

Acute effects of physical activity on hydrocortisone have been examined by several investigators. In general, hydrocortisone response slowly increases for light to moderate work and then increases sharply during hard

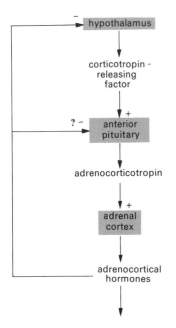

Fig. 23.7   Relation of the hypothalamus, pituitary, and adrenal cortex in regulation of adrenocortical hormones in the body. (Based on Langley, 1969.)

work (Hartley *et al.*, 1972). However, some investigators have found decreases in hydrocortisone rates during severe exercise, probably due to adrenal cortex exhaustion of the mechanisms of substrate synthesis or a general defense reaction against further depletion of the resources of the organism (Chin, 1971; Suzuki *et al.*, 1967).

Tharp and Buuck (1974) trained groups of rats on a treadmill for 2, 4, 6 and 8 weeks and reported that the adrenal cortex of trained rats progressively declined in their release of corticosterone (one of the steroids), reaching a significantly lower level than that of untrained rats at 6 and 8 weeks. They concluded that the decrease was due to adaptation of the adrenal cortex to ACTH stimulation. Others have reported similar results.

M. BRAIN ACTIVITY

The brain is constantly active, meaning that in a living organism there are millions of neurons in the brain firing at any given second. The electroencephalogram is a graph against time of rhythmic variations in the minute electrical potentials recorded between electrodes which have been placed on the scalp. These voltage waves vary in amplitude from a few microvolts up to as high as 200 microvolts, and in frequency from near 0 to 50 Hz (cycles per second).

The electroencephalogram (EEG) spectrum may be divided into bands of frequencies. Frequencies of 8-13 Hz and having rather large amplitude are called alpha waves; small amplitude frequencies from 15 to 50 Hz are beta waves. Slow waves having a frequency of below 4 Hz and generally of large amplitude are known as delta waves. The frequencies from 4 to 7 Hz are called theta waves.

Alpha waves are characteristic of a rested, relaxed person, while beta waves are common when a person is thinking or is in an excited state. Delta waves are observed during deep sleep and theta waves are associated with creative thoughts, attentive behavior, and, occasionally, anxiety. Sympathetic stimulation causes an increase in theta and beta wave activity. This probably occurs through mediating influences on the metabolic rate and through the indirect route of the reticular formation. Since reticular-formation activity is enhanced by sympathetic stimulation, the overall effect would be to excite cerebral cortex cells.

24

Arousal and Motor Behavior

All complex human behavior takes place in the presence of a certain level of arousal and it is goal-directed. The combination of arousal and direction toward a goal are integrated into what is called "motivated behavior." When we say that persons are "motivated" we mean, at least partly, that they are aroused. Emotional, tense, anxious are other adjectives that are frequently used to express the same idea by many people, and in sports "psyched up" conveys the same notion.

Arousal is a key element in motivated behavior and in this chapter we shall review the physiological mechanisms underlying this state of the individual and examine the relationship between this physical state and motor behavior.

THE CONCEPT OF AROUSAL

Arousal (activation is synonymous*) is a concept which attempts to order the intensive aspects of an individual's functioning. Elizabeth Duffy (1962), perhaps the most reknowned of arousal theorists, defines arousal as being "the extent of release of potential energy stored in the tissues of the organism, as this is shown in activity or response," and this notion that arousal refers to the degree of neural activity and behavior manifested by an individual is common to arousal theorists. An individual's state of arousal may be viewed as a continuum, with deep sleep at one end of the spectrum and

---

*Arousal and activation are used interchangeably by most motivation theorists, although there are some who have attempted to make distinctions between the two concepts. In this text, the two words will be considered to be synonymous.

intense excitement at the other end. Every person goes through a daily cycle of deep sleep (low arousal), awakening and engaging in normal behavior throughout the day (average arousal), becoming sleepy (diminished arousal), and sleep again (low arousal). While this daily cycle holds fairly constant, there are wide variations that occur throughout each day, especially in the waking hours. For example, you have to take an important examination—arousal level goes up. You have to sit through a boring lecture—arousal level goes down (sometimes so low as to cause sleep!). You have to play an intramural basketball game—arousal goes way up. Variations of arousal are different each day, and the arousal level, it may be seen, is changing moment by moment.

There are two basic tenets to arousal theory. First, there is the notion that individuals are motivated to seek arousal levels which are not too high and not too low, but are at some intermediate level between the two extremes. Some theorists have proposed that the level being sought is some optimal level based on previous experience, others have suggested that the level sought is slightly lower or higher than previous experience (Berlyne, 1960; Fiske and Maddi, 1961). What is common to all of these is the notion that individuals will engage in behavior designed to decrease arousal when it is too high and to increase it when it is too low. This drive seeking to maintain an optimal arousal level is called sensoristasis by Schultz (1965).

A second major tenet of arousal theory is that there is an optimal state of arousal for best performance, and performance is impaired when arousal is too high or too low; the greater the distance from the optimal point, the greater the impairment of performance. In brief, the hypothesized curve relating performance to arousal is that of an inverted U, and direct and indirect evidence for this relationship has been thoroughly reviewed by Duffy (1962). In this chapter we will focus our attention on this aspect of arousal theory rather than the first tenet which was described above, since it seems more pertinent to understanding motor learning and performance.

THE STUDY OF AROUSAL

The arousal concept has been an important part of psychology for the past 80 years, and it still represents a basic tenet in a diversity of areas within psychology today. This concept has been implied, if not directly used, by numerous psychological theorists since the latter years of the 19th century. William James (1890), suggested that arousal was an important dimension of emotion, while Freud (1933) employed concepts such as psychic energy and tension which clearly implied arousal, even though the word arousal was not used by Freud. Arousal theory also owes a great deal to Walter

Cannon's (1932) emergency theory of emotions, but it was Duffy's (1941, 1951) and Freeman's (1948) contention that a major dimension of emotion is arousal and energy mobilization. It was further developed by Duffy's (1962), Schlosberg's (1954), and Malmo's (1959) demonstrations that arousal can be indexed by a variety of measures and that arousal is a continuum, varying from sleep to states of high excitement. A number of recent theorists have proposed conceptual and theoretical refinements to arousal theory (Lacey, 1967; Routtenberg, 1968).

It was Moruzzi and Magoun (1949) who first identified that neuro-anatomical basis for arousal. This led to extended neuropsychological work on arousal by many scholars, especially Lindsley (1957) and Hebb (1955) who were instrumental in examining the neural correlates to arousal and the effects on behavior.

NEUROLOGICAL BASIS OF AROUSAL

Fundamental to arousal theory is the notion that there are specific structures in the nervous system which are responsible for arousal states. This "arousal system" is made up of the cerebral cortex and a series of subcortical structures in the brainstem and midbrain which project nonspecific fiber pathways into the cortex and other brain centers to produce arousal. Input to these subcortical structures comes from sensory collateral fibers which are given off by the various sensory afferents as they pass through the subcortical parts of the brain and from impulses originating in the cerebral cortex and projecting down into the subcortical areas. Thus, one source for arousal is the specialized sensory organs (the eyes, ears, skin, and proprioceptors) and another source is the cortex itself. The resultant effect of these two sources on the arousal system produces a "state of arousal."

A. THE CORTEX

The brain is constantly active, and its electrical activity (known as brain waves) may be picked up by electrodes which are either attached to the surface of the scalp or implanted in the brain. This activity may then be amplified and recorded by an electroencephalograph (EEG). As noted in a previous chapter, the brain emits characteristic wave patterns, depending upon the state of the organism. When the individual is awake, but relaxed, the wave pattern tends to be characterized by high amplitude, low frequency waves in the 8-12 Hz range, which are called alpha waves. The effect of an environmental or internal stimulus is to disrupt the alpha activity and produce a wave pattern characterized by a rapid, low amplitude, asynchronous pattern, known as beta waves. Thus, the neural correlate of arousal in the cortex is an increase in neural discharge characterized by rapid, asynchronous bursts of impulses.

B. THE RETICULAR FORMATION

The primary location of arousal structures is in the brainstem and midbrain, and the reticular formation has probably received the most attention with respect to the arousal function. As you will recall, this structure extends from the medulla up to the lower thalamus, with branches into the posterior hypothalamus. This vast network of neurons seems to function by sending diffuse fibers throughout the nervous system, especially throughout the cortex. Impulses from these fibers facilitate neuronal centers throughout the brain; some authors refer to this network as the "reticular activating system." Of course, some reticular formation fibers descend into the spinal cord to influence activity there, too.

The input to the reticular formation comes from collaterals from the various sensory modalities. Also, the cortex projects fibers to the reticular formation, so cortical activity is capable of activating reticular neurons as well as vice versa. Finally, there are cells in the reticular formation that are sensitive to epinephrine; thus, the secretion of this hormone by the adrenal medulla has the effect of heightening activity in the reticular formation.

C. THE HYPOTHALAMUS

The hypothalamus is also part of the arousal system. This structure receives input from higher brain centers as well as from other internal organs of the body. It is thus in a critical position for integrating messages from the higher nervous centers as well as those from the internal organs.

The posterior area of the hypothalamus plays a critical role in maintaining wakefulness. Over thirty years ago, Ranson (1939) reported that lesions in this area produced sleep and drowsiness in monkeys. Hess (1954) has reported that electrical stimulation applied to the posterior hypothalamus causes alertness and excitement.

The posterior area of the hypothalamus also has an important control over the sympathetic division of the ANS, so in addition to eliciting wakefulness, electrical stimulation causes the secretion of catecholamines by the adrenal medulla which in turn produces all of the autonomic responses associated with sympathetic nervous system action—increase in heartbeat, respiration increase, sweating, etc. In this context, hypothalamic influence on the adrenal gland emphasizes the biochemical component of arousal.

You will recall from the previous chapter that special motivation centers are located in the hypothalamus. Here are found centers for regulation of eating, anger and fear, sex, and pleasure motivations. Evidence from investigations where parts of the hypothalamus have been destroyed, from clinical studies, and from electrical stimulation studies have provided us with information about the functional roles of the hypothalamic nuclei.

D. THE LIMBIC SYSTEM

In recent years, neurophysiological studies using selective lesions and electrodes implanted in subcortical areas of the brain have led researchers to claim that areas in the "limbic system" are involved in the arousal process, which adds an interesting new dimension to this area. The exact way in which this limbic system subserves motivation is unknown, but it seems to be involved with the development and elaboration of emotions (Papez, 1937; MacLean, 1949).

The literature is inconsistent in the identification of the structures of the "limbic system," but the structures usually listed are: the cingulate and hippocampal gyri, hippocampus, amygdala, septum, epithalamus, and the dorsomedial and anterior thalamic nuclei (Fig. 24.1). These subcortical structures are located in the medial and ventral parts of the forebrain, between the diencephalon and cerebral cortex, and this "system" has a complex network of fiber connections with these structures. Moreover, limbic structures are interconnected with each other by fiber pathways. Finally, these structures have connections with the hypothalamus, so there is probably a functional relationship there, too.

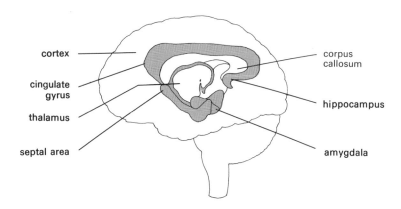

Fig. 24.1   Schematic diagram of the limbic system. (Based on Kimble, 1963.)

E. ADRENAL MEDULLA

A final structure which must be mentioned in relation to the arousal system is the adrenal medulla. Although this structure is not located in the brain, as are the other arousal mechanisms, some of the subcortical structures activate the adrenal medulla which through its secretions reactivates subcortical arousal mechanisms.

The adrenal medulla is excited by sympathetic nervous activity, which can be traced back to hypothalamic influences, and when it is excited it secretes catecholamines which circulate in the blood and act directly on smooth muscles and glands. It also provides input to the subcortical arousal system structures directly because catecholamines stimulate them. Now, since the arousal system activates the sympathetic nervous system, it may be seen that a feedback loop exists from the subcortical arousal system to the adrenal medulla and back to the arousal system. We have already discussed the cortical-to-arousal-system feedback loop; we now see that the arousal system is involved in two types of feedback loops. It is now fairly simple to see the special relation that the ANS has to arousal.

F. AROUSAL INTEGRATION

The cerebral cortex, the reticular formation, and the hypothalamus are the primary centers mediating arousal but, more important, they function in conjunction with a major component of the nervous system—the autonomic nervous system—to mobilize the body's resources. Moreover, all of these structures interact with each other, and with other systems such as the endocrine, sensory, and musculature. All in some way play a role in regulating overall arousal. On the basis of this arousal and the specific information being fed into the brain by the sensory organs, the individual prepares to respond to a stimulus situation.

AROUSAL AND EMOTION

Up to this point, very little use has been made of the word "emotion" in relation to arousal. This has been intentional. The concept of emotion is complicated by the absence of any kind of general agreement on a fundamental definition of the nature of this concept. Indeed, Duffy (1962) suggests that this concept be abandoned and replaced with "arousal" or "energy mobilization." Several other psychologists have suggested that the difference between the various emotions is to be found in differences in level of arousal. Malmo (1957), for example, indicates that the distinction between emotional and nonemotional behavior is superfluous and he suggests that intensity of motivation be equated with arousal. Many psychologists, however, believe that emotions may be differential along dimensions other than level of arousal.

Efforts to find physiological patterns characteristic of the several emotions have met with little success, and the research indicates that such differences are at best very subtle, and that the variety of emotion and feeling states is by no means matched by an equal variety of physiological patterns. This state of affairs has led some investigators to suggest that cognitive factors may be the main determinants of emotional states. Schachter and Singer (1962) write:

Cognitions arising from the immediate situation as interpreted by past experience provide the framework within which one understands and labels his feelings. It is the cognition which determines whether the state of physiological arousal will be labeled as "anger," "joy," "fear," or whatever.

This suggests that an emotional state is a function of a state of physiological arousal and of a cognition appropriate to that state of arousal. Schachter and his colleagues (Schachter and Singer, 1962; Schachter and Wheeler, 1962) have manipulated activation by employing various chemical agents and have shown that given a state of sympathetic activation, for which no immediately appropriate explanation is available, human subjects can be readily manipulated into states of euphoria, anger, and amusement. It seems, then, that while some types of internal, physiological events accompany human emotion, external stimuli and past experience also play a role.

AROUSAL AND MOTOR PERFORMANCE

We may now turn our attention to the effects of arousal on motor performance. Studies of the relationship between effort and performance carried out in the first three decades of this century demonstrated that induced tension facilitated such tasks as memorization, solving addition problems, and naming letters (Bills, 1927). But as work of this type continued, it was demonstrated that not all degrees of tension were equally effective at enhancing performance, and of special interest was the finding that behavioral efficiency increased to a maximum as tension rose to an intermediate level and then began to decline as tension continued to increase (Freeman, 1933, 1938). This work became incorporated into arousal theory and, indeed, became one of the major propositions of it under the name of "the inverted U hypothesis." The inverted U hypothesis simply proposes that

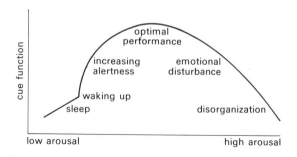

Fig. 24.2 Relationship of arousal to performance. The inverted U curve of arousal. (Based on Hebb, 1972.)

increases in arousal are accompanied by increases in the quality of performance up to a certain point, after which additional increases in arousal result in a deterioration in the quality of performance. Thus, the level of optimal arousal lies somewhere in the middle range of the arousal continuum (Fig. 24.2).

There are a number of studies which have provided support for the inverted U hypothesis, only a few of which will be mentioned here. Perhaps the best known study in which arousal was directly manipulated via reticular formation stimulation is the one by Fuster (1958). He studied the effects of electrical stimulation of the brainstem reticular formation on tachistoscopic perception* of monkeys. First, the animals were trained to discriminate between geometric objects presented in pairs, with a food reward under one of the objects in each pair. Then the animals were subjected to a series of trials where the objects were briefly exposed and the number of correct responses and reaction time were measured. Finally, with electrodes implanted in the brainstem, different intensities of electrical stimulation were applied shortly before the presentation of the discrimination task trial. Moderate intensities of stimulation increased the animal's efficiency at discrimination by improving percentage of correct responses and shortening reaction times, compared with controls. Higher intensities had a deleterious effect on the responses and reaction times. Lansing et al. (1959) and Ogawa (1963) also reported findings with reticular stimulation which support the notion that there are intensities of reticular activity which are associated with optimal performance.

Stennett (1957), in another frequently cited study, examined the relationship between auditory tracking performance of human subjects under four conditions of increasing incentive and two physiological measures of arousal (skin conductance and electromyograph (EMG) recordings). The incentive conditions varied. At one extreme subjects were under the impression that their scores were not even being recorded; at the other extreme

---

*Tachistoscopic perception is assessed by an instrument for exposing material to subjects for very brief durations of time.

subjects' scores determined whether or not they avoided a strong electric shock and earned bonus money from $2 to $5. The most efficient tracking performance was associated with intermediate EMG gradients and intermediate levels of palmar skin conductance. Performance on tracking associated with very high or lower levels of physiological functioning was inferior to tracking performance associated with moderate levels of physiological functioning.

In a study that manipulated arousal level through exercise-induced activation (EIA), Sjoberg (1968) showed a clear-cut inverted U relationship. Human subjects pedaled a bicycle ergometer at work loads of 150, 300, 450, 600, and 750 kgm/minute for 5 1/2 minutes and then performed choice reaction time trials while continuing to pedal. The work loads produced mean heart rates of 84 beats per minute (bpm) at rest to 147 bpm at the highest work load. Thus, the EIA levels ranged from low to moderately high. Best performance occurred at the 450 kgm/minute, with the mean heart rate at 121 bpm at this work load.

Although a number of other studies demonstrate similar findings utilizing other perceptual-motor tasks and other methods of producing arousal, the inverted U relationship does not appear to be clear and simple. One major weakness of much of the research on this proposition is that seldom has arousal been varied systematically from a very low to a very high degree and observation made of corresponding changes in performance. Martens (1971), in an eloquent review of anxiety and motor behavior, indicated that the evidence supporting the inverted U hypothesis is far from conclusive with regard to human motor performance. He says:

The nature of the task, the stage of practice, the inhibitory ability of the individual, and certain personality variables may separately or in combination alter the shape of the inverted U.

Nevertheless, as Martens (1974) notes in a more recent review of arousal and motor behavior:

From the limited experimental evidence testing the relationship between arousal and motor performance, the inverted U hypothesis appears to be favored.

A. OPTIMUM LEVELS OF AROUSAL

Since motor activities must frequently be performed under conditions of varying arousal levels, a fuller examination of the effects of arousal upon skill performance is necessary. Clearly, arousal channeled into goal-directed behavior is an essential condition of motor performance. Low arousal yields poor performance; but intense arousal can disrupt performance. Stage fright and "blanking out" on an examination are examples of how even well-learned responses can be impaired by high levels of arousal. The optimal degree of arousal for efficient and effective performance is probably a fluctuating one, depending upon a wide variety of factors. Some degrees of arousal may be disrupting, or disorganizing, in one task but organizing in another. For example, intense arousal, resulting in high finger tremor, would adversely affect mirror-tracing performance but not football tackling.

1. The nature of the task

The oldest notion concerning an optimal level of performance was first formulated over 60 years ago by two comparative psychologists, and it carries their names as the Yerkes-Dodson Law (1908). Simply stated, it proposes that optimal arousal for behavioral efficiency decreases with increased task difficulty of complexity (Fig. 24.3). Yerkes and Dodson found fewer errors in behavior when an electric shock of medium intensity was applied to mice than when shocks of low or high intensity were applied. When tasks were made more difficult, the optimal shock for the most efficient behavior was found to be progressively weaker.

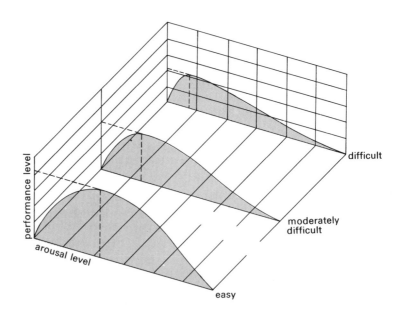

Fig. 24.3 A model illustrating the Yerkes-Dodson law. As tasks increase in difficulty, peak performance is achieved with less arousal. (Based on H.J. Eysenck, 1963.)

Although several lines of research have confirmed this "law" in the intervening years, there are several problems with this notion, the chief of which are the questions of what is a "difficult" or "complex" task and what is a "simple" task. In recent years several scholars have advanced proposals which attempt to classify tasks in an information processing framework and in the degree of inhibition required during performance. The first classifies tasks by the perceptual and cognitive demands; the greater these requirements, the more complex the task. The second classification proposes that motor tasks can be thought of in terms of the degree of inhibition required for appropriate performance. Thus, to the extent that a task involves a great deal of information processing and/or inhibition, high levels of arousal result in poor performance.

It may be inferred from the above that motor tasks requiring concentration, judgment, discrimination, and fine muscle control, such as in tracking, aiming, and steadiness, are performed best under rather low, moderate states of arousal. Conversely, motor tasks demanding strength, endurance, speed, or in which ballistic movements dominate necessitate rather high arousal levels.

The manipulation of task complexity, or difficulty, and arousal has not been a popular research topic, so there is very little empirical work on this topic, especially for motor tasks. One approach, though, that has generated some interest recently makes use of exercise-induced activation (EIA) for manipulating arousal. Arousal levels may be influenced by various stimuli, including exercise, since the proprioceptors are known to supply a rich input to the reticular formation as well as influencing other parts of the "arousal system." Thus, movement activity presumably affects arousal.

When tasks have been classified for the inhibition required for their performance, the effects of EIA on tasks at either the very high or very low ends of the inhibition continuum have resulted in rather consistent and clear-cut findings: High EIA facilitates tasks demanding little inhibition and disturbs performance of tasks requiring inhibition (Phillips, 1962, 1963; Ross et al., 1954).

Levitt (1972) assessed the effects of various arousal states, induced by exercise, on tasks of varying amounts of information processing demands. He exercised subjects on a treadmill at heart rates (HR) of about 80, 115, 145, and 175 beats per minute. After several minutes of walking at the specified HR, the subjects performed either a simple RT task, a two-choice or five-choice RT task. It was hypothesized that the optimal level of EIA would vary with the type of RT task—the higher the number of choices, the lower the optimal level of EIA. Summed over the three RT tasks, a clear inverted U curve was found, with optimal performance at HR of 115 and 145 bpm. Performance was poorer at 80 and 175 bpm. Under similar HR conditions Levitt

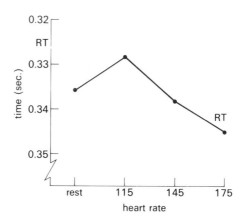

Fig. 24.4 Five-choice reaction time as a function of heart rate. (Based on Levitt and Gutin, 1971.)

and Gutin (1971) found that a five-choice RT task was performed best at 115 bpm, which may be interpreted as a rather low to moderate level of arousal, and worst performance was at 175 bpm (Fig. 24.4). In a study concerned with the effects of arousal on inhibition, Gutin and his colleagues (1974) assessed the effects of EIA on arm and hand steadiness. Unsteadiness following exercise was 35, 53, and 181 percent greater than preexercise steadiness performance for the treatments in which heart rate was raised to 100, 130, and 160 bpm, respectively.

One implication for the motor skills instructor is that in order to regulate arousal for optimal performance, an analysis of the information processing and inhibition demands of the task should be made. On the basis of this analysis, a decision may be made as to whether procedures should be taken to produce low, medium, or high states of arousal for performance. A speculation of the relationship between arousal and sports performance as a function of task characteristics was proposed by Oxendine (1970) (Fig. 24.5).

2. Skill level of the performer

Optimal arousal level seems to be sensitive to the skill level of the performer. A given level of arousal that might disrupt performance when the performer is a beginner on a task may enhance performance when the task is well learned. Put another way, the greater the level of skill, the higher the arousal can be without causing disruption in performance. Thus, the poorly skilled athlete does poorly under pressure, while the highly skilled athlete excels when the pressure is greatest.

level of arousal	sports skills
5 (extremely excited)	football blocking and tackling performance on the Rogers' PFI test running (220 yards to 440 yards) situp, pushup, or bent arm hang test
4	running long jump running very short and long races shot put swimming races wrestling and judo
3	basketball skills boxing high jumping most gymnastic skills soccer skills
2	baseball pitchers and batters fancy dives fencing football quarterback tennis
1 (slight arousal)	archery and bowling basketball free throw field goal kicking golf putting and short irons skating figure 8s
0 (normal state)	

Fig. 24.5 Optimum arousal level for some typical sports skills. (Based on Oxendine, 1970.)

Lazarus *et al.* (1952) reported that emotional "stress" introduced early in the learning process, before the skills were well learned, had a detrimental effect on performance, but stress introduced later in learning had a facilitating effect. If we assume that "stress" increases arousal, we can see the relevance of this study. Ryan (1961) also reported that stress (produced by electric shock) introduced late in learning had less disruptive effect on performance than it had when introduced early in learning. Other studies have reported similar findings.

A central topic in social psychology is called social facilitation, and research on this topic provides the most complete literature on the effects of arousal on performers of different proficiency. Social facilitation examines the consequences upon individual behavior of the sheer presence of others. Since one of the consequences of the presence of others is an increase in the individual's arousal state, arousal may be manipulated by introducing persons into a situation and observing the effects.

The first experimental studies of social facilitation go back to just before the beginning of the 20th century, and interest remained high until the late 1930s but dwindled because of the equivocal findings and the lack of a theoretical framework to explain them. But in the middle 1960s Zajonc (1965, 1966) made a careful analysis of the previous research and, drawing upon the rather extensive literature which shows that arousal, activation, and drive all enhance dominant responses, and upon the evidence that the presence of others increases an individual's arousal state, he combined all this information with the results of previous social facilitation results and proposed a general theory that an "audience enhances the emission of dominant responses."

Zajonc's theory may be explained in this way: In the early stage of learning, performers' responses are mostly incorrect ones; that is, they will emit more wrong responses than right ones; thus, wrong responses are dominant and strong during early learning. However, when individuals have mastered the task, correct responses become dominant. Now, if an audience has arousal consequences for the subject, and if arousal enhances the emission of dominant responses, it may be seen that if the dominant responses are the wrong ones, as is the case during early learning, the wrong responses will be enhanced in the presence of an audience while correct responses will be prevented. But if dominant responses are the correct ones, which is the case after mastery of a task, an audience will enhance the individuals' performance.

In general, evidence has supported Zajonc's theory. Martens (1969) reported that when subjects were in the initial stage of learning a coincident timing task (analogous to hitting a baseball), the presence of spectators impaired the subjects' performance. But after the subjects had learned the task reasonably well, in the presence of an audience they performed better than those performing alone did.

A refinement of Zajonc's original hypothesis was proposed by Cottrell (1968) to account for some studies which did not support the theory that the mere presence of others is sufficient for social facilitation to occur. Cottrell proposed that the mere presence of others is not the source of arousal in social facilitation research; instead, the source of arousal resides in the anticipation of positive or negative outcomes of performing in the presence of others. Martens and Landers (1972) had subjects learn a motor skill under one of three conditions: direct evaluation of performance, evaluation of performance outcome (indirect evaluation), and no evaluation. They found support for Cottrell's formulation, in that direct evaluation (actual observation of performance) produced much stronger effects than the other two conditions.

There is a variety of factors that are known to affect performance in the presence of others—age, sex, types of audience—and it is beyond the scope of this text to examine this extensive literature.

3. Individual differences

Individuals vary considerably in what might be called their "normal arousal state." Everyday observation confirms this; some persons seem to constantly operate in a state of excitement, anxiety, and "hustle bustle," while others go about their daily tasks in a relaxed, lethargic manner.

Instruments for assessing this "general arousal state," such as Spielberger's State-Trait Anxiety Inventory (Spielberger *et al.* 1970), confirm that indeed there are great individual differences in what Spielberger (1966) calls trait anxiety, which is a relatively stable anxiety proneness; that is, there are differences between people in the tendency to respond to situations. According to Spielberger, persons high in trait anxiety have a behavioral disposition that predisposes them to perceive a wide range of objectively nondangerous circumstances as threatening, and to respond to these with intensity disproportionate to the magnitude of the objective danger.

Differences in trait anxiety, or normal arousal levels, have been studied by several scholars and some generalizations about behavioral tendencies can be drawn from the findings: Individuals who are high in trait anxiety (sometimes called hypertense or hyperanxious persons) tend to respond with a high degree of arousal to a wide variety of situations. They tend to perform better than individuals with normally low arousal levels on very simple tasks. Thus, high normal arousal level tends to enhance performance when the task is simple. On the other hand, these "high arousal" individuals tend to do worse on complex tasks, especially if novel responses are required.

Suggestive evidence that differences in trait anxiety are related not only to general arousal but also to arousal responses to specific situational stimuli and ultimately to performance comes from the British personality theorist, Hans Eysenck (1967). He has identified what he believes are two independent dimensions of personality: (1) extraversion-introversion, (2) stable-neurotic. Extraversion refers to the outgoing, uninhibited, impulsive, and sociable person, while the typical introvert is quiet, introspective, and somewhat "nervous." There is some evidence indicating that level of arousal is related to degree of introversion, with the introvert being higher in "normal arousal" and responding with higher levels of arousal to stimuli (Corcoran, 1964; Colquhoun and Corcoran, 1964). Moreover, according to Eysenck, high neuroticism scores are indicative of emotional lability and overreactivity, and persons who are high in this dimension of personality "respond more strongly to stimuli, show greater variability of response, and take much longer to return to their prestimulation baselines."

There is an extensive literature on the issue of anxiety and performance, but it will suffice to cite only two or three studies. Stabler and Dyal (1963) reported that discrimination reaction time was slower among highly anxious subjects than among less anxious subjects early in practice, although the positions were reversed later, showing that as skill increases, higher arousal is not as disruptive to performance. Carron (1968) also reported differential performance improvement of high-anxious and low-anxious subjects on the stabilometer when an electric shock stresser was introduced early in the learning, with high-anxious subjects significantly inferior to other groups. Finally, Slevin (1971) had subjects execute a modified fencing lunge and recovery task requiring both speed and accuracy under various experimental conditions and found that the low-trait anxiety group performed significantly better under all of the different conditions than did the high-anxiety group.

4. Physical fitness

Various studies have shown that when cognitive tasks are performed immediately after or during an exercise bout the groups in better physical condition are somewhat less fatigued as a result of the exercise and tend to perform the tasks better (Gutin, 1966; Gutin and DiGennaro, 1968; Stockfelt, 1970). Stockfelt found that "well-trained" subjects performed arithmetic computations better at 25, 65, and 85 percent of previously determined maximal aerobic capacity than did "poorly trained" subjects. Thus, the "well-trained" group maintained a higher level of cognitive performance under physiological stress than the other group did.

In a series of studies Weingarten (1970; Weingarten and Alexander, 1970) tested subjects on an abstract reasoning task during physical exertion. As with other studies, he found that fit and unfit subjects performed the same under relaxed or relatively mild physical exertion, but during severe physical exertion the fit subjects performed significantly better. Weingarten (1973) summarized work on this topic in this way: "...when relatively complex problems were to be solved by physically fit and nonfit persons under stress, the fit consistently out-performed the nonfit...."

Presumably the differences in performances that have been noted during or immediately after physical exertion by physically fit and unfit subjects are related, at least in part, to the effects of the exercise on arousal levels. During physical exertion the physically fit person is probably closer to an intermediate level of arousal than the less fit, whose level of arousal is probably quite high, because the exercise does not alter the physiological mechanisms of arousal as dramatically for the fit person as for the unfit. One of the consequences of a conditioning program is physiological adaptations which make a given amount of exercise less stressful.

THEORIES OF AROUSAL AND PERFORMANCE

Theories which attempt to explain the inverted U-shaped function relating arousal and performance have been formulated by several psychologists. We shall make only a very brief examination of this literature. The improvement in performance with increasing arousal up to an optimal point and then the worsening of performance due to supraoptimal arousal levels are explained in several related ways. Hebb (1972) proposes that "with low arousal cortical transmission is poor and with high arousal it is too good permitting the occurrence of irrelevant and conflicting cortical activities; with very high arousal, too many messages get through and prevent the animal from responding selectively to any one set of stimuli." Similarly, Welford (1968b) proposes that when arousal is very low the nervous system will be inert and signals are likely to be "lost" in either the perceptual system or at some later point in the chain leading to a response. The deterioration in performance at high levels of arousal, according to Welford, is due to the cortical cells not only being facilitated but actually being fired, when the stream of impulses impinging on the cortex becomes intense. The cortex becomes "noisy" when this occurs, and signals from external stimuli or impulses from one part of the nervous system to another tend to become blurred.

Using a slightly different perspective, Esterbrook (1959) has proposed a "range of cue utilization" to relate arousal and performance. At low levels of arousal, irrelevant cues are being attended to; an increase in arousal will reduce the attention to irrelevant cues and increase attention to relevant ones, resulting in improved performance. But high levels of arousal tend to narrow the utilization of relevant cues, resulting in a decrement in quality performance.

In summary, the hypotheses relating arousal and behavior suggest that moderate arousal tends to have an organizing effect on behavior by enhancing transmission throughout the brain. On the other hand, high levels of arousal may so completely activate the brain centers that all selectivity of transmission is lost. The result may be an inability to integrate and coordinate sensory inflow and motor outflow. The individual is unable to accurately perceive the stimulus situations, and behavior may be inappropriate or even impossible. Viewed another way, the ability of specific sensory data to guide behavior is very poor if the arousal level is low or very high. When arousal is low, the cortical activity is low and sensory data are not fully processed in the cortex; when the arousal level is too high, the selectivity of the integrative functions of the cortex is disturbed. Thus cortical function is best during periods of medium arousal.

MEASUREMENT OF AROUSAL

Since the concept of arousal is closely related to nervous system function, it is obvious that assessments of such functions as the electrical activity of the brain, muscle tension, and autonomic nervous system activity, such as skin conductance, heart rate, blood pressure, respiration, temperature, and catecholamine responses would be used in measuring arousal. Indeed, a great deal of work has gone into assessing arousal by these various physiological methods, singularly and in combinations. Unfortunately, physiological measures are cumbersome to employ, and their interpretation encounters many of the same problems encountered by verbal measures. The various physiological measurements are only moderately successful in assessing arousal states and there are only moderate correlations, at best, between different measures of physiological arousal, suggesting that whatever each of these measures is measuring, each one is measuring something separate from the others in addition to measuring the commonality that exists. The best generalization seems to be that there is some degree of generality in physiological responses and some degree of particularity with respect to the stimulus situation and the individual.

One solution to the problem posed by imperfect validity of any one physiological measure is a composite index of several physiological variables. It has been proposed that this may yield a more accurate measure of arousal than any single measure. While the simultaneous measurement of several physiological arousal variables does provide a somewhat more accurate means of measuring arousal, it certainly restricts activation assessment to laboratory situations. This limitation of arousal assessment to circumstances which permit the use of elaborate and bulky measurement apparatus seems especially unfortunate to the motor skills instructor who would like to make assessments in the dynamic situation.

Another method of assessing arousal makes use of a simple self-report of arousal. Thayer (1967, 1970) developed the Activation-Deactivation Adjective Check List (AD-ACL) and reported that it correlated more highly with a physiological composite of heart rate and skin conductance than these two physiological measures correlated with each other. Others have found similar results when arousal was estimated in a general subjective sense (Dermer and Berscheid, 1972). These techniques provide an alternative to the physiological assessment procedures for measuring arousal.

Even though there are physiological and self-report techniques for measuring arousal, valid measurement remains a problem. As Martens (1974) says, "At present this measurement problem is the severest limitation to the utility of arousal as a psychological or physiological concept." But, as Duffy (1962) suggested a number of years ago:

It is evident that the measurement of activation presents many problems [but]. . . . It would be unwise . . . to permit either the complexity of the problem or the inadequacy of our present information to obscure the fact that the level of activation is a basic aspect of behavior, which, even with the present imperfect means of measurement, shows relationships with stimulus situations and with other aspects of behavior.

AROUSAL AND SPORTS PERFORMANCE

Studies of the effects of arousal on sports skill performance are quite rare. Harmon and Johnson (1952), using physiological indicators (galvanic skin response, blood pressure, and pulse rate), found a close relationship between college football players' level of arousal prior to a game and their actual game performance. The higher the level of arousal, the higher the quality of performance. Basler and Fisher (1974) studied the relationship between arousal (assessed by pulse rate and sweat rate), anxiety (using Spielberger's State-Trait Anxiety Inventory), and past performance, on collegiate gymnasts' performance. They found low correlations between arousal and anxiety measures and gymnastic performance, and in attempting to statistically predict gymnastic performance from the various variables, arousal and anxiety measures were of relative unimportance.

It is clear that the research on the topic of arousal and sports performance is much too sparse to draw any kind of conclusions or inferences at this time, but an interesting study reported by Lloyd Percival (1971b), the Technical Director, Coaching Association of Canada, suggests that coaches need to be more sensitive to the arousal states of their athletes. In a study of over 380 athletes representing 24 sports and ranging from youth age-group to professional competitive levels, he asked the athletes for an opinion of their psychological states just before competition. The athletes indicated that in a great many cases they felt that they were too aroused (Fig. 24.6).

The implication of Percival's study suggests that "pep talks" and other techniques commonly employed before contests in an effort to "motivate" or "psyche up" athletes may be counterproductive. In many cases, the athletes

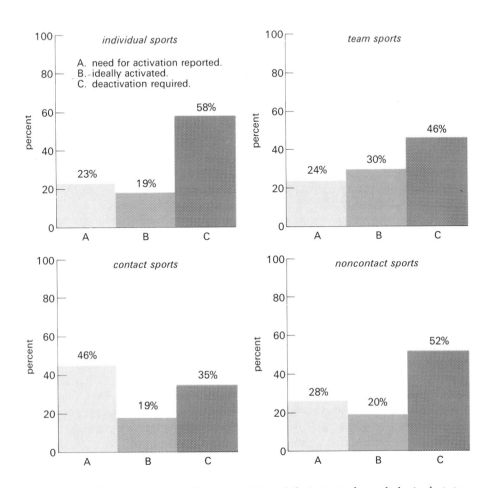

Fig. 24.6 Athletes were asked for an opinion of their typical psychological state just before competition. (Based on Percival, 1971.)

may need to have their arousal states reduced. Of course, since there are so many factors which affect arousal levels, and rather imperfect methods for assessing activation, the job of manipulating arousal states for optimal performance is quite difficult. One thing is clear—attempts to "psyche up" a team will have varying effects on the athletes. As Cratty (1971) says:

> ...attempts to activate a group of...athletes prior to important contests is likely to have mixed results. Those in the group who are already at their optimum levels may be overactivated, and their performances will thus suffer, while those who may be underaroused prior to being given a "pep talk" may

perform better. However, a helpful strategy on the part of the coach is to treat each athlete as an individual prior to competition, attempting to adjust each level of activation he perceives in each athlete either upward or downward as indicated.

MANIPULATING AROUSAL

Controlling or manipulating arousal levels is more of an intuitive art form than a science at this time, but nevertheless motor skills directors have at their disposal a number of ways to deal with arousal phenomena.

A. DETERMINING AROUSAL LEVEL

In an earlier section of this chapter it was noted that the measurement of arousal states is difficult, especially if one is seeking a precise assessment. On the other hand, if one is seeking a "rough" measure of arousal, several indices may be used. Observation of the following things provides an indication of arousal: (1) Hand tremor, (2) Body perspiration, (3) Eye dilation, and (4) Restless and random fine and gross body movements. Another assessment that can be made without elaborate equipment is heart rate. Self-report inventories, such as the State-Trait Anxiety Inventory may be used.

B. INCREASING AROUSAL

A state of high arousal is best attained and sustained under conditions of stimulus variety and intensity. In situations where stimuli are monotonous and unchanging, arousal level wanes and, if alertness is needed to perform in this situation, performance will decline. For example, numerous studies have shown that if subjects worked at monotonous, boring tasks for long periods of time, their performance deteriorated in direct proportion to the time spent on the task. Thus, if individuals must monitor a radar scope or watch for defective parts on an assembly line, their chances of making correct responses decline in proportion to the time spent on the job.

Visual stimulation, such as bright, blinking, and moving lights will enhance arousal, as will intense and varying auditory stimuli. The proprioceptors provide a rich source of input to the reticular formation, so movement increases arousal.

Since cerebral cortical impulses activate the arousal system, cognitive content, such as appeals to survival, pride, self-esteem ("Get this one for the Gipper!") increases arousal, as do incentives, rewards, and punishment.

C. REDUCING AROUSAL

Very little attention has been given to reducing arousal in motor learning and performance. Coaching manuals are filled with ways to "motivate" players, but motivation in this context invariably refers to increasing the arousal level. The fact that overarousal may disrupt performance does not seem to be known or appreciated by most physical educators and coaches.

Just as sensory variety and stimulus intensity are useful in enhancing arousal, low levels of stimuli are effective in reducing arousal. Cognitive content designed to distract the performer from arousal-inducing content and content aimed at placing competition and performance in the context of the "larger picture" of the world may reduce arousal. One coach before an important contest told his athletes: "Less than one percent of the entire world's population knows we are even playing today!"

There are some techniques for systematically developing arousal control; several of these are used in medicine and psychotherapy, but they are capable of being employed in other situations. Over 40 years ago Edmund Jacobson (1938) developed a method of relaxation, which he called Progressive Relaxation. This relaxation technique has been used extensively in clinical settings. The basic principle of this method rests upon persons developing a kinesthetic awareness of tension in their various muscles. The method requires the individual to learn to tense and relax specific muscle groups, gradually relaxing the entire musculature of the body. Since it is true that the proprioceptors play a prominent role in activating the arousal system via their collaterals which innervate the reticular formation, Jacobson's method of neuromuscular relaxation does provide a means for reducing arousal. Once having learned to relax, the person is capable of relaxing in arousal-inducing situations. A similar technique called "autogenic training" was developed in Europe and has been frequently used by athletes on the continent (Schultz, 1956).

Biofeedback training provides a potential technique for teaching people to reduce arousal. Biofeedback is the instantaneous presentation of information to an individual about ongoing physiological processes such as muscle tension, heart rate, temperature, brain waves, etc. The physiological processes are typically recorded by specially designed electrical equipment and fed back to the individual by visual or auditory means, i.e., lights, sounds. With this immediate and objective feedback, a person can learn to regulate these normally involuntary processes.

Biofeedback research has demonstrated that persons can be taught to self-regulate numerous physiological processes, especially the processes which control arousal states. Once having learned to regulate these processes with the aid of the biofeedback equipment, the individual retains the ability to control these processes without the equipment, and upon command.

Although biofeedback training has been employed primarily in medicine and psychotherapy up to now, there is every reason to believe that its use will become quite widespread, and its potential for use in teaching motor activities is already being explored (Gallagher, 1974).

The notion of reducing arousal has occasionally been promoted by mystics and oriental religions. Usually the approach is to some kind of "mind-over-matter" concepts. Transcendental Meditation (TM) is currently the most popular of the various meditation techniques. As described by Maharishi (1969), TM is a systematic procedure of "turning the attention inwards towards the subtler levels of thought until the mind transcends the experiences of the subtlest state of thought and arrives at the source of thought. This expands the conscious mind and at the same time brings it in contact with the creative intelligence that gives rise to every thought."

TM meditators report improvement in tension reduction in stressful situations, and increased psychomotor function. Much of the TM research is still in its infancy but that which has been published is sufficient to establish that the psychophysiological effects during and after TM are real and unique in their degree of integration (Wallace and Benson, 1972; *Fundamentals of Progress*, 1974; Smith, 1975).

Although the idea of using hypnosis to control arousal states may strike some as being "far out," this technique has been frequently employed in medicine and dentistry. Few persons realize that it is also occasionally used in motor behavior. Mitchell (1972) has discussed in some detail the use of hypnosis in sports. The competence of the hypnotist and the ethical and legal issues of using this technique with motor performers are beyond the scope of this text; suffice to say that these considerations should be fully explored before hypnosis is employed.

Because of the inherent ethical questions, little use has been made of depressants or tranquilizers with motor performers. With the increasing use of drugs, though, the coming years may witness their use to control arousal. The uncertain effects of these pharmaceuticals make their use undesirable in industry and education at this time.

AROUSAL AND MOTOR LEARNING

Throughout this chapter emphasis has been on the effects of arousal on performance; no mention has been made of the effects of arousal on learning. This has been intentional because the effects of arousal on motor learning are more confused than the effects on motor performance are, despite considerable interest in this topic extending over the past four decades. Over 30 years ago Bills (1927), Freeman (1931, 1933), and others found that the learning of various tasks was improved if, during performance, tension was induced in irrelevant muscles of the body—for example, squeezing a hand dynamometer improved the rate of learning. More recently several investigators have found that enhanced arousal states facilitate learning rate, and they propose that consolidation memory theory may be employed to explain the underlying mechanism of this phenomenon (Walker and Tarte, 1963; Weiner, 1966, 1967; Weiner and Walker, 1966). Walker and Tarte (1963) suggest that the neural memory trace established by practice will be more "robust" under high arousal, and, since this neural trace is essential for the production of a structural modification in the nervous system (represented as a long-term memory) the higher arousal during the practice period will produce greater long-term memory. Weiner (1966) suggests that differences in recall between motivational and nonmotivational conditions "are not caused by differential rehearsal of stimuli." For Weiner, incentive effects are attributed to some as yet unspecified arousal function so that "augmented motivation during trace formation makes...the trace more resistant to interference" or, possibly, more resistant to decay.

Although a number of studies have found that "arousal" conditions enhance learning, certain methodological problems exist which need to be resolved before definitive statements can be made about this phenomenon. One such problem is the question of whether or not the agent or instrument employed to induce arousal actually does in fact produce an increase in arousal. Generally, experimenters have used a procedure in which arousal is induced via application of electric shock. The assumption is made that the electric shock produces an increase in arousal; this assumption may or may not be true. For example, Marteniuk and Wenger (1970) administered electric shock to a "related arousal" group immediately after a trial if their performance did not improve by 5 percent, and a "unrelated arousal" group was administered shock randomly following certain trials regardless of their performance. A possible weakness in their investigation was that they did not ascertain whether the administration of shock was indeed arousal producing for their subjects. This weakness could have been overcome by the use of some instrument for assessing arousal during the practice trials.

A second problem area is related to individual differences in "normal arousal level," or trait anxiety. There is empirical support for individual differences in trait anxiety and these differences are important for learning and performance. Several studies have shown that more anxious subjects learn better than less anxious subjects do, when the new task does not conflict with associations induced by previous tasks. Thus, control of this variable would seem to be critical when conducting research on arousal and learning and performance (Martens, 1971).

A third problem in this area of research is the question of whether arousal affects learning or whether it affects performance. This distinction has not been used consistently in research on this topic.

A final area of concern is related to whether the arousal-inducing stimuli are related or unrelated to performance of the task. Marteniuk and Wenger (1970) suggest that the reason that some studies have found no significant effects from arousal-inducing stimuli may have been the result of using task-unrelated types of arousal inducement. In the Marteniuk and Wenger study two types of shock were used—one related and the other unrelated to the demands of the task. They found no reliable differences on either learning or performance according to whether the shock was related or unrelated.

Sage and Bennett (1973) examined the effects of induced arousal on motor learning, while attempting to control for the methodological problems

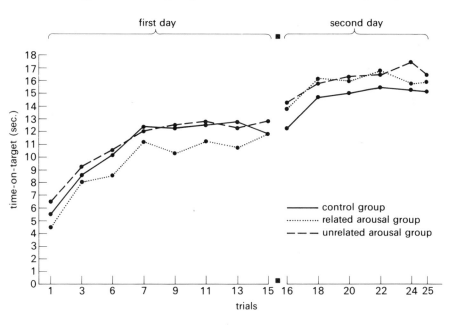

Fig. 24.7   Mean performance scores for three groups over two days of practice. Twenty-four hours of rest were interpolated between trials 15 and 16. (Based on Sage and Bennett, 1973.)

discussed above. Subjects were administered practice on a pursuit-rotary task over two days. Fifteen trials were given on the first day and 10 trials were administered 24 hours later. Subjects were randomly assigned to one of three conditions: related arousal, unrelated arousal, and control. Arousal was enhanced by administering electric shock during trials 6-15 on the first day. Subjects in the related arousal group received shock if their performance did not reach an established criterion, whereas subjects in the unrelated arousal group received shock on a random schedule regardless of their performance. The control group received no shock. To determine if the induced-arousal was anxiety evoking, the A-State form of the State-Trait Anxiety Inventory was administered. Analysis of the results indicated that electric shock administration significantly enhanced arousal of the related arousal group over the control group but not the unrelated arousal group. Learning rate was significantly enhanced in the related arousal group over the control group but not in the unrelated arousal group compared with the control group (Fig. 24.7).

The exact relationship between arousal and motor learning will have to await further research. As with other conditions related to learning, a variety of environmental and personal differences undoubtedly combine with arousal states to influence the learning that occurs.

25

The Direction
of Motivation

We have examined the arousal function of motivation. Now we shall consider the second basic function of motivation, which is the integrative and directive function. In the arousal function, the individual is prepared for action—energized—in the directive function, specific behavior is selected.

As we noted in Chapter 22, the subject of motivation is too immense for us to enter into a full examination of its literature; indeed, entire books are devoted to this single topic. Thus, only selected parts of the directive aspects of behavior are examined here.

THE DIRECTION OF BEHAVIOR

The direction of behavior may be viewed as either moving toward or away from a stimulus situation, and the behavior may occur at any of many possible degrees of intensity, frequency, and duration. The directional aspect of motivation derives from the fact that behavior typically exhibits selectivity; that is, the individual approaches certain objects, situations, persons, or certain aspects of them, and withdraws from others. Behavior, therefore, may be described as directed toward or away from various stimuli.

Behavior is normally channeled toward a goal. The individual's responses are directed toward bringing about a particular condition—be it more of a certain thing or less of it. The goal of motivated behavior is the meeting of some need or needs which the individual has. The individual approaches or withdraws from a certain person, object, or situation as he or she interprets it as a means to the end of achieving his or her goal and meeting a need.

While it seems fairly simple and straightforward to say that behavior is directed toward achieving some goal, and thus meeting or satisfying some need, the "need structure" of an individual cannot be directly viewed, so any effort to describe a certain behavior as meeting a specific need or attempting to structure conditions so as to get a person to behave in the service of meeting a need is fraught with difficulties. In the first place individuals vary considerably in their "need structure"; second, it is changing from moment to moment, although there are underlying persistent needs; third, individuals themselves may not be consciously aware of their own needs. Finally, sometimes behavior is not immediately need satisfying. For example, the soldier who goes into battle and risks being killed is certainly not gratifying some immediate need. So things that bring immediate pleasure are not necessarily need satisfying, while things that bring immediate pain are not necessarily dissatisfying or punishing. The human gives "meaning" to an event or behavior and thus it takes on need-meeting characteristics.

A. NEURAL BASIS OF DIRECTED BEHAVIOR

Basic physiological processes can go a long way toward explaining certain types of human motivated behavior, but they fall short of providing an adequate account of normal human motivation, especially complex games, sports, dance, and occupational behavior. Hunger, thirst, aggression, and sex are not the dominant motives in our ordinary daily life. Achievement of success in schoolwork and motor skills, recognition and approval from peers, popularity, these are a few of our more common motives, and they are social; they derive, at least in part, from our relations with other persons.

Much is known about such aspects of motivation as hunger, thirst, aggression, and sex partly because it is easy to observe and measure their behavioral expressions—eating, drinking, and so forth. There is little useful work linking brain structures to specific types of motor behavior found in games, sports, and other complex motor skills.

CATEGORIES OF NEEDS

One of the most frustrating problems for motivation researchers has been the identification of human needs. For many, it has seemed essential to catalog needs because once this is done it is believed that greater understanding of human behavior will emerge, and for those who are interested in controlling the behavior of others, conditions might be manipulated in such a way that persons will behave in the service of meeting needs.

Human needs have been classified into two general categories: biological and social. Although there is considerable disagreement in the psychology literature as to exactly how many needs there are in each category and in which category certain needs fit, there is agreement that the biological needs are unlearned, that they fulfill a survival function, and that the social needs are learned by particular interactions with the environment. It is further agreed that, although social needs would not occur in the absence of learning, once they are learned, they may be as essential to the maintenance of the normal health of an individual as biological needs. A state of motivation, then, may be triggered by biological needs, such as hunger, thirst, need for oxygen, temperature regulation, elimination, etc., or by acquired needs, such as achievement, self-respect, security, recognition, etc.

In the process of fulfilling needs (biological or social), we learn to associate specific responses with those needs. For example, going to a restaurant and ordering food is a learned response for the hunger needs. Working on a job to earn money is a learned response for security and other social needs. Every need has various learned responses associated with it. The presence of, or the absence of, something in the body or in the environment acts as a stimulus to a tendency to respond.

A. BIOLOGICAL NEEDS

One perspective of motivation limits biological needs to such tissue requirements as the need for nutrition, water, oxygen, elimination, temperature regulation, and perhaps sex; all other needs are held to be learned through associations rewarded by food, water, and so forth. However there is considerable evidence that motivated behaviors ranging from exploration, manipulation, and curiosity to affection and certain other social behaviors are not learned from eating, drinking, etc. In fact many of these more complex needs have significant aspects that are not learned at all. While we cannot devote any extensive space to an identification and examination of all of these needs, we shall discuss several of them that have been identified because of their relation to motor performance.

To the basic biological needs we may add an exploratory need, which is widespread in primates and humans. In humans this tendency is often called a curiosity need. Experimental psychologists, working with various animal species, have confirmed the fact that the animals will seek out novel, strange, and complex stimuli many times for no particular reward (Butler, 1954). Developmental psychologists relate that human infants prefer novel and complex stimuli over the common and simple. Young children's activities are replete with exploratory behavior.

Another need that may be added is the manipulative need. There is considerable evidence that primates and humans engage in manipulative behavior for its own sake. Harlow (1950) reported that monkeys will work for hours attempting to solve simple mechanical problem puzzles for no reward other than the satisfaction derived from solving the problem (Fig. 25.1). Growing children will run, climb, throw, jump, and perform many other activities without any extrinsic rewards. Indeed, their efforts to learn to walk may be accompanied by pain when they fall and, in some cases, parental disapproval, but this seldom deters them from the task.

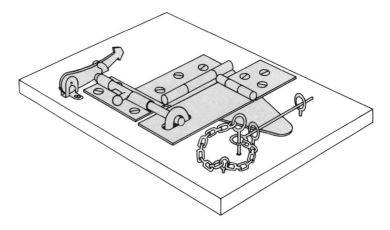

Fig. 25.1 A six-part mechanical puzzle used in studying manipulatory motivation in monkeys. Monkeys work at this puzzle without extrinsic reward. (Based on Harlow, 1950.)

Another need that seems to be closely related to the exploratory and manipulative needs is the need for sensory stimulation. When the environment is devoid of sensory stimulation, individuals seek out stimuli. In sensory deprivation studies done at McGill University, Heron (1957) paid subjects $20 per day for remaining in a comfortable bed with all of their senses restricted in some way—blindfolds on the eyes, cardboard cuffs over the hands, sounds muffled, etc. They had to do nothing. Most subjects could not continue for more than two or three days. They simply could not take life without sensory stimulation (Fig. 25.2).

B. SOCIAL NEEDS

Various efforts have been made to catalog social needs with little success or agreement among those who have compiled lists. Regardless of the number and names of the social needs, it appears that each person comes to have a

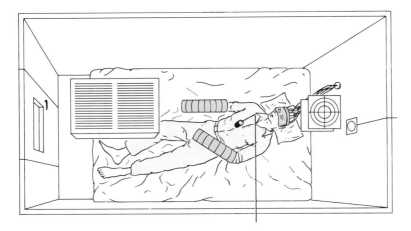

Fig. 25.2 Subject in a sensory deprivation study. Cuffs on hands and arms prevent somesthetic perception. Eye shields admit light but prevent pattern vision; ears are covered to prevent perception of sound. Air conditioner shown in left center picture is actually on ceiling of chamber. Just above subject's chest is a microphone by which he could report his experiences. (Based on Heron, 1957.)

considerable number of them. They may emerge as a result of random interaction with the environment; that is, they may develop even though there is no conscious effort by anyone to force the acquisition of them on the individual. They may develop through an unstructured culturalization process. On the other hand, social needs may be developed through a conscious manipulation of the environment by someone. In schools and business there are constant attempts to manipulate the environment in an effort to produce and control social needs.

MOTIVATION TECHNIQUES

Regardless, of the need structure, various manipulations and controls can be administered to get an individual to perform, or behave, in a certain way to satisfy a need. Commonly used motivational techniques are the employment of incentives and reinforcements (sometimes called "motivators").

In the motivation literature, complex semantic problems surround the concepts of incentive and reinforcement, and some writers have written elaborate explanations differentiating the two. As we shall use it here, incentives are objects, conditions, or stimuli external to individuals which produce a state of arousal in individuals so that they will be energized to approach or withdraw from an object, condition, or persons; concomitantly it produces actual responses to approach or withdraw from the incentive. It may be seen, then, that incentives are of two basic types: positive incentives, which individuals tend to approach, and negative incentives, which they tend to avoid. In both, incentives enhance some measure of performance such as speed, accuracy, or effort. The final point, with regard to an incentive, is that it is in some sense the *promise* which produces changes in behavior before any reward or other reinforcement is given (Cofer, 1972). Thus persons will work hard to obtain food (an incentive) to satisfy a need.

Any event which modifies the strength of some response is called a reinforcer, and the operation of providing for the occurrence of the reinforcer is called reinforcement. Like incentives, reinforcers are either positive or negative. Any event that increases the probability of a recurrence of some response is a positive reinforcer, while any event which decreases the probability of recurrence of some response is a negative reinforcer. The reinforcing effect refers to the role of a reinforcer producing more or less permanent behavior changes (Annett, 1969). The critical temporal aspect of reinforcement is that it is administered *after* the behavior, and its application is contingent upon specific, appropriate behavior.

A. EFFECTIVENESS OF MOTIVATORS

Incentives and reinforcers are both powerful means for influencing behavior, but before discussing the application of incentives and reinforcers, it may be well to examine a number of well-known factors which influence the effectiveness of these "motivators." The person who is employing the motivators is known to be important. Incentives and reinforcers successfully used by coaches are frequently ineffective when used by parents and classroom teachers. In general, motivators are more effective when used by persons who are highly esteemed and respected by an individual or a group.

Receptiveness to motivators varies with age. Young children are more receptive to verbal incentives and reinforcements than older ones. What is effective for one age group may strike another as "corny." There are also sex differences in that several studies have found that females are more responsive to verbal exhortations than males are, which is probably related to parental socialization practices in which girls are talked to more than boys beginning in infancy (Lewis, 1972).

Since lower social class child rearing practices differ from those of the middle and upper classes, differential responses to incentives and reinforcements may be expected, and indeed have been documented. This same notion probably cuts across racial and ethnic backgrounds.

These are only a few of the numerous factors that influence the effectiveness of motivators. Recognizing this, one principle of human motivation should become quite clear: individuals cannot be treated alike if one wishes to motivate them! What will be effective for one person will not be effective for another; what may have been effective at one time for an individual may not be effective at another time. The extreme complexity of motivating factors makes it impossible to set forth definite statements about which motivating techniques are the "best." Successful instructors or coaches must be aware of all these factors and use techniques which fit the different needs of the students as well as their own personalities. We shall now examine some of the motivational methods that have been studied.

B. INCENTIVES

In a previous section of this chapter an incentive was described as either material or symbolic object, condition, or stimulus which energizes an individual to approach or withdraw from it. Although an incentive is viewed as a promise of a reward, previous experiences which involved reward affect present performance because, after rewards have been employed, the individual acquires an *expectancy* that certain responses will be followed by a reward. The expected reward provides an incentive to perform those responses which will lead to the reward, or expected goal. Incentive theories assume that behavior is primarily energized by anticipation of reward or punishment consequences.

In the sense that incentives satisfy needs they have a positive function and cause approach behavior, leading to pleasure. Objects which are unpleasant have an opposite effect, so we tend to withdraw from them. They are said to be negative incentives. These do not satisfy needs, unless we take the view that the body has a need to escape unpleasantness, or pain. Since persons tend to move toward positive incentives and away from negative incentives, they may be viewed as being pulled toward certain things and pushed away from others.

Many incentives have been used to get persons to perform. In industry, workers are constrained to work by the promise of more money or better working conditions; in school, students are enticed by the promise of good grades for high performance. Athletes may be promised medals, trophies, or public recognition for outstanding performances. In all cases, though, it appears that an essential condition for incentives to affect behavior is that the individual recognize and evaluate the incentive and generate goal and/or intentions in response to the evaluation.

What are the most effective incentives for enhancing motor behavior? In the sense of attempting to establish an initial set for effort, incentives have been the subject of several studies.

Perhaps the most frequently used incentive in motor skills instructional settings is verbal exhortation. The verbal learning literature is replete with studies showing that verbal exhortation is useful in bringing about enhanced verbal performance and learning, but there is a scarcity of research on the incentive effects of verbal exhortation in motor behavior; consequently there are wide differences of opinion regarding this topic. Oxendine (1968) states, "There can be little doubt that the pep talk and other precontest techniques have often been effective in motivating young people to greater effort." In contrast, Tutko and Ogilvie (1967) state ". . . the belief that a pep talk sparks a team to victory or that the coach ignites a team with a few well-chosen words is simply a myth." A study by Fleishman (1958) is particularly relevant to motor performance. Using an airplane control simulator as the skill, Fleishman found that strong verbal encouragement as an incentive produced superior performance results only among the better half of the experimental group, compared to the control group.

It seems likely that the exact benefits of verbal exhortations will vary with the situation. In many situations it will enhance learning and performance; in some cases it will have little or no effect. It is probable that teachers or coaches should not rely too heavily on verbal encouragement if they wish to evoke maximum performance.

Some investigators have used verbal exhortations in conjunction with other incentives or they have used material incentives of some kind. Caskey (1968) compared verbal to visual incentives on broad-jump performance of children in grades one, two, and three. One incentive involved the use of verbal encouragement, one visual incentive utilized the visualization of previous efforts in regard to lines on the jumping circle, while the second visual incentive involved visually relating performance to the child's height which was marked on the jumping surface. The visual incentives positively affected the standing broad-jump performance.

In one study, Nelson (1962) used ten incentive conditions on 250 male students from physical education classes at the University of Oregon. The three incentive conditions using verbal instruction and encouragement produced the lowest improvement means of all ten situations. The highest improvement was in incentive conditions that emphasized ego-involvement and individual competition.

We have emphasized that many different incentives are effective for producing effective learning and performance. Although this basic fact is true, apparently incentives do not produce improved performance on all tasks. Various studies could be cited to show that the incentives used in the experiments did not produce performance improvement, but we shall identify only one as an illustration. The following example was chosen because the experimental task involved motor performance.

Ryan (1961b) studied the effects of four types of "motive-incentive" conditions on performance on grip strength. The experimental conditions were:

1. Instructions to do as well as possible.
2. Verbal exhortations to improve.
3. Subjects provided with results of preliminary test and permission to watch dial during retest trial.
4. Threat of electric shock for failure to improve.

He reported no differences in performance between groups at the different performance levels and no differences between the four "motive-incentive" conditions. He suggested that in testing strength no additional incentives are necessary, as long as the subjects understand the importance of giving a maximum effort.

1. Competition as an incentive

Competition has been found to be a powerful incentive, and physical educators, coaches, and employers have used it as a favorite incentive technique. Competition serves as an incentive because its outcomes meet a variety of individual needs, especially in a society whose core value orientation is the exaltation of the "successful" competitor—the winner. Studies of the effects of competition upon motor performance have shown that competition between individuals and groups tends to enhance performance in a variety of tasks and for various age groups (Higgs, 1972; Mortier, 1971; Nelson, 1962; Strong, 1963).

These results have led to a general assumption that competition is a reliable means of improving performance, but there is the disturbing fact that in some cases competition has not improved performance (Voor, Lloyd, and Cole, 1969; Lloyd and Voor, 1973). There are a number of possible reasons why competition may not enhance performance—indeed, may even reduce performance efficiency. There is neurophysiological evidence that competition tends to increase arousal; whether the competition enhances or decreases performance will depend on the level of arousal it produces. If the increased arousal produces a state near the optimal level for performance of that task, performance will be enhanced; on the other hand, if it pushes the arousal state beyond optimal for performance on that task, a decrement in performance will occur.

Competition is an effective incentive if the participants believe that they have a chance to win; if they do not believe they have a chance to win, it frequently is not an effective incentive because the participants may either refuse to compete or compete in a halfhearted fashion. Competition among persons or groups of nearly equal skill produces better performance than among persons or groups of unequal skill. If winning is a matter of skill, interest and effort decline rapidly when the same person or group wins consistently. Moreover, persistent losing in a competitive situation may be reflected in a significant decline in both positive self-concept and favorable body-image (Read, 1969).

The incentive effects of competition have complex dimensions to which we cannot devote space in this volume, but one final aspect of competition as an incentive deserves note. Competition in a sport setting often takes the performers' attention from the main purpose of performing a task well and focuses it upon an outside goal—winning at any cost. Documentation for this can be seen in many organized sports programs.

2. Threats of force as an incentive

Physical educators and coaches have used threats of force on their students in several ways. Coaches have threatened to drop a player from the team, or threatened to demote a player to the bench, in order to bring the players to do what they demand. There is no question that threats of force serve as powerful incentives to conform, and there are situations where they may properly be used. An athlete who will not show up for practice or will not execute plays correctly cannot be given a starting position on a team without disrupting the total team effort. Although forceful actions are usually unpleasant, they are sometimes unavoidable.

Two potential outcomes of this method of incentive are frequently evident. First, it often creates an overdependence on the instructor. Some students may function in such a state of fear of the instructor that they cease to show initiative and imagination for fear that the leader may disapprove and punish them. These students rarely perform with a spontaneous enthusiasm for the activity. Second, the method of threat tends to create resentment. Invariably, the individuals believe that they have been unfairly disciplined and cooperation is difficult to obtain. So if threat of force is to be used, it must be used wisely and discreetly.

3. Goal setting and incentives

Goals or objectives serve as incentives and persons will expend great effort to achieve them. There are two basic ways in which goals may be set: They may be set by someone other than the person performing the task, in which case they are called "other-identified performance goals," or they may be set by the performer or a group of performers, in which case they are called "self-identified performance goals." In both cases there is considerable evidence to support the view that goals and intentions are important determinants of task performance (Locke, 1968).

Locke and Bryan (1966a, 1966b) had subjects produce a pattern of display lights with a corresponding pattern produced by a moving joystick and a foot-pedal control. Subjects were either simply allowed to "do their best" or given a target goal corresponding to their previous test score plus a fixed increment above the subjects' best previous score. Their findings showed that the setting of a specific standard ("hard goals") led to both a faster rate of improvement and an overall higher standard. Church and Camp (1965), in a reaction time study, observed similar effects when hard goals based on previous performance scores were used. In another study, Bryan and Locke (1967) also found that specific other-identified performance goals may be used to motivate persons who have a low degree of motivation.

It is generally agreed by psychologists that the best method of motivating people is to attempt to get them to perform because they want to, not because they have to or because a material incentive is held out before them. That is to say, they are motivated because they have identified goals for themselves and/or for the group, which they want to accomplish for their own self-edification. Thus, it is most effective if people perform because this seems like a good goal for themselves, not because of threat of force if they do not perform, nor because of a material incentive.

Although it has rarely been used in physical education and athletics, participation in setting goals appears to be an effective incentive in motivating behavior. Several industrial studies have shown that when workers are asked to establish their own goals they set higher goals than management expected, and they reached those goals at a better rate than management-established goals (Taylor, 1972). If, for example, an individual or group is encouraged to establish a suitable goal, the "goal striving" will spur the individual or group toward improved performance. The goal serves as an incentive for better performance, and when the goal is achieved it is quite rewarding.

In terms of meeting needs, participation in goal setting seems to involve two of the strongest social needs—self-esteem and social approval. Self-esteem comes into play when individuals feel that they are respected enough to be consulted about group decisions. Social approval acts through persons feeling that their roles are important cogs in the group's activity.

Using participation in self-identified and group identified goals sometimes conflicts with the traditional viewpoints which many teachers and coaches have regarding their assigned role and that of their students, which is that teachers and coaches often want students to do as they are told rather than use their initiative. But the implications of work on self-identified and group-identified goals suggest that if individuals choose their own goals, they may produce better performance than when goals are set for them. Moreover, studies suggest that when persons perceive themselves as voluntarily undertaking arduous tasks in order to achieve a goal, they tend to evaluate the tasks more highly than if they feel themselves to be coerced into performing the tasks (Brehm and Cohen, 1962).

4. Level of aspiration

Closely related to the topic of goal setting is "level of aspiration." Here self-identified performance goals are set by the performer, but the specific unique concern is with previous performance on subsequent performance goals that is of interest. A great deal of the incentive which motivates persons comes from the consequences of their own behavior. When behavior leads to successful accomplishment of a goal, or at least closely approaches the goal, it can serve to sustain the same behavior at a subsequent time when the task must be performed. Level of aspiration refers to the goal level individuals (or groups) set for themselves on a particular task—the belief that persons (or groups) have concerning their potential for performance. Investigations of level of aspiration usually involve two basic considerations: First, comparisons of the effects of success or failure on estimations of future performance; second, comparisons between individuals' (or groups') estimation of their performance and their actual performance.

Although it is not possible to always predict how success and failure will affect a person's aspiration about future performance, Cofer and Appley (1964) have proposed the most generally accepted generalizations. Simply stated, aspiration level is affected by past experience; successful performance tends to lead to an increase in the level of aspiration, or standard of excellence; failure tends to lead to a decrease in aspiration level; and persons with high aspirations perform at high levels. These generalizations have been confirmed with academic tasks (Worell, 1959), with individuals on a wide variety of motor tasks (Clawson, 1965; Harari, 1969; Price, 1960; Clarke and Clarke, 1961), and with selected groups (Zander, 1971).

In addition to the basic effects of success and failure on aspiration level, several other factors have been identified which seem to be important too. In general, boys have a higher aspiration level than girls (Walter and Marzolf, 1951), the social setting affects aspiration (Hilgard et al., 1940), parental aspiration levels are related to level of aspiration of their children (Rosen and D'Andrade, 1959).

Helson (1964) has proposed a "hypothesis of par" or "tolerance" to account for the relationship between aspiration and performance. Basically, the hypothesis is that for most tasks individuals establish some standard of excellence for themselves and are content to achieve, but not really to strive to exceed, this standard. Mostly, this "level of aspiration" is set lower than the performance level which the person is capable of reaching. Although this hypothesis is capable of describing the aspiration and behavior of many individuals, there are individuals to whom it cannot be applied. Nevertheless, it is a useful device with which to confront a particular student who is reluctant to perform to capability.

The implications of the findings on aspiration level for teaching motor skills are rather clear. Regular opportunities for success are necessary if steady progress is to be expected. Setting goals just slightly above the learner's capabilities is one way of providing frequent success. When performers must compete against others, it would be wise to schedule contests so success is attained regularly. When a player or team is constantly overmatched, the aspiration, and hence performances, will diminish. Of course, total and constant success becomes boring and motivation may wane. It is apparent that an important job of the teacher or coach is to manipulate the environment so success can be used as an incentive to improve performances.

C. REINFORCEMENT

The basis of reinforcement theory goes back to E. L. Thorndike's (1911) proposal which is known as the "Law of Effect." This "law" postulates that those responses that occur in a situation and which lead to "satisfaction" will tend to be repeated when the situation recurs, whereas those responses that do not lead to satisfaction will not be strengthened. Other Behaviorists in psychology refined reinforcement theory during the first half of this century, but it was B. F. Skinner, of Harvard, who extended and elaborated Thorndike's Law of Effect into what has become known as operant psychology, a modern reinforcement theory.

The basic notion behind reinforcement theory is that reinforcement produces a repetition in the response on subsequent occasions; when this happens, the reinforcer is said to be a positive reinforcer. When the reinforcement produces a cessation of a response, it is said to be a negative reinforcer. Thus, in the sense that reinforcements lead to meeting certain needs, they have a positive or attractive influence and lead to satisfaction; on the other hand, reinforcements may have a negative influence, and cause the individual to move away from them. Negative reinforcements satisfy needs in the sense that the body has a need to escape painful or unpleasant stimuli. Since we tend to move toward positive reinforcers and away from negative reinforcers, we may view ourselves as being drawn toward certain behaviors and pushed away from others. There are, then, two ways of influencing behavior with reinforcers—one associated with reward and another with punishment. Positive and negative reinforcers are either material or symbolic objects that are given *after* certain behavior has been emitted.

1. Positive reinforcers

It is necessary to note at the outset of this section that no effort will be made to discuss the reinforcement effects of feedback on motor behavior. This was covered in Chapter 20.

One of the most frequently employed types of reinforcement is positive reinforcers, which may be social, i.e., praise, smiles, or material, i.e., money, candy, trophies, and they are commonly referred to as rewards. Typically, the reinforcer is applied immediately after a response and it is, of course, contingent upon appropriate behavior. Extensive programs employing reinforcement techniques have been employed in clinical psychology, schools, mental hospitals, and prisons under the label of "behavior modification" programs, and many remarkable stories have been recounted about the successes in using various kinds of positive reinforcers. Behavioral modification techniques have recently been introduced into physical education programs (Siedentop and Rife, 1975). Rushall and Siedentop (1972) have published a book on the applications of operant psychology for teaching physical activities.

Motor behavior is affected by an array of social influence processes, one of which is social reinforcement. Tangible, or material, reinforcement is also influential in altering motor behavior. Both social and material reinforcement research on verbal behavior has been much more prevalent than studies examining the effect of reinforcement on motor behavior. Of those studies which have been done with motor behavior they tend to be limited by two characteristics: Most have used young children as subjects; the tasks used were rather simple.

Positive social and tangible reinforcement of various types has been found to be effective in enhancing the response rate of subjects performing tasks that emphasize speed, rate, and other "quantitiative" responses, but studies in which tasks emphasizing accuracy, fine motor control, and other "qualitative" responses were used have found that reinforcement, either positive or negative, had little influence on the early performance trials of these tasks. Martens and his colleagues (1972) have suggested three possible reasons for this: (1) Performance on quantitative motor tasks soon loses its appeal and becomes boring since the tasks are not intrinsically motivating, while the performance of qualitative tasks is challenging and possesses high levels of intrinsic motivation. (2) Performance of quantitative tasks requires little learning, the skills necessary for task performance were previously acquired by the subjects. This is typically not true of qualitative tasks. (3) In the studies using quantitative motor tasks a clear goal was not present from the task itself, thus information to modify behavior was heavily dependent on the reinforcement provided. It appears that the reinforcement acted to change the motive state. On the other hand, in studies with qualitative tasks the information was available to the subjects in the form of knowledge of results. Martens *et al.* concluded that since little learning is required on quantitative tasks and because it was generally difficult for the subjects to ascertain what good or poor performance was, reinforcements have enhanced motor behavior. Conversely, since qualitative tasks have typically required learning to a criterion, provided knowledge of results as part of the performance, and in general were intrinsically motivating, reinforcement had little effect in the early performance trials. Martens and his colleagues hypothesized that once a qualitative motor task had been well learned the influence of reinforcement would be similar to that of quantitative tasks, since the challenge to learn the task is gone and motivation to perform well wanes. They found support for their proposition.

Although little in the way of specific conclusions can be drawn from the studies of positive reinforcement, in terms of its effects on motor behavior, it is clear that supportive and encouraging signs by an instructor create a favorable interpersonal atmosphere among participants and instructor. This social environment is rarely measured in laboratory studies but it is present, and important, in dynamic settings where motor tasks are performed. And there is evidence that where a favorable social climate exists participants enjoy their experiences and wish to continue their relationship with persons in that group (Berscheid and Walster, 1969).

Positive material reinforcers, too, can be effective in producing feelings of satisfaction and pleasure on the part of the recipient of these rewards. However, there is always the danger that when the reinforcers which have been employed to reward appropriate behavior are withdrawn, the appropriate behavior may cease. This will be discussed in more detail in a later section of this chapter entitled "Intrinsic and Extrinsic Motivation."

Reward techniques may also lead to resentment. When individuals are performing in response to rewards that are manipulated by a leader, they frequently come to understand that they are actually being tricked into performing—much like the dog who sits up for a morsel of food. Although dogs never seem to resent this trickery, humans do because they perceive this form of "behavior control" as an insinuation that they are unintelligent and naive. Many instructors fail to understand this phenomenon and are completely at a loss to understand why individuals or teams sometimes suddenly lose enthusiasm or fail to perform at all in response to rewards that are being offered.

2. Negative reinforcers

A negative reinforcer decreases the probability of recurrence of a response. The word punishment is often used in place of negative reinforcement and behaviorists define a punisher as any stimulus that reduces the frequency of the behavior that precedes it. Like positive reinforcers, negative reinforcers may be social, i.e., reproof, frowns, or material, i.e., physical assault, shock, etc. Negative reinforcement is a common technique in behavior control but it is also the most controversial and complex of the reinforcement methods when used on humans.

Research on the effects of negative reinforcement on behavior has produced very confusing findings. Two reviews on the effects of social reinforcement reported almost opposite conclusions. Kennedy and Willcutt (1964) concluded that positive social reinforcement facilitates learning more than negative reinforcement, while Marshall (1965) concluded virtually the opposite. More recently, Parke (1969), after review of the literature on the use of punishment (verbal harangue, physical punishment, withholding certain things, electric shock) stated:

Punishment can be an effective means of controlling behavior. The operation of punishment, however, is a complex process and its effects are quite varied and highly dependent on such parameters as timing, intensity, consistency, and affectional and/or status relationship between the agent and recipient of punishment, and the kind of cognitive structuring accompanying the punishment stimulus.

Aside from the issue of the effects of punishment on learning and performance, this form of reinforcement has the potential for a number of unintended consequences. Fear and phobias may be produced by punishers which produce a great deal of pain, for example. In addition, a regular program of negative reinforcement is likely to foster resentment on the part of the recipient of the punishment against the person doing the punishing. In this case, while remarkable behavioral control may be maintained by an instructor through the employment of punishers, this may produce dislike on the part of the performer, not only for the administrator of the punishment but also for the entire activity or situation in which it occurs. Thus, physical educators and coaches who resort to frequent use of negative reinforcers to control performers' behavior may indirectly produce a general dislike for physical educators and coaches as well as an abhorrence for the motor skills they are teaching.

While positive reinforcers are typically employed in a rational way, negative reinforcers are frequently employed irrationally without any consideration to their potential effects; in an instructional situation they are often employed when instructors are frustrated because the students have not performed up to the instructor's expectations. Frustration often leads to aggressive behavior, and punishment is a form of aggressive behavior that persons use to allievieate their frustrations. Unfortunately, when punishment is used this way it may merely frustrate and anger the persons being punished rather than motivate them toward appropriate behavior.

Of course, there are occasions when punishment may have to be used. Persons of all ages continually explore limits; if there are none, behavior may get out of hand. The teacher and coach cannot permit students to get away with violations of viable rules and policies and they cannot put up with lackadaisical effort on the part of students. Rushall and Siedentop (1972) suggest a guideline for the application of punishment: "When punishment must be used it should be specific, have minimal emotionality attached to it, should be relatively severe, and should always be applied consistently." It might also be added that punishment highlights what *not* to do, so when punishment is used a good teaching procedure is to describe an alternative response which would be appropriate, since punishment itself does not specify what is the appropriate response.

3. Vicarious reinforcement

Vicarious reinforcement occurs when the behavior of an individual is influenced as a result of observing someone else's behavior and the reinforcement that follows. This kind of social influence has been found to be important in directing behavior of the observer. People, especially young persons, model their behavior after others, and a number of researchers have shown that children and youths imitate the behaviors of adults. It is common to see, for example, youngsters imitate the techniques of successful performers, i.e., the Fosbury flop.

One of the critical factors which affects the degree of imitation of a model that takes place by young observers is the consequences of the model's behavior. In general, if the model is given positive reinforcement for his or her behaviors, young observers tend to emulate these same behaviors, when given the chance; on the other hand, when the model receives negative reinforcers, these behaviors are suppressed by those witnessing them. Another important factor affecting the influence that an adult model has on a young observer is the perceived power and prestige of the model. In general, the greater these perceived characteristics, the greater the imitation that takes place (Bandura and Walters, 1963).

Instructors of motor behavior need to be aware that their own behavior is being observed closely by those whom they are instructing, and since they are perceived as powerful and prestigious persons by young persons, their behaviors will be emulated. While the cliche, "Don't do as I do, do as I say," may give an instructor a convenient excuse for not setting a good example, it is not likely to be heeded. "Teaching by example rather than by precept" seems to be a more appropriate teaching model in terms of what is known about vicarious reinforcement.

INTRINSIC AND EXTRINSIC MOTIVATION

Motivation to perform an activity may be divided into two broad classes: intrinsic motivation and extrinsic motivation. One is intrinsically motivated if one performs an activity for no apparent reward except the activity itself. Extrinsic motivation, on the other hand, refers to the performance of an activity because it leads to rewards, i.e., money, trophies, passing grades. Several investigators have proposed that when material rewards are given for an intrinsically motivated task, persons perceive that the locus of control or the knowledge or feeling of personal causation shifts to an external source, causing the individuals to feel that they are "pawns" to the source of external rewards. Their behavior then becomes motivated by the external reward rather than by their intrinsic interest (deCharms, 1968). Festinger (1967) proposed that external rewards influence individuals' perception of why they are working and their attitude toward the work. Reasoning from his theory of cognitive dissonance,* Festinger (1957) also predicted that external rewards should decrease intrinsic motivation.

Deci (1971, 1972) conducted a series of studies to investigate the effects of externally mediated rewards on intrinsic motivation. Subjects were given tasks to perform which were intrinsically interesting. One group was given extrinsic rewards for performing the tasks while a second group was not given any extrinsic rewards. After a period of time, the group that had been receiving extrinsic rewards for task performance no longer got the rewards. Both groups were then observed for continued participation with the tasks. The group that had received no extrinsic motivation continued to perform the tasks to a much greater extent than the group that had received the extrinsic rewards. The experiments suggest that when material rewards are used for some activity, the subjects lose intrinsic motivation for it. This work was extended by Greene and Lepper (1974) with essentially the same results. They say:

Powerful and salient extrinsic rewards will be . . .effective so long as the reward system is in operation. At the same time, the more powerful and salient the rewards, the more likely they are to undermine the child's intrinsic motivation in the absence of these rewards.

Apparently, positive social reinforcement does not produce the same decrement in intrinsic motivation that material reinforcers do. Deci (1972) found that when verbal encouragement and other social approval measures

---

*Cognitions are said to be in a dissonant relationship whenever they are incompatible. According to cognitive dissonance theory, the presence of dissonance gives rise to pressures to reduce or eliminate the dissonance and to avoid an increase in dissonance.

were used, the subjects intrinsic motivation seemed to increase. He proposed that social reinforcers do not seem to affect one's phenomenology in the same way as material reinforcers do. Social reinforcers are less likely to be perceived by performers as controlling their behavior.

The findings of these studies suggest that one who is interested in developing and enhancing intrinsic motivation in children, employees, athletes, etc. should not concentrate on external control, such as material reinforcers, which are linked to performance but, instead, should concentrate on structuring situations so as to capitalize upon intrinsic interest, and then be interpersonally supportive toward the persons in the situation.

Such attempts at motivation have their limitations, too. First it may not be possible to get persons to perceive the situation in a way in which intrinsic motivation is created. A second problem with this technique is that it may breed a spirit of self-determination and independence, which can be disruptive to any sort of team endeavor. If individuals are encouraged to perform on the basis of their perceived goals, they may develop and assert ideas that are not productive of a normative standard of high performance. Furthermore, due to rapidly changing moods and attitudes, internalized motivation varies dramatically from day to day. Thus, performance is likely to vary, too. Thus, this method of motivation also has inherent problems. At the same time, it has great potential. It is an important method for developing judgment, resourcefulness, leadership, and real enthusiasm for an endeavor.

.

References

Adams, G.L. 1965. Effect of eye dominance on baseball batting. *Res. Quart.* **36**: 3–9.

Adams, J.A., E.T. Goetz, and P.H. Marshall 1972. Response feedback and motor learning. *J. Exp. Psychol.* **92**: 391–397.

_____ 1971. A closed-loop theory of motor learning. *J. Motor Behavior* **3**: 111–150.

_____ 1967. *Human memory.* New York: McGraw-Hill.

_____, and S. Dijkstra 1966. Short-term memory for motor responses. *J. Exp. Psychol.* **71**: 314–318.

_____, and L.R. Creamer 1962. Anticipatory timing of continuous and discrete responses. *J. Exp. Psychol.* **63**: 84–90.

_____, and L.E. Hufford 1962. Contributions of a part-task trainer to the learning and relearning of a time-shared flight maneuver. *Human Factors* **4**: 159–170.

Adey, W.R., J.P. Segundo, and R.B. Livingston 1957. Corticofugal influences on intrinsic brainstem conduction in cat and monkey. *J. Neurophysiol.* **20**: 1–16.

Agranoff, B.W. 1967. Memory and protein synthesis. *Sci. Am.* **216** (June): 115–122.

Albe-Fessard, D., and J. Liebeskind 1966. Origin des messages somato-sensitifs activant les cellules du cortex moteur chez le singe. *Exp. Brain Res.* **1**: 127–146.

Alderfer, C.P. 1969. An empirical test of a new theory of human needs. *Organ. Behav. and Human Perf.* **4**: 142–175.

Alderman, R.B. 1965. Influence of local fatigue on speed and accuracy in motor learning. *Res. Quart.* **36**: 131–140.

Alderson, G.J.K. 1972. Variables affecting the perception of velocity in sports situations. In H.T.A. Whiting (ed.), *Readings in sports psychology.* London: Henry Kimpton, pp. 116–155.

Alexander, L.T. 1951. Knowledge of results and the temporal gradient of reinforcement. *Am. J. Psychol.* **6**: 292–293. (Abstract.)

Ammons, R.B. 1958. Le mouvement. In G.H. Seward and J.P. Seward (eds.), *Current psychological issues*. New York: Holt.

_____ 1956. Effects of knowledge of performance: a survey and tentative theoretical formulation. *J. Gen. Psychol.* **54**: 279–299.

_____ 1947. Acquisition of motor skills: II. Rotary-pursuit performance with continuous practice before and after a single rest. *J. Exp. Psychol.* **37**: 393–411.

Annett, J. 1969. *Feedback and human behavior*. Baltimore: Penguin.

Astrand, P., and K. Rodahl 1970. *Textbook of work physiology*. New York: McGraw-Hill.

Averback, E., and G. Sperling 1961. Short-term storage of information in vision. In C. Cherry (ed.), *Information theory*. London: Butterworth, pp. 196–211.

Bachman, J.C. 1961. Specificity vs. generality in learning and performing two large muscle motor tasks. *Res. Quart.* **32**: 3–11.

Bahrick, H.P., M.E. Noble, and P.M. Fitts 1954. Extratask performance as a measure of learning a primary task. *J. Exp. Psychol.* **48**: 298–302.

Ballard, P.B. 1913. Obliviscence and reminiscence. *Brit. J. Psychol. Monograph, Suppl.* **1** (No. II): 1–73.

Bandura, A. 1965. Vicarious processes: a case of no-trial learning. In L. Berkowitz (ed.), *Advances in experimental social psychology*. Vol. 2. New York: Academic Press, pp. 1–55.

_____, and R.H. Walters 1963. *Social learning and personality development*. New York: Holt, Rinehart and Winston.

Bartlett, F.C. 1958. *Thinking*. London: Unwin.

_____ 1932. *Remembering: a study in experimental and social psychology*. Cambridge: Cambridge University Press.

Bartley, S.H. 1969. *Principles of perception*. (2nd ed.) New York: Harper & Row.

Basler, M.L., and A.C. Fisher 1974. Prediction of gymnastic performance from arousal and anxiety measures. Paper presented at the AAHPER convention, Anaheim.

Beeby, C.E. 1930. An experimental investigation into the simultaneous constituents in an act of skill. *Brit. J. Psychol.* **20**: 336–353.

Beecher, H.K. 1959. *Measurement of subjective responses*. Oxford: Oxford University Press.

Beer, M. 1966. *Leadership, employee needs, and motivation*. Columbus: The Ohio State University, Bureau of Business Research.

Beise, D., and V. Peaseley, 1937. The relation of reaction time—speed and agility of big muscle groups to certain sport skills. *Res. Quart.* **8** (March): 133–142.

Bell, V.L. 1968. Augmented knowledge of results and its effect upon acquisition and retention of a gross motor skill. *Res. Quart.* **39**: 25–30.

Berlyne, D. 1960. *Conflict, arousal and curiosity.* New York: McGraw-Hill.

Bernstein, N. 1967. *The coordination and regulation of movement.* New York: Pergamon.

Berscheid, E., and E.H. Walster 1969. *Interpersonal attraction.* Reading, Mass.: Addison-Wesley.

Bertelson, P. 1961. Sequential redundancy and speed in a serial two-choice responding task. *Quart. J. Exp. Psychol.* **13**: 90–102.

Bessou, P., and E.R. Perl 1969. Response of cutaneous sensory units with unmyelinated fibers to noxious stimuli. *J. Neurophysiol.* **32**: 1025–1043.

Bills, A.G. 1927. The influence of muscular tension on the efficiency of mental work. *Am. J. Psychol.* **38**: 227–251.

Bilodeau, E.A. 1969. Retention under free and stimulated conditions. In E.A. Bilodeau and I. McD. Bilodeau (eds.), *Principles of skill acquisition.* New York: Academic Press, pp. 171–203.

———— (ed.) 1966. *Acquisition of skill.* New York: Academic Press.

————, and C.M. Levy 1964. Long-term memory as a function of retention time and other conditions of training and recall. *Psychol. Rev.* **71**: 27–41.

————, and I. McD. Bilodeau 1961. Motor-skills learning. In P. Farnsworth (ed.), *Annual Rev. Psychol.* **12**: 243–280.

————, I. McD. Bilodeau, and D.A. Schumsky 1959. Some effects of introducing and withdrawing knowledge of results early and late in practice. *J. Exp. Psychol.* **58**: 142–144.

————, and I. McD. Bilodeau 1958a. Variable frequency of knowledge of results and the learning of a simple skill. *J. Exp. Psychol.* **55**: 379–383.

————, and I. McD. Bilodeau 1958b. Variation of temporal intervals among critical events in five studies of knowledge of results. *J. Exp. Psychol.* **55**: 603–612.

Bilodeau, I. McD. 1969. Information feedback. In E.A. Bilodeau (ed.), *Principles of skill acquisition.* New York: Academic Press, pp. 255–287.

———— 1956. Accuracy of a simple positioning response with variation in the number of trials by which knowledge of results is delayed. *Am. J. Psychol.* **69**: 434–437.

Black, J. 1949. *An experimental study of the learning of a fine motor skill.* Unpublished master's thesis. University Park, Pa.: The Pennsylvania State University.

Blick, K.A., and E.A. Bilodeau 1963. Interpolated activity and the learning of a simple skill. *J. Exp. Psychol.* **65**: 515–519.

Bliss, J.C., H.D. Crane, P.K. Mansfield, and J.T. Townsend 1966. Information available in brief tactile presentations. *Percept. and Psychophysics* 1: 273–283.

Boring, E.G. 1942. *Sensation and perception in the history of experimental psychology.* New York: Appleton-Century-Crofts.

Bossom, J., and A.K. Ommaya 1968. Visuo-motor adaptation (to prismatic transformation of the retinal image) in monkeys with bilateral dorsal rhizotomy. *Brain* **91**: 161–172.

Boswell, J.J., and E.A. Bilodeau 1964. Short-term retention of a simple motor task as a function of interpolated activity. *Percept. and Motor Skills,* **18**: 227–230.

Botwinick, J., and L.W. Thompson 1966. Premotor and motor components of reaction time. *J. Exp. Psychol.* **71**: 9–15.

Boucher, J.L. 1974. Higher processes in motor learning. *J. Motor Behavior* **6**: 131–137.

Boulter, L.R. 1964. Evaluation of mechanisms in delay of knowledge of results. *Can. J. Psychol.* **18**: 281–291.

Bower, T.G. 1966. The visual world of infants. *Sci. Am.* **215** (December): 80–92.

Boyd, L.P. 1969. *A comparative study of the effects of ankle weights on vertical jumping ability.* Unpublished master of science thesis. Springfield, Mass.: Springfield College.

Brace, D.K. 1941. Studies in the rate of learning gross bodily motor skills. *Res. Quart.* **12**: 181–185.

———— 1927. *Measuring motor ability.* New York: A.S. Barnes.

Brehm, J.W. and A.R. Cohen 1962. *Explorations in cognitive dissonance.* New York: Wiley.

Broer, M. 1958. Effectiveness of a general basic skills curriculum for junior high school girls. *Res. Quart.* **29**: 379–388.

Brose, D.E., and D.L. Hanson 1967. Effects of overload training on velocity and accuracy of throwing. *Res. Quart.* **38**: 528–533.

Broughton, B., and D.O. Nelson 1967. Verbal conditioning in selected skills. *Scholastic Coach* **37** (November): 38–40, 44 *et seq.*

Brown, I.D. 1960. Many messages from few sources. *Ergonomics* **3**: 159–168.

Brown, J.S. 1949. A proposed program of research on psychological feedback (knowledge of results) in the performance of psychomotor tasks. In *Research Planning Conference on Perceptual and Motor Skills,* AFHRRC Conference Report, Rept. 49-2, 81–87 (U.S. Air Force, San Antonio, Texas, 1949).

Brown, P.K., and G. Wald 1964. Visual pigments in single rods and cones of the human retina. *Sci.* **144**: 45–52.

Browne, K., J. Lee, and P.A. Ring. 1954. The sensation of passive movement at the metatarso-phalangeal joint of the great toe in man. *J. Physiol.* **126**: 448–458.

Bryan, J.F., and E.A. Locke 1967. Goal setting as a means of increasing motivation. *J. Appl. Psychol.* **51**: 274–277.

Bryan, W.L., and N. Harter 1899. Studies on the telegraphic language: the acquisition of a hierarchy of habits. *Psychol. Rev.* **6**: 345–375.

Buckfellow, W.F. 1954. *Peripheral perception and reaction time of athletes and nonathletes.* Unpublished master's thesis. Urbana, Ill.: University of Illinois.

Burdeshaw, D., J.E. Spragens, and P.A. Weis 1970. Evaluation of general versus specific instruction of badminton skills to women of low motor ability. *Res. Quart.* **41**: 472–477.

Burg, A., and S. Hulbert 1961. Dynamic visual acuity as related to age, sex, and static acuity. *J. Appl. Psychol.* **45**: 111–116.

Burgess, P.R., and J.F. Clark 1969. Characteristics of knee joint receptors in the cat. *J. Physiol.* **203**: 317–335.

_____, and E.R. Perl 1967. Myelinated afferent fibers responding specifically to noxious stimulation of the skin. *J. Physiol.* **190**: 541–562.

Burpee, R.H., and W. Stroll 1936. Measuring reaction time of athletes. *Res. Quart.* **7** (March): 110–118.

Butler, R.A. 1954. Curiosity in monkeys. *Sci. Am.* **190** (February).

_____ 1953. Discrimination learning by Rhesus monkeys to visual-exploration motivation. *J. Comp. Physiol. Psychol.* **46**: 95–98.

Cameron, D.E., and L. Solyom 1961. Effects of RNA on memory. *Geriat.* **16**: 74–81.

Camhi, J.M. 1971. Flight orientation in locusts. *Sci. Am.* **225** (August): 74–81.

Cannon, W.B. 1932. *The wisdom of the body.* New York: Norton.

Caplan, C.S. 1970. The influence of physical fatigue on massed versus distributed motor learning. Paper presented at the AAHPER convention, Seattle, Washington.

Carreras, M., and S.A. Andersson 1963. Functional properties of neurons of the anterior ectosylvian gyrus of the cat. *J. of Neurophysiol.* **26**: 100–126.

Carroll, J. 1972. Deception in games-playing. In H.T.A. Whiting (ed.), *Readings in sport psychology.* London: Henry Kimpton, pp. 238–246.

Carron, A.V. 1972. Motor performance and learning under physical fatigue. *Medicine and Science in Sports* **4**: 101–106.

_____, and A.D. Ferchuk 1971. The effect of fatigue on learning and performance of a gross motor task. *J. Motor Behav.* **3**: 62–68.

_____ 1969. Performance and learning in a discrete motor task under massed vs. distributed practice. *Res. Quart.* **40**: 481–489.

_____ 1968. Motor performance under stress. *Res. Quart.* **39**: 463–469.

Casey, K.L. 1973. Pain: a current view of neural mechanisms. *Am. Scientist* **61**: 194–200.

Caskey, S.R. 1968. Effects of motivation on standing broad jump performance of children. *Res. Quart.* **39**: 54–59.

Catalano, J.F. 1967. Arousal as a factor in reminiscence. *Percept. and Motor Skills* **24**: 1171–1180.

_____, and P.M. Whalen 1967. Factors in recovery from performance decrement: activation, inhibition, warm-up. *Percept. and Motor Skills* **24**: 1223–1231.

Chang, H.T. 1955. Activation of internuncial neurons through collaterals of pyramidal fibers at cortical level. *J. Neurophysiol.* **18**: 452–471.

Chapanis, A. 1964. Knowledge of performance as an incentive in repetitive monotonous tasks. *J. Appl. Psychol.* **48**: 263–267.

Chase, R.A. 1965a. An information-flow model of the organization of motor activity Part II: Sampling, central processing, and utilization of sensory information. *J. Nerv. and Ment. Disease* **140**: 334–350.

_____ 1965b. Information system analysis of organization of motor activity. In P.H. Hock and J. Zubin (eds.), *Psychopathology of perception*. New York: Grune and Stratton, pp. 83–103.

_____, S. Harvey, S. Standfast, I. Rapin, and S. Sutton 1961a. Studies on sensory feedback I. Effect of delayed auditory feedback on speech and keytapping. *Quart. J. Exp. Psychol.* **13**: 141–152.

_____ *et al.* 1961b. Sensory feedback influences on motor performance. *J. Audit. Res.* **1**: 212–223.

_____ *et al.* 1961c. Studies on sensory feedback II. Sensory feedback influence on keytapping motor tasks. *Quart. J. Exp. Psychol.* **13**: 153–167.

Cherry, C., 1953. Some experiments on the recognition of speech with one and with two ears. *J. Acoust. Soc. Amer.* **25**: 975–979.

Chew, R.A. 1974. Verbal, visual, and kinesthetic error feedback in the learning of a simple motor task. Paper presented at the AAHPER Convention, Anaheim.

Chin, A., and E. Evonuk 1971. Changes in plasma catecholamine and corticosterone levels after muscular exercise. *J. Appl. Physiol.* **30**: 205–207.

Christina, R.W. 1973. Influence of enforced motor and sensory sets on reaction latency and movement speed. *Res. Quart.* **44**: 483–487.

_____ 1970. Minimum visual feedback processing time for amendment of an incorrect movement. *Percept. and Motor Skills* **31**: 991–994.

_____ 1967. The side-arm positional test of kinesthetic sense. *Res. Quart.* **38**: 177–183.

Church, R.M., and D.S. Camp 1965. Change in reaction time as a function of knowledge of results. *Am. J. Psychol.* **78**: 102–106.

_____ 1962. The effects of competition on reaction time and palmar skin conductance. *J. Ab. Soc. Psychol.* **65**: 32–40.

Clark, L.V. 1960. Effect of mental practice on the development of a certain motor skill. *Res. Quart.* **31**: 560–569.

Clarke, H.A., and D.H. Clarke 1961. Relationships between level of aspiration and selected physical factors of boys aged nine years. *Res. Quart.* **32**: 12–19.

Clawson, A.L. 1965. *The effect of three types of competitive motivating conditions upon the scores of archery students.* Unpublished doctoral dissertation. Austin, Tex.: University of Texas.

Cleghorn, T.E., and H.D. Darcus 1952. The sensibility to passive movement of the human elbow joint. *Quart. J. Exp. Psychol.* **4**: 66–77.

Cobb, R.A. 1969. *Effects of selected visual conditions on throwing accuracy.* Unpublished doctoral dissertation. Springfield, Mass.: Springfield College.

_____ 1967. *A comparative study of color recognition in the peripheral field of vision of participants in selected sports.* Unpublished master's thesis. Springfield, Mass.: Springfield College.

Cofer, C.N. 1972. *Motivation and emotion.* Glenview, Ill.: Scott Foresman.

_____, and M.H. Appley 1964. *Motivation: theory and research.* New York: Wiley.

Coleman, D.M. 1967. *The effect of a unit of movement education upon the level of achievement in the specialized skill of bowling.* Unpublished doctoral dissertation. Denton, Tex.: Texas Women's University.

Colquhoun, W.P., and D.W.J. Corcoran 1964. The effects of time of day and social isolation on the relationship of temperament to performance. *Brit. J. Soc. Clin. Psychol.* **3**: 226–231.

Connolly, K., and B. Jones 1970. A developmental study of afferent-reafferent integration. *Brit. J. Psychol.* **61**: 259–266.

Considine, W.J. 1966. *Reflex and reaction times within and between athletes and nonathletes.* Unpublished master's thesis. Normal, Ill.: Illinois State University.

Cook, T.W. 1933. Studies in cross-educational mirror tracing the star-shaped maze. *J. Exp. Psychol.* **16**: 144–160.

Cooper, J.H. 1955. *An investigation of the relationship between reaction time and speed of movement.* Unpublished doctoral dissertation. Bloomington, Ind.: University of Indiana.

Corbin, C.B. 1972. Mental practice. In W.P. Morgan (ed.), *Ergogenic aids and muscular performance.* New York: Academic Press, pp. 93–118.

_____ 1967a. Effects of mental practice on skill development after controlled practice. *Res. Quart.* **38**: 534–538.

_____ 1967b. The effects of covert rehearsal on the development of a complex motor skill. *J. Gen. Psychol.* **76**: 143–150.

Corcoran, D.W.J. 1964. The relationship between introversion and salivation. *Am. J. Psychol.* **77**: 298–300.

Cotten, D.J., J.R. Thomas, W.R. Spieth, and J. Biasiotto 1972. Temporary fatigue effects in a gross motor skill. *J. Motor Behavior* **4**: 217–222.

Cottrell, N.B. 1968. Performance in the presence of other human beings: mere presence audience, and affiliation effects. In E.C. Simmel, R.A. Hoppe, and G.A. Milton (eds.), *Social facilitation and imitative behavior.* Boston: Allyn and Bacon, pp. 91–110.

Coville, F.H. 1957. The learning of motor skills as influenced by knowledge of mechanical principles. *J. Educ. Psychol.* **48**: 321–327.

Cozens, F.W. 1929. *The measurement of general athletic ability in college men.* Eugene, Ore.: University of Oregon Press.

Craik, K.J.W. 1948. Theory of the human operator in control systems II. Man as an element in a control system. *Brit. J. Psychol.* **38**: 142–148.

Cratty, B.J. 1973. *Movement behavior and motor learning.* (3rd ed.) Philadelphia: Lea and Febiger.

_____ 1971. Activation and athletic endeavor. In J.W. Taylor (ed.), *Proceedings of the first international symposium on the art and science of coaching.* Willowdale, Ontario: F.I. Productions, pp. 235–242.

_____ 1969. *Perceptual-motor behavior and educational processes.* Springfield, Ill.: Charles C. Thomas.

_____ 1964. *Movement behavior and motor learning.* Philadelphia: Lea and Febiger.

_____, and R.S. Hutton 1964. Figural aftereffect, resulting from gross action patterns. *Res. Quart.* **35**: 147–160.

_____ 1963. Recency vs. primacy in a complex gross motor task. *Res. Quart.* **34**: 3–8.

_____ 1962. Transfer of small-pattern practice to large-pattern learning. *Res. Quart.* **33**: 523–535.

Creamer, L.R. 1963. Event uncertainty, psychological refractory period, and human data processing. *J. Exp. Psychol.* **66**: 187–194.

Cronbach, L.J. 1960. *Essentials of psychological testing.* (2nd ed.) New York: Harper & Row.

Crossman, E.R.F. 1959. A theory of the acquisition of speed-skill. *Ergonomics* **2**: 153–166.

Crouch, J.E. 1965. *Functional human anatomy.* Philadelphia: Lea and Febiger.

Cureton, T. 1951. *Physical fitness of champion athletes.* Urbana, Ill.: University of Illinois Press.

Darwin, C. 1859. *Origin of species.* (New York: Modern Library, 1936.)

Davis, K. 1947. Final note on a case of extreme isolation. *Am. J. Soc.* **52**: 432–437.

_____ 1940. Extreme social isolation of a child. *Am. J. Soc.* **45**: 554–565.

Davis, R. 1959. The role of "attention" in the psychological refractory period. *Quart. J. Exp. Psychol.* **11**: 211–220.

_____ 1957. The human operator as a single channel information system. *Quart. J. Exp. Psychol.* **9**: 119–129.

de Charms, R. 1968. *Personal causation: the internal affective determinants of behavior.* New York: Academic Press.

Deci, E.L. 1972. Intrinsic motivation, extrinsic reinforcement, and inequity. *J. Person. Soc. Psychol.* **22**: 113–120.

_____ 1971. Effects of externally mediated rewards on intrinsic motivation. *J. Person. Soc. Psychol.* **18**: 105–115.

DeCoursey, R.M. 1968. *The human organism.* (3rd ed.) New York: McGraw-Hill.

Deese, J. 1967. *General psychology.* Boston: Allyn and Bacon.

Delgado, J.M.R., W.W. Roberts, and N.E. Miller 1954. Learning motivated by electrical stimulation of the brain. *Am. J. Physiol.* **179**: 587–593.

Del Rey, P. 1971. Effects of videotaped feedback on form, accuracy, and latency in an open and closed environment. *J. Motor Behav.* **3**: 281–288.

Dennis, W. 1960. Causes of retardation among institutional children: Iran. *J. Genet. Psychol.* **96**: 47–59.

Dermer, M., and E. Berscheid 1972. Self-report of arousal as an indicant of activation level. *Behav. Sci.* **17**: 420–429.

Deutsch, J.A. 1971. The cholinergic synapse and the site of memory. *Sci.* **174**: 788–794.

_____, and D. Deutsch 1966. *Physiological psychology.* Homewood, Ill.: The Dorsey Press.

de Vries, H. 1972. Flexibility, an overlooked but vital factor in sports conditioning. In L. Percival (ed.), *International symposium on the art and science of coaching.* Volume 1. Willowdale, Ontario: F.I. Productions, pp. 209–217.

Dickinson, J. 1968. The training of mobile balancing under a minimal visual cue situation. *Ergonomics* **11**: 69–75.

Dickson, J.F. 1953. *The relationship of depth perception to goal shooting in basketball.* Unpublished doctoral dissertation. Iowa City, Iowa: State University of Iowa.

Digman, J.M. 1959. Growth of a motor skill as a function of distribution of practice. *J. Exp. Psychol.* **57**: 310–316.

Dingman, W., and M. Sporn 1964. Molecular theories of memory. *Sci.* **144**: 26–29.

Dodt, E. 1956. Centrifugal impulses in a rabbit's retina. *J. Neurophysiol.* **19**: 301–307.

Donders, F.C. 1969. On the speed of mental processes, 1868. In W.G. Koster (ed. and trans.), *Acta Psychol.* **30**: 412–431.

Dore, L.R., and E.R. Hilgard 1938. Spaced practice as a test of Snoddy's two processes in mental growth. *J. Exp. Psychol.* **23**: 359–374.

Drowatzky, J.N., and R.M. Schwartz 1971. Effect of physical work on static depth perception. *Int. J. Sport Psychol.* **2**: 135.

Duffy, E. 1962. *Activation and behavior.* New York: Wiley.

_____ 1951. The concept of energy mobilization. *Psychol. Rev.* **58**: 30–40.

_____ 1941. An explanation of "emotional" phenomena without the use of the concept "emotion." *J. Gen. Psychol.* **25**: 283–293.

Duncan, C.P. 1953. Transfer in motor learning as a function of degree of first-task learning and intertask similarity. *J. Exp. Psychol.* **45**: 1–11.

Durentini, C.L. 1967. *The relationship of a purported measure of kinesthesis to the learning of a simple motor skill, the basketball free throw, projected with and without vision.* Unpublished master's thesis. Amherst, Mass.: University of Massachusetts.

Dyal, J.A. 1966. Effects of delay of knowledge of results and subject response bias on extinction of a simple motor skill. *J. Exp. Psychol.* **71**: 559–563.

_____ 1964. Effects of delay of knowledge of results in a line-drawing task. *Percept. and Motor Skills* **19**: 433–434.

Eccles, J.C. 1973. *The understanding of the brain.* New York: McGraw-Hill.

———— 1965. The synapse. *Sci. Am.* **212** (January): 56–66.

———— 1964. *The physiology of synapses.* New York: Academic Press.

———— 1953. *The neurophysiological basis of mind.* New York: Oxford University Press.

Eckert, H.M. 1964. Linear relationships of isometric strength to propulsive force, angular velocity, and angular acceleration in the standing broad jump. *Res. Quart.* **35**: 298–306.

Egstrom, G.H. 1964. Effects of an emphasis on conceptualizing techniques during early learning of a gross motor skill. *Res. Quart.* **35**: 472–481.

Elbel, E.R. 1940. A study of reaction time before and after strenuous exercise. *Res. Quart.* **11**: 86–95.

Eldred, E. 1965. The dual sensory role of muscle spindles. In *The child with central nervous system deficit.* Washington, D.C., United States Government Printing Office.

Ellis, W.D. 1938. *A source book of Gestalt psychology.* London: Routlege and Kegon Paul, New York: Harcourt Brace.

Ellison, K., and J. Freischlag 1975. Pain tolerance, arousal, and personality relationships of athletes and nonathletes. *Res. Quart.* **46**: 250–255.

Ells, J.G. 1969. *Attentional requirements of movement control.* Unpublished doctoral dissertation. Eugene, Ore.: University of Oregon.

Elwell, J.L., and G.C. Grindley 1938. The effect of knowledge of results on learning and performance. I. A coordinated movement of the two hands. *Brit. J. Psychol.* **29**: 39–53.

Eriksen, C.W., and J.F. Collins 1968. Sensory traces versus the psychological moment in the temporal organization of form. *J. Exp. Psychol.* **77**: 376–382.

Espenschade, A. 1958. Kinesthetic awareness in motor learning. *Percept. and Motor Skills* **8**: 142.

Essman, W.B. 1966. Effect of tricyanoaminopropene on the amnesic effect of electroconvulsive shock. *Psychopharmacologia* **9**: 426–433.

———— 1965. Facilitation of memory consolidation by chemically induced acceleration of RNA synthesis. *Abstr. 23rd Intern. Congr. Physiol. Sci.* Tokyo.

Esterbrook, J.A. 1959. The effect of emotion on cue utilization and the organization of behavior. *Psychol. Rev.* **66**: 183–201.

Evans, F.J. 1974. The power of the sugar pill. *Psychol. Today* **7** (April): 54–59.

Evarts, E.V. 1973. Brain mechanisms in movement. *Sci. Am.* **229** (July): 96–103.

————, E. Bizzi, R.E. Burke, M. De Long, and W.T. Thach 1971. Central control of movement. *Neuroscience Research Program Bulletin* **9**: 1–170.

Eysenck, H.J. 1967. *The biological basis of personality.* Springfield, Ill.: Charles C. Thomas.

———— 1965. A three-factor theory of reminiscence. *Brit. J. Psychol.* **56**: 163–181.

———— 1963. The measurement of motivation. *Sci. Am.* **208** (May): 130–140.

Fantz, R.L. 1966. Pattern discrimination and selective attention as determinants of perceptual development from birth. In A.H. Kidd and J.L. Rivoire (eds.), *Perceptual development in children*. New York: International Universities Press.

_____ 1961. The origin of form perception. *Sci. Am.* **204** (May): 66–72.

Farber, I.E., and K.W. Spence 1956. Effects of anxiety, stress, and task variables on reaction time. *J. of Person.* **25**: 1–18.

Fentress, J.C. 1973. Development of grooming in mice with amputated forelimbs. *Science* **179**: 704–705.

Festinger, L. 1967. The effect of compensation on cognitive processes. Paper presented at the McKinsey Foundation Conference on Managerial Compensation, Tarrytown, New York, March.

_____ 1957. *A theory of cognitive dissonance*. Evanston, Ill.: Row, Peterson.

Fiske, D.W., and S.R. Maddi 1961. *The functions of varied experience*. Homewood, Ill.: The Dorsey Press.

Fitts, P.M., and M.I. Posner 1967. *Human performance*. Belmont, Calif.: Brooks/Cole.

_____ 1966. Cognitive aspects of information processing. III. Set for speed vs. accuracy. *J. Exp. Psychol.* **71**: 849–857.

_____ 1965. Factors in complex skill training. In R. Glasser (ed.), *Training research and education*. New York: Wiley, pp. 177–197.

_____ 1964. Perceptual-motor skill learning. In A.W. Melton (ed.), *Categories of human learning*. New York: Academic Press, pp. 243–285.

_____, J.R. Peterson, and G. Wolpe 1963. Cognitive aspects of information processing. II. Adjustments to stimulus redundancy. *J. Exp. Psychol.* **65**: 423–432.

_____, and J.A. Leonard 1957. Stimulus correlates of visual pattern recognition—a probability approach. *Final Report*, Contract No. NONR-495 (02), Columbus, Ohio: The Ohio State University Research Foundation, October.

_____ 1951. Engineering psychology and equipment design. In S.A. Stevens (ed.), *Handbook of experimental psychology*. New York: Wiley, pp. 1237–1340.

Fleishman, E.A. 1972. Structure and measurement of psychomotor abilities. In R.N. Singer (ed.), *The psychomotor domain: movement behavior*. Philadelphia: Lea and Febiger, pp. 78–106.

_____ 1967. Performance assessment based on an empirically derived task taxonomy. *Human Factors* **9**: 349–366.

_____ 1966. Human abilities and the acquisition of skill. In E.A. Bilodeau (ed.), *Acquisition of skill*. New York: Academic Press, pp. 147–167.

_____ 1964. *The structure and measurement of physical fitness*. Englewood Cliffs, N.J.: Prentice-Hall.

_____, and S. Rich 1963. Role of kinesthetic and spatial-visual abilities in perceptual-motor learning. *J. Exp. Psychol.* **66**: 6–11.

_____, and J.F. Parker, Jr. 1962. Factors in the retention and relearning of perceptual-motor skill. *J. Exp. Psychol.* **64**: 215–226.

_____ 1958. A relationship between incentive motivation and ability level in psycho-motor performance. *J. Exp. Psychol.* **56**: 78–81.

_____, and W.E. Hempel, Jr. 1955. The relation between abilities and improvement with practice in a visual discrimination reaction task. *J. Exp. Psychol.* **49**: 301–312.

_____, and W.E. Hempel, Jr. 1954. Changes in factor structure of a complex psycho-motor test as a function of practice. *Psychometrika* **18**: 239–252.

Flexner, J.B., L.B. Flexner, and E. Stellar 1963. Memory in mice as affected by intra-cerebral puromycin. *Sci.* **141**: 57–59.

Fox, M.G., and E. Lamb 1962. Improvement during a nonpractice period in a selected physical education activity. *Res. Quart.* **33**: 381–385.

_____, and V.P. Young 1962. Effect of reminiscence on learning selected badminton skills. *Res. Quart.* **33**: 386–394.

_____ 1957. Lateral dominance in the teaching of bowling. *Res. Quart.* **28**: 327–331.

Francis, C.C. 1964. *Introduction to human anatomy.* (4th ed.) St. Louis: C.V. Mosby.

Freeman, G.L. 1948. *The energetics of human behavior.* Ithaca: Cornell University Press.

_____ 1940. The relationship between performance level and bodily activity level. *J. Exp. Psychol.* **26**: 602–608.

_____ 1938. The optimal muscular tensions for various performances. *Am. J. Psychol.* **51**: 146–150.

_____ 1933. The facilitative and inhibitory effects of muscular tension. *Am. J. Psychol.* **45**: 17–52.

_____ 1931. Mental activity and the muscular processes. *Psychol. Rev.* **38**: 428–449.

Freud, S. 1938. *The basic writings of Sigmund Freud.* New York: Random House.

_____ 1933. *New introductory lectures on psychoanalysis.* New York: Norton.

Fulton, R.E. 1942. Speed and accuracy in learning a ballistic movement. *Res. Quart.* **13**: 30–36.

Fundamentals of progress, 1974. Scientific Research on Transcendental Meditation. Maharishi International University.

Funkenstein, D.H. 1955. The physiology of fear and anger. *Sci. Am.* **192** (May): 74–80.

Fuster, J.M., and A. Uyeda 1962. Facilitation of tachistoscopic performance by stimu-lation of midbrain segmental points in the monkey. *Experimental Neurology* **6**: 384–406.

_____ 1958. Effects of stimulation of brainstem on tachistoscopic perception. *Science* **127**: 150.

Gagne, R.M., and E.A. Fleishman 1959. *Psychology and human performance.* New York: Holt, Rinehart and Winston.

_____, and H. Foster 1949. Transfer of training from practice on components in a motor skill. *J. Exp. Psychol.* **39**: 47–68.

Galambos, R. 1956. Suppression of auditory nerve activity by stimulation of efferent fibers to cochlea. *J. of Neurophysiol.* **19**: 438–445.

Gallagher, K.A. 1974. Biofeedback and related training: potential for physical education. In G.H. McGlynn (ed.), *Issues in physical education and sports*. Palo Alto: National Press Books, pp. 56–60.

Gallon, A.J. 1962. Use of weighted shoes in basketball conditioning. Paper presented at CAHPER Southern District Meeting, Santa Barbara, California.

Gardner, E. 1963. *Fundamentals of neurology*. (4th ed.) Philadelphia: W.B. Saunders.

Gardner, E.B. 1969. Proprioceptive reflexes and their participation in motor skills. *Quest* **12**: 1–25.

Gardner, W.J., J.C. Licklider, and A.Z. Weisz 1960. Suppression of pain by sound. *Sci.* **132**: 32–33.

Garry, R. 1963. *The psychology of learning*. Washington: The Center for Applied Research in Education.

Gazzaniga, M.S. 1967. The split brain in man. *Sci. Am.* **217** (August): 24–29.

Gelfan, S., and S. Carter 1967. Muscle sense in man. *Exp. Neurol.* **18**: 469–473.

Genasci, J.E. 1966. A study of the effect of menstruation on total body reaction time. Unpublished research paper. Springfield, Mass.: Springfield College.

_____ 1960. A study of the effect of participation in physical education activities and athletics on reaction time and movement time. Unpublished doctoral dissertation. Greeley, Colo.: University of Northern Colorado.

Gentile, A.M. 1972. A working model of skill acquisition with application to teaching. *Quest* **17**: 3–23.

George, C. 1972. Facilitative and inhibitory effects of the tonic neck reflex upon grip strength of right- and left-handed children. *Res. Quart.* **43**: 157–166.

_____ 1970. Effects of the asymmetrical tonic neck posture upon grip strength of normal children. *Res. Quart.* **41**: 361–364.

George, F.H. 1952. Errors of visual recognition. *J. Exp. Psychol.* **43**: 202–206.

Gibbs, C.B. 1970. Servo-control systems in organisms and the transfer of skill. In D. Legge (ed.), *Skills*. Middlesex: Penguin, pp. 221–226.

_____, and I.D. Brown 1955. increased production from the information incentive in a repetitive task. *Medical Research Council, Appl. Psychological Res. Unit.* Great Britain, No. 230, March.

Gibson, E.J. 1969. *Principles of perceptual learning and development*. New York: Appleton-Century-Crofts.

_____, and R.D. Walk 1960. The visual cliff. *Sci. Am.* **202** (April): 64–71.

_____, and R.B. Bergman 1954. The effect of training on absolute estimation of distance over the ground. *J. Exp. Psychol.* **48**: 473–482.

Gibson, J.J. 1966. *The senses considered as perceptual systems*. Boston: Houghton Mifflin.

_____ 1933. Adaptation, aftereffect and contrast in the perception of curved lines. *J. Exp. Psychol* **16**: 1–31.

Gill, D.L. 1975. Knowledge of results precision and motor skill acquisition. *J. Motor Behav.* **7**: 191–198.

_____ 1955. *The effect of practice on peripheral vision reaction time.* Unpublished master's thesis. Urbana, Ill.: University of Illinois.

Gire, E., and A. Espenschade 1942. Relationship between measures of motor educability and learning of specific motor skills. *Res. Quart.* **13**: 43–56.

Glencross, D.J. 1973. Response complexity and the latency of different movement patterns. *J. Motor Behav.* **5**: 95–104.

_____ 1972. Latency and response complexity. *J. Motor Behav.* **4**: 251–256.

_____ 1970. Serial organization and timing in a motor skill. *J. Motor Behav.* **2**: 229–237.

Glidewell, W.F. 1964. *An investigation of various warm-up procedures in relation to physical performance.* Doctoral dissertation. Austin, Tex.: University of Texas.

Godwin, M.A., and R.A. Schmidt 1971. Muscular fatigue and learning a discrete motor skill. *Res. Quart.* **42**: 374–382.

Goldscheider, A. 1899. Untersuchungen über den Muskelsinn. *Arch. Anat. Physiol.* (Lpz.): 392–502.

Goodenough, F.L. 1935. The development of the reactive process from early childhood to maturity. *J. Exp. Psychol.* **18**: 431–450.

Goodwin, G.M., D.I. McCloskey, and P.B.C. Matthews 1972. Proprioceptive illusions induced by muscle vibration: contribution by muscle spindles to perception? *Sci.* **175**: 1382–1384.

Gottsdanker, R., and G.E. Stelmach 1971. The persistence of psychological refractoriness. *J. Motor Behav.* **3**: 301–312.

Gramza, A., and P.A. Witt 1969. Choices of colored blocks in the play of preschool children. *Percept. and Motor Skills* **29**: 783–787.

Granit, R. 1955. Centrifugal and antidromic effects on ganglion cells on the retina. *J. Neurophysiol.* **18**: 388–411.

_____, and B.R. Kaada 1952. Influence of stimulation of central nervous structures on muscle spindles in cat. *Acta Physiol. Scand.* **27**: 130–160.

Graybiel, A., E. Jokl, and C. Trapp 1955. Russian studies of vision in relation to physical activity and sports. *Res. Quart.* **26**: 480–485.

Greene, D., and M.T. Lepper 1974. How to turn play into work. *Psychol. Today* **8** (September): 49–54.

Greenspoon, J., and S. Foreman 1956. Effects of delay of knowledge of results on learning a motor task. *J. Exp. Psychol.* **51**: 226–228.

Greenwald, A.G. 1970. Sensory feedback mechanisms in performance control: with special reference to the ideo-motor mechanism. *Psychol. Rev.* **77**: 73–99.

Gregory, R.L., and J.G. Wallace 1963. Recovery from early blindness: a case study. *Exp. Psychol. Soc. Monogr.*, No. 2.

Grossman, S.P. 1967. *A textbook of physiological psychology*. New York: Wiley.

Guilford, J.P. 1958. A system of psychomotor abilities. *Am J. Psychol.* **71**: 164–174.

Guthrie, E.R. 1935. *The psychology of learning*. New York: Harper & Row.

Gutin, B., R.K. Fogle, J. Meyer, and M. Jaeger 1974. Steadiness as a function of prior exercise. *J. Motor Behav.* **6**: 69–76.

_____ 1970. Effect of systemic exertion on rotary pursuit and maze performance and learning. In G.S. Kenyon (ed.), *Contemporary psychology of sport*. Chicago: The Athletic Institute, pp. 565–575.

_____, and J. DiGennaro 1968. Effect of one-minute and five-minute step-ups on performance of simple addition. *Res. Quart.* **39**: 81–85.

_____ 1966. Effect of increase in physical fitness and mental ability following physical and mental stress. *Res. Quart.* **37**: 211–220.

Guyton, A.C. 1966. *Textbook of medical physiology*. (3rd ed.) Philadelphia: W.B. Saunders.

_____ 1964. *Function of the human body*. (2nd ed.) Philadelphia: W.B. Saunders.

Haas, M.A. 1966. *The relationship of kinesthetic acuity to bowling performance for beginners*. Unpublished doctoral dissertation. Iowa City, Iowa: State University of Iowa.

Hagbarth, K.E., and D.I.B. Kerr 1954. Central influences on spinal afferent conduction. *J. of Neurophysiol.* **17**: 295–307.

Haith, M.M. 1966. The response of the human newborn to visual movement. *J. Exp. Child Psychol.* **3**: 235–243.

Halstead, W., and W. Rucker 1968. Memory: a molecular maze. *Psychol. Today* **2** (June): 38–41.

Hamilton, E.L. 1929. The effect of delayed incentive on the hunger drive of the white rat. *Genetic Psychol. Monographs* **5**: 131–207.

Hampton, G. 1970. *The effects of manipulating two types of feedback, knowledge of performance and knowledge of results in learning a complex skill*. Unpublished doctoral dissertation. Teachers College, Columbia University.

Hanawalt, N.G. 1942. The effect of practice upon the perception of simple designs masked by more complex designs. *J. Exp. Psychol.* **31**: 134–148.

Hanley, E.A., B.H. Massey, C.A. Morehouse, and H.B. White, Jr. 1971. Skill acquisition by two body parts with concurrent practice. *Res. Quart.* **42**: 383–390.

Harari, H. 1969. Level of aspiration and athletic performance. *Percept. and Motor Skills* **28**: 519–524.

Hardy, J.D., H.G. Wolff, and H. Goodell 1952. *Pain sensations and reactions*. Baltimore: Williams and Wilkins.

Harlow, H.F. 1950. Learning and satiation of response in intrinsically motivated complex puzzle performance by monkeys. *J. Comp. Physiol. Psychol.* **43**: 289–294.

_____ 1949. The formation of learning sets. *Psychol. Rev.* **56**: 51–65.

Harmon, J.M., and J.B. Oxendine 1961. Effect of different lengths of practice periods on the learning of a motor skill. *Res. Quart.* **32**: 34–41.

_____, and W.R. Johnson 1952. The emotional reactions of college athletes. *Res. Quart.* **23**: 391–397.

_____, and A.G. Miller 1950. Time patterns in motor learning. *Res. Quart.* **21**: 182–187.

Hartley, L.H., J.W. Mason, R.P. Hogan, L.G. Jones, T.A. Kotchen, E.H. Mougey, F.E. Wherry, L.L. Pennington, and P.T. Ricketts 1972. Multiple hormonal responses to prolonged exercise in relation to physical training. *J. Appl. Physiol.* **33**: 607–610.

Haubenstricker, J.L., and D.C. Milne 1974. The relationship of selected measures of proprioception to physical growth, motor performance, and academic achievement in young children. Paper presented at AAHPER Convention, Anaheim.

Haywood, K.M., and H.L. Glad 1974. Relative effects of three knowledge of results treatments on the ability to perform a coincidence-anticipation task. Paper presented at the AAHPER Convention, Anaheim.

Hebb, D.O. 1972. *Textbook of psychology.* (3rd ed.) Philadelphia: W.B. Saunders.

_____ 1966. *A textbook of psychology.* (2nd ed.) Philadelphia: W.B. Saunders.

_____ 1955. Drives and C.N.S. (Conceptual nervous system). *Psychol. Rev.* **62**: 243–254.

_____ 1949. *The organization of behavior.* New York: Wiley.

Heider, F. 1958. *The psychology of interpersonal relations.* New York: Wiley.

Heimerer, E.M. 1968. *A study of the relationship between visual depth perception and general tennis ability.* Unpublished master's thesis. Greensboro, N.C.: University of North Carolina.

Held, R. 1965. Plasticity in sensory-motor systems. *Sci. Am.* **213** (November): 84–94.

_____, and S. Freedman 1963. Plasticity in human sensorimotor control. *Sci.* **142**: 455–462.

_____, and A. Hein 1963. Movement-produced stimulation in the development of visually guided behavior. *J. Comp. Physiol. Psychol.* **56**: 872–876.

Hellebrandt, F., and J. Waterland 1962. Expansion of motor patterning under exercise stress. *Am. J. Phys. Med.* **41**: 56–66.

_____, M. Schade, and M. Carns 1962. Methods of evoking the tonic neck reflexes in normal human subjects. *Am. J. Phys. Med.* **41**: 90–139.

Helson, J. 1964. *Adaptation-level theory.* New York: Harper & Row.

Hendrickson, G., and W.H. Schroeder 1941. Transfer of training in learning to hit a submerged target. *J. Educ. Psychol.* **32**: 205–213.

Henry, F.M. 1970. Individual differences in motor learning and performance. In L.E. Smith (ed.), *Psychology of motor learning*. Chicago: Athletic Institute, pp. 243–256.

_____, and J.S. Harrison 1961. Refractoriness of a fast movement. *Percept. and Motor Skills* **13**: 351–354.

_____, and L.E. Smith 1961. Simultaneous vs. separate bilateral muscular contractions in relation to neural overflow theory and neuromotor specificity. *Res. Quart.* **32**: 42–46.

_____ 1960. Influence of motor and sensory sets on reaction latency and speed of discrete movements. *Res. Quart.* **31**: 459–468.

_____, and D.E. Rogers 1960. Increased response latency for complicated movements and a memory drum theory of neuromotor reaction. *Res. Quart.* **31**: 448–458.

_____ 1958. Specificity vs. generality in learning motor skills. *61st Proceedings of the NCPEAM*, pp. 126–128.

_____ 1956. Coordination and motor learning. *59th Proceedings of the NCPEAM*, pp. 68–75.

_____ 1952. Force-time characteristics of the sprint start. *Res. Quart.* **23**: 301–318.

Hernandez-Peon, R., H. Scherrer, and M. Jouvet 1956. Modification of electric activity in cochlear nucleus during "attention" in unanesthetized cats. *Sci.* **123**: 331–332.

Heron, W. 1957. The pathology of boredom. *Sci. Am.* **196** (January): 52–56.

Hess, R. 1954. *Diencephalon—autonomic and extra-pyramidal functions*. New York: Grune and Stratton.

Hick, W.E. 1952. On the rate of gain of information. *Quart. J. Exp. Psychol.* **4**: 11–26.

_____ 1949. Reaction time for the amendment of a response. *Quart. J. Exp. Psychol.* **1**: 175–179.

Higgins, J.D., B. Tursky, and G.E. Schwartz 1971. Shock-elicited pain and its reduction by concurrent tactile stimulation. *Sci.* **172**: 866–867.

Higgins, J.R., and R.K. Spaeth 1972. Relationship between consistency of movement and environmental condition. *Quest* **17**: 61–69.

_____, and R.W. Angle 1970. Correction of tracking errors without sensory feedback. *J. Exp. Psychol.* **84**: 412–416.

Higgs, S.L. 1972. The effect of competition upon the endurance performance of college women. *Int. J. Sport Psychol.* **3**: 128–140.

Hilgard, E.R. 1957. *Introduction to psychology*. New York: Harcourt, Brace.

_____, E.M. Sait, and G.A. Margaret 1940. Level of aspiration as affected by relative standing in an experimental social group. *J. Exp. Psychol.* **27**: 411–421.

Hinrichs, J.R. 1970. Ability correlates in learning a psychomotor task. *J. Appl. Psychol.* **54**: 56–64.

Hodgkins, J. 1963. Reaction time and speed of movement in males and females of various ages. *Res. Quart.* **34**: 335–343.

_____ 1962. Influence of age on the speed of reaction and movement in females. *J. Geront.* **17**: 385–389.

Holding, D.H. 1965. *Principles of training.* New York: Pergamon Press.

_____ 1962. Transfer between difficult and easy tasks. *Brit. J. Psychol.* **53**: 397–407.

Holmes, G. 1939. The cerebellum in man. *Brain* **62**: 21–30.

Holson, R., and M.T. Henderson 1941. A preliminary study of visual fields in athletes. *Iowa Academy of Science* **48**: 331–337.

Holzman, P.S., and G.S. Klein 1954. Cognitive system—principles of leveling and sharpening: individual differences in assimilation effects in visual time-error. *J. Psychol.* **37**: 105–122.

Hopek, R. 1967. *Effect of overload on the accuracy of throwing a football.* Unpublished master's thesis. Charleston, Ill.: Eastern Illinois University.

Hopson, J., R. Cogan, and D. Batson 1971. Color preference as a function of background and illumination. *Percept. and motor skills* **33**: 1083–1088.

Hornak, J.E. 1971. *The effects of three methods of teaching on the learning of a motor skill.* Unpublished doctoral dissertation. Greeley, Colo.: University of Northern Colorado.

Houk, J., and E. Henneman 1967. Responses of Golgi tendon organs to active contractions of the soleus muscle of the cat. *J. of Neurophysiol.* **30**: 466–481.

Howard, I.P. 1968 Displacing the optical array. In S.J. Freedman (ed.), *The neuropsychology of spatially oriented behavior.* Homewood, Ill.: The Dorsey Press, pp. 19–36.

_____, and W.B. Templeton 1966. *Human spatial orientation.* New York: Wiley.

Howell, M.T. 1956. Use of force-time graphs for performance analysis in facilitating motor learning. *Res. Quart.* **27**: 12–22.

Hubbard, A.W., and C.M. Seng 1954. Visual movements of batters. *Res. Quart.* **25**: 42–57.

Hull, C. 1952. *A behavior system: an introduction to behavior theory covering the individual organism.* New Haven: Yale University Press.

_____ 1943. *Principles of behavior.* New York: Appleton-Century-Crofts.

Hunt, V. 1964. Movement behavior: a model for action. *Quest* **2**: 69–91.

Hutton, R.S. 1972. Neurosciences: mechanisms of motor control. In R.N. Singer (ed.), *The psychomotor domain: movement behavior.* Philadelphia: Lea and Febiger, pp. 349–384.

_____, J.L. Stevens, and F. Stevens 1972. The effect of strenuous and exhaustive exercise on learning: a theoretical note and preliminary findings. *J. Motor Behav.* **4**: 207–216.

Hyden, H. 1965. Activation of nuclear RNA in neurons and glia in learning. In D.P. Kimble (ed.), *The anatomy of memory.* Palo Alto, Calif.: Science and Behavior Books, pp. 178–239.

Hyman, R. 1953. Stimulus information as a determinant of reaction time. *J. Exp. Psychol.* **45**: 188–196.

Hymovitch, B. 1952. The effects of experimental variations on problem solving in the rat. *J. Comp. and Physiol. Psychol.* **45**: 313–320.

Irion, A.L. 1949. Reminiscence in pursuit-rotor learning as a function of length of rest and amount of prerest practice. *J. Exp. Psychol.* **39**: 492–499.

Ismail, A.H., J. Kane, and D.R. Kirkendall, 1969. Relationships among intellectual and nonintellectual variables. *Res. Quart.* **40**: 83–92.

_____, and J.J. Gruber 1967. *Motor aptitude and intellectual performance.* Columbus, Ohio: Charles E. Merrill.

Jabbur, S.J., S.F. Atweh, G.F. To'mey and N.R. Banna 1971. Visual and auditory inputs into the cuneate nucleus. *Sci.* **174**: 1146–1147.

Jacobs, B.L., and C.A. Sorenson 1969. Memory disruption in mice by brief posttrial immersion in hot or cold water. *J. Comp. and Physiol. Psychol.* **68**: 239–244.

Jacobson, E. 1938. *Progressive relaxation.* (2nd ed.) Chicago: University of Chicago Press.

_____ 1930. Electrical measurements of neuromuscular states during mental activities. II. Imagination and recollection of various muscular acts. *Am. J. Physiol.* **94**: 22–34.

Jahnke, J.C., and C.A. Duncan 1956. Reminiscence and forgetting in motor learning after extended rest intervals. *J. Exp. Psychol.* **52**: 273–282.

James, W. 1890. *The principles of psychology.* (2 vols.) New York: Holt.

Jansen, J.K.S., and T. Rudjord 1964. On the silent period and Golgi tendon organs of the soleus muscle of the cat. *Acta Physiol. Scand.* **62**: 364–379.

Jenkins, W.O., and J.C. Stanley, Jr. 1950. Partial reinforcement: a review and critique. *Psychol. Bull.* **47**: 193–234.

Jensen, B.E. 1975. Pretask speed training and movement complexity as factors in rotary-pursuit skill acquisition. *Res. Quart.* **46**: 1–11.

John, E.R. 1967. *Mechanisms of memory.* New York: Academic Press.

Johnson, B.L., Q.A. Christian, and T.W. Arterbury 1968. The effect of varied degrees of fatigue upon static balance performance. Paper presented at the AAHPER Convention, St. Louis.

Johnson, G.B. 1932. Physical skill tests for sectioning classes into homogeneous units. *Res. Quart.* **3** (March): 128–136.

Johnson, W.G. 1952. *Peripheral perception of athletes and nonathletes and the effect of practice.* Unpublished master's thesis. Urbana, Ill.: University of Illinois.

Jokl, E. 1958. *The clinical physiology of physical fitness and rehabilitation.* Springfield, Ill.: Charles C. Thomas.

Jones, B. 1974. The role of central monitoring of efference in short-term memory for movements. *J. Exp. Psychol.* **102**: 37–43.

Jordan, W.L. 1966. *The results of speed and accuracy emphases on the learning of a selected motor skill in golf.* Unpublished doctoral dissertation. Minneapolis: University of Minnesota.

Judd, C.H. 1908. The relation of special training to general intelligence. *Educ. Rev.* **36**: 28–42.

Kao, Dji-Lih 1937. Plateaus and the curve of learning in motor skills. *Psychol. Monographs* **49** (3): 1–81.

Kay, H. 1957. Information theory in the understanding of skills. *Occupat. Psychol.* **31**: 218–224.

Keele, S.W. 1973. *Attention and human performance.* Pacific Palisades, Calif.: Goodyear.

_____ 1968. Movement control in skilled motor performance. *Psychol. Bull.* **70**: 387–403.

_____, and M.I. Posner 1968. Processing of visual feedback in rapid movements. *J. Exp. Psychol.* **77**: 155–158.

_____ 1967. Compatibility and time-sharing in serial reaction time. *J. Exp. Psychol.* **75**: 529–539.

Keller, F.S. 1958. The phantom plateau. *J. Exp. Anal. Behav.* **1**: 1–13.

Keller, L.F. 1942. The relation of quickness of bodily movements to success in athletics. *Res. Quart.* **13**: 146–155.

Kelso, J.A.S., G.E. Stelmach, and W.M. Wanamaker 1974. Behavioral and neurological parameters of the nerve compression block. *J. Motor Behav.* **6**: 179–190.

Kennedy, D. 1967. Small systems of nerve cells. *Sci. Am.* **216** (May): 44–52.

Kennedy, W.A., and H.C. Willcutt 1964. Praise and blame as incentives. *Psychol. Bull.* **62**: 323–332.

Kerr, B.A. 1966. Relationship between speed of reaction and movement in a knee extension movement. *Res. Quart.* **37**: 55–60.

Kerr, D.I.B., and K.E. Hagbarth 1955. An investigation of olfactory centrifugal fiber system. *J. Neurophysiol.* **18**: 362–374.

Kientzle, M.J. 1946. Properties of learning curves under varied distributions of practice. *J. Exp. Psychol.* **36**: 187–211.

Kimble, D.P. 1963. *Physiological psychology: a unit for introductory psychology.* Reading, Mass.: Addison-Wesley.

Kimble, G.A. 1949. An experimental test of a two-factor theory of inhibition. *J. Exp. Psychol.* **39**: 15–23.

Klemmer, E.T. 1957. Simple reaction time as a function of time uncertainty. *J. Exp. Psychol.* **54**: 195–200.

Knapp, B.N. 1961. A note on skill. *Occupat. Psychol.* **35**: 76–78.

Knapp, C.G., and W.R. Dixon 1952. Learning to juggle. II. A study of whole and part methods. *Res. Quart.* **23**: 398–401.

Kohler, I. 1962. Experiments with goggles. *Sci. Am.* **206** (May): 62–72.

Kolers, P.A., and D.L. Zink 1962. Some aspects of problem solving: sequential analysis of the detection of embedded patterns. Technical Documentary Report No. AMRL-TDR-62-148, Project No. 7183, Task No. 718303, Wright-Patterson Air Force Base, Ohio.

Konorski, J. 1967. *Integrative activity of the brain.* Chicago: University of Chicago Press.

Korman, A.K. 1974. *The psychology of motivation.* Englewood Cliffs, N.J.: Prentice-Hall.

Kuypers, H.G.J.M. 1960. Central cortical projections to motor and somatosensory cell groups. *Brain* **83**: 161–184.

LaBarba, R. 1967. Differential response efficiency to simple kinesthetic and tactile stimuli. *Res. Quart.* **38**: 420–429.

Lacey, J.I. 1967. Somatic response patterning and stress: some revisions of activation theory. In M.H. Appley and R. Trumbull (eds.), *Psychological stress: issues in research.* New York: Appleton-Century-Crofts, pp. 14–37.

Lakatos, J.S. 1968. Eye dominance in batting performance. *Athl. J.* **49** (November): 76.

Landers, D., and D.M. Landers 1973. Teacher versus peer models: effects of model's presence and performance level on motor behavior. *J. Motor Behav.* **5**: 129–139.

Langley, L.L., I.R. Telford, and J.B. Christensen 1969. *Dynamic anatomy and physiology.* (3rd ed.) New York: McGraw-Hill.

Lansing, R.W., E. Schwartz, and D. Lindsley 1959. Reaction time and EEG activation under alerted and nonalerted conditions. *J. Exp. Psychol.* **58**: 1–7.

Larre, E.E. 1961. *Interpolated activity before and after knowledge of results.* Unpublished doctoral dissertation. New Orleans: Tulane University of Louisiana.

Lashley, K.S. 1951. The problem of serial order in behavior. In L.A. Jeffress (ed.), *Cerebral mechanisms in behavior.* New York: Wiley.

_____ 1950. In search of the engram. *Symp. Soc. Exp. Bio.* **4**: 454–483.

_____ 1917. The accuracy of movement in the absence of excitation from the moving organ. *Am. J. Physiol.* **43**: 169–194.

Laszlo, J.I., and P.J. Bairstow 1971. Accuracy of movement, peripheral feedback, and efference copy. *J. Motor Behav.* **3**: 241–252.

_____ 1967. Training of fast tapping with reduction of kinesthetic, tactile, visual, and auditory sensations. *Quart. J. Exp. Psychol.* **19**: 344–349.

_____ 1966. The performance of a simple motor task with kinesthetic sense loss. *Quart. J. Exp. Psychol.* **18**: 1–8.

Lavery, J.J. 1964. The effect of one-trial delay in knowledge of results on the acquisition and retention of a tossing skill. *Amer. J. Psychol.* **77**: 437–443.

_____, and F.H. Suddon 1962. Retention of simple motor skills as a function of the number of trials by which KR is delayed. *Percept. and Motor Skills* **15**: 231–237.

Lawler, E., and J.C. Suttle 1972. A causal correlational test of the need hierarchy concept. *Organ. Behav. and Human Perform.* **7**: 265–287.

Lawther, J.D. 1972. *Sport psychology.* Englewood Cliffs, N.J.: Prentice-Hall.

Lazarus, R.S., J. Deese, and S.F. Osler 1952. The effects of psychological stress upon performance. *Psychol. Bull.* **49**: 293–317.

Leonard, J.A. 1959. Tactual choice reactions: Part 1. *Quart. J. Exp. Psychol.* **11**: 76–83.

Lersten, K.C. 1969. Retention of skill on the rho apparatus after one year. *Res. Quart.* **40**: 418–419.

_____ 1968. Transfer of movement components in a motor learning task. *Res. Quart.* **39**: 575–581.

Levitt, M., M. Carreras, C.N. Liu, and W.W. Chambers 1964. Pyramidal and extra-pyramidal modulation of somatosensory activity in gracile and cuneate nuclei. *Arch. Ital. Biol.* **102**: 197–229.

Levitt, S. 1972. *The effects of exercise-induced activation upon simple, two-choice, and five-choice reaction time and movement time.* Unpublished doctoral dissertation. New York: Teachers College, Columbia University.

_____, and B. Gutin 1971. Multiple choice reaction time and movement time during physical exertion. *Res. Quart.* **42**: 405–410.

Lewellen, J.O. 1951. *A comparative study of two methods of teaching beginning swimming.* Unpublished doctoral dissertation. Stanford University.

Lewis, M. 1972. Culture and gender roles: there's no unisex in the nursery. *Psychol. Today* **5** (May): 54–57.

Li, Ch-L. 1958. Activity of interneurons in the motor cortex. In H.H. Jasper, L.D. Proctor, R.S. Knighton, W.C. Norsbay, and R.T. Costello (eds.), *Reticular formation of the brain.* Boston: Little, Brown.

Liebowitz, H.W., and S. Appelle 1969. The effect of a central task on luminance thresholds for peripherally presented stimuli. *Human Factors* **11**: 387–392.

Lincoln, R.S. 1956. Learning and retaining a rate of movement with the aid of kines-thetic and verbal cues. *J. Exp. Psychol.* **51**: 199–204.

Lindeburg, F.A., and J.E. Hewitt 1965. Effect of oversized basketball on shooting abil-ity and ball handling. *Res. Quart.* **36**: 164–167.

_____ 1949. A study of the degree of transfer between quickening exercises and other coordinated movements. *Res. Quart.* **20**: 180–195.

Lindsley, D.B. 1951. Emotion. In S.S. Stevens (ed.), *Handbook of experimental psy-chology.* New York: Wiley, pp. 473–516.

_____ 1957. Psychophysiology and motivation. In M.R. Jones (ed.), *Nebraska sym-posium on motivation.* Lincoln, Neb.: University of Nebraska Press, pp. 44–105.

Llewellyn, J.H. 1972. Effects of hand and eye dominance combinations on hitting per-formance. *VAHPER Research Journal* **1** (1): 8–11.

Llina, R.R. 1975. The cortex of the cerebellum. *Sci. Am.* **232** (January): 56–71.

Lloyd, A.J., and L.S. Caldwell 1965. Accuracy of active and passive positioning of the leg on the basis of kinesthetic cues. *J. Comp. Physiol. Psychol.* **60**: 102–106.

Lloyd, A.J., and J.H. Voor 1973. The effect of training on performance efficiency during a competitive isometric exercise. *J. Motor Behav.* **5**: 17–24.

Locke, E.A. 1968. Toward a theory of task motivation and incentives. *Organ. Behav. and Human Perform.* **3**: 157–189.

_____, N. Cartledge, and J. Koeppel 1968. Motivational effects of knowledge of results: a goal-setting phenomenon? *Psychol. Bull.* **70**: 474–485.

_____ 1967. Motivational effects of knowledge of results: knowledge or goal setting? *J. Appl. Psychol.* **51**: 324–329.

_____, and J.F. Bryan 1966a. Cognitive aspects of psychomotor performance: the effects of performance goals on level of performance. *J. Appl. Psychol.* **50**: 286–291.

_____, and J.F. Bryan 1966b. The effects of goal setting, rule learning, and knowledge of score on performance. *Am. J. Psychol.* **79**: 451–457.

Lockhart, A. 1966. Communicating with the learner. *Quest* **6**: 57–67.

Lordhal, D.S., and E.J. Archer 1958. Transfer effects on a rotary-pursuit task as a function of first task difficulty. *J. Exp. Psychol.* **56**: 421–426.

Lorge, I., and E.L. Thorndike 1935. The influence of delay in the aftereffect of a connection. *J. Exp. Psychol.* **18**: 186–194.

_____ 1930. *Influence of regularly interpolated time intervals upon subsequent learning.* Teachers College Contributions to Education, No. 438.

Lotter, W.S. 1961. Specificity or generality of speed of systematically related movements. *Res. Quart.* **32**: 55–62.

_____ 1960. Interrelationships among reaction times and speeds of movement in different limbs. *Res. Quart.* **31**: 147–155.

Loucks, J., and H. Thompson 1968. Effect of menstruation on reaction time. *Res. Quart.* **39**: 407–408.

Low, F.N. 1946. Some characteristics of peripheral visual performance. *Am. J. Physiol.* **146**: 573–584.

Ludvigh, E., and J.W. Miller 1958. Study of visual acuity during the ocular pursuit of moving test objects. I. Introduction. *J. Opt. Soc. Amer.* **48**: 799–802.

Lund, F.H. 1932. The dependence of eye-hand coordinations upon eye dominance. *Am. J. Psychol.* **44**: 756–762.

Luria, A.R. 1970. Functional organization of the brain. *Sci. Am.* **222** (March): 66–78.

_____ 1966. *Human brain and psychological processes.* New York: Harper & Row.

Lykken, D.T. 1968. Neuropsychology and psychophysiology in personality research. In E.F. Borgatta and W.W. Lambert (eds.), *Handbook of personality theory and research.* Chicago: Rand McNally, pp. 413–509.

Lynn, R.W. 1971. *Effects of massed and distributed practice on rate of learning of a fine and a gross perceptual-motor skill.* Unpublished master's thesis. University of Toledo.

McCloy, C.H. 1937. An analytical study of the stunt type test as a measure of motor educability. *Res. Quart.* **8** (Oct.): 46–55.

McConnel, J.K. 1957. Muscular co-ordination and the fear of pain. *Physiotherapy* **43**: 270–271.

McConnell, J.V. 1964. Cannibalism and memory in flatworms. *New Scientist* **21**: 465–468.

_____ 1962. Memory transfer through cannibalism in planarians. *J. Neuropsychiat.* **3** (Suppl. 1): 542–548.

McCoy, K.W. 1968. *The effect of varied speed and accuracy training upon a gross motor skill.* Unpublished doctoral dissertation. Laramie, Wyo.: University of Wyoming.

McDougall, W. 1912. *An introduction to social psychology.* (2nd ed.) London: Methuen.

McGaugh, J.C. 1965. Facilitation and impairment of memory storage processes. In D.P. Kimble (ed.), *The anatomy of memory.* Palo Alto, Calif.: Science and Behavior Book, pp. 240–291.

McGonnigal, J.D., and D.L. Santa Maria 1974. The effects of shock arousal upon fractionated reaction time. Paper presented at the AAHPER Convention, Anaheim.

McGuigan, F.J. 1959. The effect of precision, delay, and schedule of knowledge of results on performance. *J. Exp. Psychol.* **58**: 79–84.

McIntyre, J.S., W. Mostoway, R.A. Stojak, and M. Humphries 1972. Transfer of work decrement in motor learning. *J. Motor Behav.* **4**: 223–229.

McNaught, A.B., and R. Callander 1963. *Illustrated physiology.* Baltimore: Williams and Wilkins.

MacLean, P.D. 1949. Psychosomatic disease and the "visceral brain." *Psychosom. Med.* **11**: 338–353.

Magill, R.A. 1975. The effect of the length of and activity during the post-knowledge of results interval on the acquisition of a serial-motor task. Paper presented at the AAHPER Convention, Atlantic City, N.J.

_____ 1973. The post-KR interval: time and activity effects and the relationship of motor short-term memory theory. *J. Motor Behav.* **5**: 49–56.

Maharishi Mahesh Yogi 1969. *Maharishi Mahesh Yogi on the Bhagavad Gita: a new translation and commentary.* Baltimore: Penguin.

Mahut, H. 1964. The effects of subcortical electrical stimulation on discrimination learning in cats. *J. Comp. Physiol. Psychol.* **58**: 390–395.

Mail, P.D. 1965. *The influence of binocular depth perception in the learning of a motor skill.* Unpublished master's thesis. Northampton, Mass.: Smith College.

Malina, R.M. 1969. Effects of varied information feedback practice conditions on throwing speed and accuracy. *Res. Quart.* **40**: 134–145.

Malmo, R.B. 1959. Activation: a neuropsychological dimension. *Psychol. Rev.* **66**: 367–386.

_____ 1957. Anxiety and behavioral arousal. *Psychol. Rev.* **64**: 276–287.

Manolis, G.G. 1955. Relation of charging time to blocking performance in football. *Res. Quart.* **26**: 170–178.

Marshall, H.H. 1965. The effect of punishment on children: a review of the literature and a suggested hypothesis. *J. Gen. Psychol.* **106**: 23–33.

Marteniuk, R.G., and H.A. Wenger 1970. Facilitation of pursuit motor learning by induced stress. *Percept. and Motor Skills* **31**: 471–477.

_____ 1969a. Generality and specificity of learning and performance on two similar speed tasks. *Res. Quart.* **40**: 518–522.

_____ 1969b. Differential effects of shock arousal on motor performance. *Percept. and Motor Skills* **29**: 443–447.

Martens, R. 1974. Arousal and motor performance. In J.H. Wilmore (ed.), *Exercise and sport science reviews.* (Vol. 2.) New York: Academic Press, pp. 155–188.

_____, L. Burwitz, and K.M. Newell 1972. Money and praise: do they improve motor learning and performance? *Res. Quart.* **43**: 429–442.

_____, and D.M. Landers 1972. Evaluation potential as a determinant of coaction effects. *J. Exp. Soc. Psychol.* **8**: 347–359.

_____ 1971. Anxiety and motor behavior: a review. *J. Motor Behav.* **3**: 151–179.

_____ 1969. Effect of an audience on learning and performance of a complex motor skill. *J. of Pers. and Soc. Psychol.* **12**: 252–260.

Martin, W. 1970. What the coach should know about vision. Paper presented at the 3rd Annual Sports Medicine Seminar, Seattle.

Maslow, A.H. 1970. *Motivation and personality.* (2nd ed.) New York: Harper & Row.

Matthews, P.B.C. 1972. *Mammalian muscle receptors and their central actions.* Baltimore: Williams and Wilkins.

Matzl, N.R. 1966. *Response comparisons of football players, tennis players, and nonathletes.* Unpublished master's thesis. Normal, Ill.: Illinois State University.

Mayer, D.J., T.L. Wolfle, H. Akil, B. Carder, and J.C. Liebeskind 1971. Analgesia from electrical stimulation in the brainstem of the rat. *Sci.* **174**: 1351–1354.

Meday, H.W. 1952. *The influence of practice on kinesthetic discrimination.* Unpublished master's thesis. University of California.

Mednick, S.A. 1964. *Learning.* Englewood Cliffs, N.J.: Prentice-Hall.

Meek, F.L. 1970. *Relationship of motor performance and field independence of girls as measured by the rod and frame test.* Unpublished master's thesis. Santa Barbara: University of California.

Melnick, M.J. 1971. Effects of overloading on the retention of a gross motor skill. *Res. Quart.* **42**: 60–69.

Melzack, R. 1973. *The puzzle of pain.* New York: Basic Books.

_____, and K.L. Casey 1967. Sensory, motivational, and central control determinants of pain. In D.R. Kenshalo (ed.) *International symposium on skin senses.* Springfield, Ill.: Charles C. Thomas, pp. 423–439.

_____, and P.D. Wall 1965. Pain mechanisms: a new theory. *Science* **150**: 971–979.

Mengelkoch, R.F., J.A. Adams, and C.A. Gainer 1971. The forgetting of instrument flying skills. *Human Factors* **13**: 397–405.

Merton, P.A. 1972. How we control the contraction of our muscles. *Sci. Am.* **226** (May): 30–37.

_____ 1964. Human position sense and sense of effort. *Symposium Soc. Exp. Biol.* **18**: 387–400.

Merkel, J. 1885. Die zeitlichen Verhältnisse der Willensthaligkeit. *Philos. St.* **2**: 73–127.

Meyers, C., W. Zimmerli, S.D. Farr, and N.A. Baschnagle 1969. Effect of strenuous physical activity upon reaction time. *Res. Quart.* **40**: 332–337.

Meyers, J.L. 1967. Retention of balance coordination learning as influenced by extended layoffs. *Res. Quart.* **38**: 72–78.

Miles, W.R., and B.C. Graves 1931. Studies in exertion. III Effect of signal variation on football charging. *Res. Quart.* **2** (Oct.): 14–31.

Miller, D.M. 1960. *The relationship between some visual-perceptual factors and the degree of success realized by sports performers.* Unpublished doctoral dissertation. Los Angeles: University of Southern California.

Miller, G.A., R. Galanter, and K.H. Pribram 1960. *Plans and the structure of behavior.* New York: Holt.

Miller, J.W. and E.J. Ludvigh 1962. The effect of relative motion on visual acuity. *Surv. Ophth.* **7**: 83–116.

Miller, N.E., and J. Dollard 1941. *Social learning and imitation.* New Haven: Yale University Press.

Milner, B. 1964. Some effects of frontal lobectomy in man. In J.M. Warren and K. Akert (eds.), *The frontal granual cortex and behavior.* New York: McGraw-Hill, pp. 313–334.

Milner, P.M. 1970. *Physiological psychology.* New York: Holt, Rinehart and Winston.

Mitchell, W.M. 1972. *The use of hypnosis in athletics.* Printed by Valley Oaks Printers, Stockton, Calif.

Mohr, D.R., and M.E. Barrett 1962. Effect of knowledge of mechanical principles in learning to perform intermediate swimming skills. *Res. Quart.* **33**: 574–580.

_____ 1960. The contributions of physical activity to skill learning. *Res. Quart.* **31**: 321–350.

Montebello, R.A. 1953. *The role of stereoscopic vision in some aspects of baseball playing ability.* Unpublished master's thesis. Columbus: The Ohio State University.

Montgomery, R.A. 1961. *The effects of knowledge and application of the mechanical principles of force and projection upon selected physical performance test items.* Unpublished doctoral dissertation. Greeley, Colo.: University of Northern Colorado.

Moray, N. 1970. *Attention: selective processes in vision and hearing.* London: Hutchinson.

Morehouse, L.E. and P.J. Rasch 1963. *Sports medicine for trainers.* (2nd ed.) Philadelphia: W.B. Saunders.

Morgan, W.P. 1974. Selected psychological considerations in sport. *Res. Quart.* **45**: 374–390.

Morrell, F. 1961. Lasting changes in synaptic organization produced by continuous neuronal bombardment. In J.F. Delafresnaye (ed.), *Brain mechanisms and learning.* Blackwell: Oxford.

Morris, G.S. 1974. *The effects ball color and background color have upon the catching performance of second, fourth, and sixth grade youngsters.* Unpublished doctoral dissertation. Eugene, Ore.: University of Oregon.

Mortier, L.C. 1971. *The effects of praise and punishment motivation as evidenced by college football athletes in tension-producing situations involving competition on a gross motor task.* Unpublished master's thesis. Macmob, Ill.: Western Illinois University.

Moruzzi, G., and H.W. Magoun 1949. Brainstem reticular formation and activation of the EEG. *Electroencephalog. and Clin. Neurophysiol.* **1**: 455–473.

Mott, F.W., and C.S. Sherrington 1895. Experiments upon the influence of sensory nerves upon movement and nutrition of the limbs: preliminary communication. *Proceedings of the Royal Society of London* **57**: 481–488.

Mowbray, G.H. 1960. Choice reaction times for skilled responses. *Quart. J. Exp. Psychol.* **12**: 193–202.

_____, and M.V. Rhoades 1959. On the reduction of choice reaction time with practice. *Quart J. Exp. Psychol.* **11**: 16–23.

Mowrer, O.H. 1960. *Learning theory and behavior.* New York: Wiley.

Müller, G.E., and A. Pilzecker 1900. Experimentelle Beiträge zur Legre vom Gedächtniss. *Zeitschrift für Psychologie und Physiologie der Sinnesorgane,* Erganzungsband **1**: 1–288.

Müller, J. 1842. *Elements of physiology.* Taylor.

Mumby, H.H. 1953. Kinesthetic acuity and balance related to wrestling ability. *Res. Quart.* **24**: 327–334.

Munn, N.L. 1932. Bilateral transfer of learning. *J. Exp. Psychol.* **15**: 343–353.

Munro, S.J. 1951. The retention of the increase in speed of movement transferred from a motivated simpler response. *Res. Quart.* **22**: 229–233.

Namikas, G., and E.J. Archer 1960. Motor skill transfer as a function of intertask interval and pretransfer task difficulty. *J. Exp. Psychol.* **59**: 109–112.

Nance, R.D. 1946. *The effects of pacing and distribution on intercorrelations of motor abilities.* Unpublished doctoral dissertation. Iowa City: Iowa State University.

Naylor, J.C., and G.E. Briggs 1961. Long-term retention of learned skills, and review of the literature. *Lab. of Aviation Psychology,* Ohio State University Research Foundation.

Nelson, D.O. 1957a. Effect of swimming on the learning of selected gross motor skills. *Res. Quart.* **28**: 374–378.

_____ 1957b. Study of transfer of training in gross motor skills. *Res. Quart.* **28**: 364–373.

Nelson, J.K. 1962. *An analysis of the effects of applying various motivational situations to college men subjected to a stressful physical performance.* Unpublished doctoral dissertation. Eugene, Ore.: University of Oregon.

Nelson, R.C., and R.A. Fahrney 1965. Relationships between strength and speeds of elbow flexion. *Res. Quart.* **36**: 455–463.

———, and M.R. Nofsinger 1965. Effect of overload on speed of elbow flexion and the associated aftereffects. *Res. Quart.* **36**: 174–182.

Nessler, J. 1973. Length of time necessary to view a ball while catching it. *J. Motor Behavior* **5**: 179–185.

Newell, A., J.D. Shaw, and H.A. Simon 1958. Elements of a theory of human problem solving. *Psychol. Rev.* **65**: 151–166.

Newell, K.M. 1974. Knowledge of results and motor learning. *J. Motor Behavior* **6**: 235–244.

Niemeyer, R.K. 1959. Part versus whole methods and massed versus distributed practice in the learning of selected large muscle activities. *62nd Proceedings of the NCPEAM*, pp. 122–125.

Nissen, H.W., K.L. Chow, and J. Semmes 1951. Effects of restricted opportunity for tactual, kinesthetic, and manipulative experience on the behavior of chimpanzees. *Amer. J. Psychol.* **64**: 485–507.

Nixon, J.E., and L.F. Locke 1973. Research on teaching physical education. In R.M.W. Travers (ed.), *Second handbook of research on teaching.* Chicago: Rand McNally, pp. 1210–1242.

Noback, C.R. 1967. *The human nervous system.* New York: McGraw-Hill.

Noble, C.E. 1966. Selection learning. In E.A. Bilodeau (ed.), *Acquisition of skill.* New York: Academic Press, pp. 47–97.

Noble, D. 1966. Unpublished data, Loughborough University of Technology. Reported in H.T.A. Whiting, *Acquiring ball skill.* Philadelphia: Lea and Febiger, 1969.

Norrie, M.L. 1967. Practice effects on reaction latency for simple and complex movements. *Res. Quart.* **38**: 79–85.

Nunney, D.N. 1963. Fatigue, impairment, and psychomotor learning. *Percept. and Motor Skills* **16**: 369–375.

Ogawa, T. 1963. Midbrain reticular influences upon single neurons in lateral geniculate nucleus. *Sci.* **139**: 343–344.

Olds, J.S. 1956. Pleasure centers in the brain. *Sci. Am.* **195** (October): 105–116.

———, and P. Milner 1954. Positive reinforcement produced by electrical stimulation of septal area and other regions of the rat brain. *J. Comp. Physiol. Psychol.* **47**: 419–427.

Olsen, E.A. 1956. Relationship between psychological capacities and success in college athletics. *Res. Quart.* **27**: 79–89.

Oscarsson, O., and I. Rosen 1966. Short latency projections to the cat's cerebral cortex from skin and muscle afferents in the contralateral forelimb. *J. Physiol.* **182**: 164–184.

_____, and I. Rosen 1963. Projection to cerebral cortex of large muscle afferents in forelimb nerves of the cat. *J. Physiol.* **169**: 924–945.

Osgood, C.E., and P.H. Tannenbaum 1955. The principle of congruity in the prediction of attitude change. *Psychol. Rev.* **62**: 42–55.

Overton, D. 1969. High education. *Psychol. Today* **3** (November): 48–51.

Oxendine, J.B. 1970. Emotional arousal and motor performance. *Quest* **13**: 23–32.

_____ 1969. Effect of mental and physical practice on the learning of three motor skills. *Res. Quart.* **40**: 755–763.

_____ 1968. *Psychology of motor learning.* New York: Appleton-Century-Crofts.

_____ 1967. Generality and specificity in the learning of fine and gross motor skills. *Res. Quart.* **38**: 86–94.

_____ 1965. Effect of progressively changing practice schedules on the learning of a motor skill. *Res. Quart.* **36**: 307–315.

Pack, M., D.J. Cotten, and J. Biasiotto 1974. Effect of four fatigue levels on performance and learning of a novel dynamic balance skill. *J. Motor Behavior* **6**: 179–190.

Paillard, J., and M. Brouchon 1968. Active and passive movements in the calibration of position sense. In S.J. Freedman (ed.), *The neuropsychology of spatially oriented behavior.* Homewood, Ill.: The Dorsey Press, pp. 37–55.

_____ 1960. The patterning of skilled movements. In J. Field (ed.), *Handbook of physiology: neurophysiology*, Section 1, Volume III. Washington: American Physiological Society.

Palermo, D.S. 1961. Relation between anxiety and two measures of speed in a reaction time task. *Child Dev.* **32**: 401–408.

Papcsy, F.E. 1968. *The effect of understanding a specific mechanical principle upon learning a physical education skill.* Unpublished doctoral dissertation. New York University.

Papez, J.W. 1937. A proposed mechanism of emotion. *Arch. Neurol. Psychiat.* **38** (Chicago): 725–743.

Parke, R.D. 1969. Some effects of punishment on children's behavior. *Young Children* **24**: 225–240.

Parker, J.F., and E.A. Fleishman 1961. Use of analytical information concerning task requirements to increase the effectiveness of skill training. *J. Appl. Psychol.* **45**: 295–302.

Patrick, J. 1971. The effect of interpolated motor activities in short-term motor memory. *J. Motor Behavior* **3**: 39–48.

Payne, R. 1970. Factor analysis of a Maslow-type need satisfaction questionnaire. *Personnel Psychol.* **23**: 251–268.

Penfield, W. 1958. *The excitable cortex in conscious man.* Liverpool: Liverpool University Press.

Percival, L. 1971a. The coach from the athlete's viewpoint. In J.W. Taylor (ed.), *Proceedings of the first international symposium on the art and science of coaching.* Willowdale, Ontario: F.I. Productions, pp. 285–326, 350.

_____ 1971b. Question clinic and commentary on Part 2. In J.W. Taylor (ed.), *Proceedings of the first international symposium on the art and science of coaching.* Willowdale, Ontario: F.I. Productions.

Petrie, A. 1967. *Individuality in pain and suffering.* Chicago: University of Chicago Press.

Pew, R.W. 1966. Acquisition of hierarchical control over the temporal organization of a skill. *J. Exp. Psychol.* **71**: 764–771.

Phillips, B.E. 1941. The relationship between certain phases of kinesthesis and performance during the early stages of acquiring two perceptuo-motor skills. *Res. Quart.* **12**: 571–586.

Phillips, M., and D. Summers 1954. Relation of kinesthetic perception to motor learning. *Res. Quart.* **25**: 456–469.

Phillips, M.I. 1972. Pain tolerance and personality in athletes. *Medicine and Science in Sports* **4** (Winter): 7.

Phillips, W.H. 1963. Influence of fatiguing warm-up exercises on speed of movement and reaction latency. *Res. Quart.* **34**: 370–378.

_____ 1962. *The effects of physical fatigue on two motor learning tasks.* Unpublished doctoral dissertation. University of California.

Pick, A.D. 1965. Improvement of visual and tactual form discrimination. *J. Exp. Psychol.* **69**: 331–339.

Picton, T.W., S.A. Hillyard, R. Galambos, and M. Schiff 1971. Human auditory attention: a central or peripheral process? *Sci.* **173**: 351–353.

Pierson, W.R., and P.S. Rasch 1959. Determination of representative score for simple reaction and movement time. *Percept. and Motor Skills* **9**: 107–110.

Pineda, A., and M. Adkisson 1961. Electroencephalographic studies in physical fatigue. *Texas Reports in Biology and Medicine* **19**: 332–342.

Poortmans, J.R. 1969. *Biochemistry of exercise.* New York: S. Karger.

Poppelreuter, A. 1928. Analysis der Erziehung zur Exaktheitsarbeit nach experimental-psychologischer Methode. *Zeitschrift für Angewandte Psychologie, Band* **29**.

Posner, M.I., and S.W. Keele 1973. Skill learning. In R.M. Travers (ed.), *Second handbook of research on teaching.* Chicago: Rand McNally, pp. 805–831.

_____ 1967. Characteristics of visual and kinesthetic memory codes. *J. Exp. Psychol.* **75**: 103–107.

_____, and A.F. Konick 1966. Short-term retention of visual and kinesthetic information. *Organizational Behav. and Human Perf.* **1**: 71–86.

_____, and E. Rossman 1965. Effect of size and location of informational transforms upon short-term memory. *J. Exp. Psychol.* **70**: 496–505.

Poulton, E.C. 1965. Skill in fast ball games. *Bio. and Human Affairs* **3**: 1–5.

_____ 1957. On prediction in skilled movements. *Psychol. Bull.* **54**: 467–478.

Powers, W.T. 1973. Feedback: beyond behaviorism. *Sci.* **179**: 351–356.

Price, N. 1960. *The relationship between the level of aspiration and performance in selected motor tasks.* Unpublished master's thesis. Women's College, University of North Carolina.

Provins, K.A., and D.J. Glencross 1968. Handwriting, typewriting, and handedness. *Quart. J. Exp. Psychol.* **20**: 282–289.

Puni, A.T. 1956. Problem of voluntary regulation of motor activity in sports. In A. Ferruccio (ed.), *Proceedings of the 1st international congress of sport psychology.* pp. 103–113.

Purdy, B.J., and A. Lockhart 1962. Retention and relearning of gross motor skills after long periods of no practice. *Res. Quart.* **33**: 265–272.

Putnam, P. 1972. Experience may not be necessary. *Sports Illustrated* **37** (August 28): 36–39.

Ragsdale, E.C. 1930. *The psychology of motor learning.* Ann Arbor, Mich.: Edward Bros.

Ranson, S.W. 1939. Somnolence caused by hypothalamic lesions in the monkey. *Arch. Neurol. Psychiat.* **41**: 1–23.

Read, D.A. 1969. *The influence of competitive and noncompetitive programs of physical education on body-image and self-concept.* Unpublished doctoral dissertation. Boston University.

Reynolds, B., and J.A. Adams 1953. Motor performance as a function of click reinforcements. *J. Exp. Psychol.* **45**: 315–320.

Richardson, A. 1967a. Mental practice: a review and discussion, part I. *Res. Quart.* **38**: 95–107.

_____ 1967b. Mental practice: a review and discussion, part II. *Res. Quart.* **38**: 263–273.

Ridini, L.M. 1968. Relationships between psychological functions tests and selected sports skills of boys in junior high school. *Res. Quart.* **39**: 674–683.

Riesen, A.H., R.L. Ramsay, and P.D. Wilson 1964. Development of visual acuity in Rhesus monkeys deprived of patterned light during early infancy. *Psychon. Sci.* **1**: 33–34.

_____ 1960. The effects of stimulus deprivation on the development and atrophy of the visual sensory system. *Am. J. Orthopsychiat.* **30**: 23–36.

Robb, M.D. 1972. *The dynamics of motor-skill acquisition.* Englewood Cliffs, N.J.: Prentice-Hall.

_____ 1968. Feedback and skill learning. *Res. Quart.* **39**: 175–184.

Roberts, W.H. 1930. The effect of delayed feeding on white rats in a problem cage. *J. Genet. Psychol.* **37**: 35–58.

Robinson, E.S. 1927. The "similarity" factor in retroaction. *Am. J. Psychol.* **39**: 297–312.

Robinson, J.S. 1955. The effect of learning verbal labels for stimuli on their later discrimination. *J. Exp. Psychol.* **49**: 112–114.

Rock, I., and C.S. Harris 1967. Vision and touch. *Sci. Am.* **216** (May): 96–104.

Rogers, C.A., Jr. 1974. Feedback precision and postfeedback interval duration. *J. Exp. Psychol.* **102**: 604–608.

Roloff, L. 1953. Kinesthesis in relation to the learning of selected motor skills. *Res. Quart.* **24**: 210–217.

Rose, J.E., and V.B. Mountcastle 1959. Touch and kinesthesis. In J. Field (ed.), *Handbook of physiology: neurophysiology*, Section I (Vol. I). Washington, D.C. American Physiological Society, pp. 387–429.

Rose, M.C., and H.L. Glad 1974. Relationship of some traditional methods and a unique procedure for measuring kinesthesis. Paper presented at AAHPER Convention, Anaheim.

Rosen, B.C., and R. D'Andrade 1959. The psychosocial origins of achievement motivation. Sociometry **22**: 185–218.

Rosenzweig, M.R., E.L. Bennett, and M.C. Diamond 1972. Brain changes in response to experience. *Sci. Am.* **226** (February): 22–29.

Ross, S., T.A. Hussman, and T.G. Andrews 1954. Effects of fatigue and anxiety on certain psychomotor and visual functions. *J. of Appl. Psychol.* **38**: 119–125.

Rothstein, A.L. 1973. Effect on temporal expectancy of the position of a selected foreperiod within a range. *Res. Quart.* **44**: 132–139.

Routtenberg, A. 1968. The two-arousal hypothesis: reticular formation and limbic system. *Psychol. Rev.* **75**: 51–80.

Rubin, E. 1958. Figure and ground. In D.C. Beardslee and M. Wertheimer (eds.), *Readings in perception*, Princeton: Van Nostrand, pp. 194–203.

Ruch, T.C., and J.F. Fulton (eds.) 1960. *Medical physiology and biophysics.* (18th ed.) Philadelphia: W.B. Saunders.

_____ 1951. Motor systems. In S.S. Stevens (ed.), *Handbook of experimental psychology*. Wiley, pp. 154–208.

Rushall, B.S., and D. Siedentop 1972. *The development and control of behavior in sport and physical education*. Philadelphia: Lea and Febiger.

Russell, W.R. 1959. *Brain: memory and learning*. London: Oxford University Press.

Ryan, E.D. 1969. Perceptual characteristics of vigorous people. In B.J. Cratty and R.C. Brown (eds.), *New perspectives of man in action*. Englewood Cliffs, N.J.: Prentice-Hall, pp. 88–101.

_____, and R. Foster 1967. Athletic participation and perceptual augmentation and reduction. *J. Personality and Soc. Psychol.* **6**: 472–476.

_____, and R.C. Kovacic 1966. Pain tolerance and athletic participation. *Percept. and Motor Skills* **22**: 383–390.

_____ 1965. Retention of stabilometer performance over extended periods of time. *Res. Quart.* **36**: 46–51.

_____ 1962. Retention of stabilometer and pursuit-motor skills. *Res. Quart.* **33**: 593–598.

_____ 1961a. Motor performance under stress as a function of the amount of practice. *Percept. and Motor Skills* **13**: 103–106.

_____ 1961b. Effect of differential motive-incentive conditions on physical performance. *Res. Quart.* **32**: 83–87.

Sackett, G.P. 1965. Effects of rearing conditions upon the behavior of Rhesus monkeys. *Child Devel.* **36**: 855–868.

Sage, G.H., and B. Bennett 1973. The effects of induced arousal on learning and performance of a pursuit motor skill. *Res. Quart.* **44**: 140–149.

Salmoni, A.G. 1975. Attention demands of a linear motor response. Unpublished study. Reported in R.A. Schmidt (ed.), *Motor skills*. New York: Harper & Row.

Samuels, I. 1959. Reticular mechanisms and behavior. *Psychol. Bull.* **56**: 1–25.

Sartain, A.Q., A.J. North, J.R. Strange, and H.M. Chapman 1962. *Psychology: understanding human behavior*. (2nd ed.) New York: McGraw-Hill.

Scannell, R.J. 1968. Transfer of accuracy training when difficulty is controlled by varying target size. *Res. Quart.* **39**: 341–350.

Schachter, S., and L. Wheeler 1962. Epinephrine, chlorpromazine, and amusement. *J. Abn. Soc. Psychol.* **56**: 121–128.

_____, and J.E. Singer 1962. Cognitive, social, and physiological determinants of emotional state. *Psychol. Rev.* **69**: 379–399.

Schildkraut, J. J., and S. S. Kety 1967. Biogenic amines and emotion. *Sci.* **156**: 21–30.

Schlesinger, H.J. 1954. Cognitive attitudes in relation to susceptibility to interference. *J. Personality* **22**: 354–374.

Schlosburg, H. 1954. Three dimensions of emotion. *Psychol. Rev.* **61**: 81–88.

Schmidt, R.A. 1975. *Motor skills*. New York: Harper & Row.

_____, and J.L. White 1972. Evidence for an error detection mechanism in motor skills: a test of Adams's closed-loop theory. *J. Motor Behav.* **4**: 143–153.

_____ 1972. Experimental psychology. In R.N. Singer (ed.), *The psychomotor domain: movement behavior*. Philadelphia: Lea and Febiger, pp. 18–55.

_____ 1971. Retroactive interference and amount of original learning in verbal and motor tasks. *Res. Quart.* **42**: 314–326.

_____ 1969. Performance and learning of a gross motor skill under conditions of artificially induced fatigue. *Res. Quart.* **40**: 185–190.

Schramm, V. 1967. *An investigation of the electromyographic responses obtained during mental practice*. Master's thesis. Madison, Wisc.: University of Wisconsin.

Schultz, D.D. 1965. *Sensory restriction: effects on behavior*. New York: Academic Press.

Schultz, J.A. 1956. *Das autogenne training, Konzentrative Selbstentspannung* (The self-training, the concentrative self-relaxation). Stuttgart, West Germany.

Schwartz, R.M. 1968. *The effects of various degrees of muscular work upon depth perception*. Unpublished master's thesis. University of Toledo.

Schwartz, S. 1972. A learning-based system to categorize teacher behavior. *Quest* **17**: 52–55.

Schwarz, D.W.F., and J.M. Fredrickson 1971. Rhesus monkey vestibular cortex: a bimodal primary projection field. *Sci* **172**: 280–281.

Scott, M.G. 1955. Measurement of kinesthesis. *Res. Quart.* **26**: 324–341.

_____ 1954. Learning rate of beginning swimmers. *Res. Quart.* **25**: 91–99.

Seashore, R.J., B.J. Underwood, R. Houston, and L. Berks 1949. The influence of knowledge of results on performance. Unpublished manuscript. See B.J. Underwood, *Experimental psychology*. New York: Appleton-Century-Crofts.

Semmes, J. 1965. A nontactual factor in asterognosis. *Neuropsychologia* **3**: 295–315.

_____, S. Weinstein, L. Ghent, and H.L.Teuber 1955. Spatial orientation in man after cerebral injury. I. Analysis by locus of lesion. *J. Psychol.* **39**: 227–244.

Shaffer, L.J., and J. Hardwick 1968. Typing performance as a function of text. *Quart. J. Exp. Psychol.* **20**: 360–369.

Shay, C.T. 1934. The progressive-part versus the whole method of learning motor skills. *Res. Quart.* **5** (Dec.): 62–67.

Shea, J.B. 1975. Interresponse interval length and the development of an error detection mechanism: a test of Adams's closed-loop theory of motor learning. Paper presented at the AAHPER Convention, Atlantic City, N.J.

Sherrington, C.S. 1906a. On the proprioceptive system, especially in its reflex aspect. *Brain* **29**: 467–482.

_____ 1906b. *The integrative action of the nervous system*. New Haven: Yale University Press.

Shick, J. 1971. Relationship between depth perception and hand-eye dominance and freethrow shooting in college women. *Percept. and Motor Skills* **33**: 539–542.

_____ 1970. Effects of mental practice on selected volleyball skills for college women. *Res. Quart.* **41**: 88–94.

Shimazu, H., N. Yanagisawa, and B. Garoutte 1965. Corticopyramidal influences on thalamic somatosensory transmission in the cat. *Japanese J. Physiol.* **15**: 101–124.

Siedentop, D., and F. Rife 1975. Behavior management skills for physical education teachers. *78th Proceedings of the NCPEAM*, pp. 167–174.

Sills, R.D., and D.C Troutman 1966. Peripheral vision and accuracy in shooting a basketball. *69th Proceedings of the NCPEAM*, pp. 112–114.

Sinclair, C.B., and I.M. Smith 1957. Laterality in swimming and its relationship to dominance of hand, eye, and foot. *Res. Quart.* **28**: 395–402.

Singer, R.N. 1968a. Interrelationship of physical, perceptual-motor, and academic achievement variables in elementary school children. *Percept. and Motor Skills* **27**: 1323–1332.

_____ 1968b. Sequential skill learning and retention effects in volleyball. *Res. Quart.* **39**: 185–194.

_____, and J.W. Brunk 1967. Relation of perceptual-motor ability and intellectual ability in elementary school children. *Percept. and Motor Skills* **24**: 967–970.

_____ 1966. Transfer effects and ultimate success in archery due to degree of difficulty of the initial learning. *Res. Quart.* **37**: 532–539.

_____ 1966. Interlimb skill ability in motor skill performance. *Res. Quart.* **37**: 406–410.

_____ 1965. Massed and distributed practice effects on the acquisition and retention of a novel basketball skill. *Res. Quart.* **36**: 68–77.

Sjoberg, H., 1968. Relations between different arousal levels induced by graded physical work and psychological efficiency. Report from the Psychological Laboratories, No. 251, University of Stockholm, Sweden, April.

Skinner, B.F. 1938. *The behavior of organisms.* New York: Appleton-Century-Crofts.

Skoglung, S. 1956. Anatomical and physiological studies of knee joint innervation in the cat. *Acta Physiol. Scand.* **36** (suppl. 124): 1–101.

Slater-Hammel, A.T. 1955. Reaction time to light stimulus in the peripheral visual field. *Res. Quart.* **26**: 82–87.

Slevin, R.L. 1971. The influence of trait and state anxiety upon the performance of a novel gross motor task under conditions of competition and audience. Paper presented at the AAHPER Convention, Detroit.

Smith, A. 1975. Sport is a Western yoga. *Psychol. Today* **9** (October): 48–51, 74–76.

Smith, E.E. 1968. Choice reaction time: an analysis of the major theoretical positions. *Psychol. Bull.* **69**: 77–110.

Smith, J.L. 1969. Kinesthesis: a model for movement feedback. In R.C. Brown and B.J. Cratty (eds.), *New perspectives of man in action.* Englewood Cliffs, N.J.: Prentice-Hall, pp. 31–50.

Smith, K.U. 1966. Cybernetic theory and analysis of learning. In E.A. Bilodeau (ed.), *Acquisition of skill.* New York: Academic Press, pp. 425–482.

_____ 1962. *Delayed sensory feedback and behavior.* Philadelphia: W.B. Saunders.

_____, and W.M. Smith 1962. *Perception and motion.* Philadelphia: W.B. Saunders.

Smith, L.E. 1961. Reaction time and movement time in four large muscle movements. *Res. Quart.* **32**: 88–92.

Smith, P.E. 1968. *Investigation of total body and arm measures of reaction time, movement time, and completion time for twelve-, fourteen-, and seventeen-year-old athletes and nonparticipants.* Doctoral dissertation. Eugene, Ore.: University of Oregon.

Smith, W.M. 1972. Feedback: real-time delayed vision of one's own tracking behavior. *Sci.* **176**: 939–940.

Smode, A. 1958. Learning and performance in a tracking task under two levels of achievement information feedback. *J. Exp. Psychol.* **56**: 297–304.

Smoll, F.L. 1972. Effects of precision of information feedback upon acquisition of a motor skill. *Res. Quart.* **43**: 489–493.

Snoddy, G.S. 1926. Learning and stability. *J. Appl. Psychol.* **10**: 1–36.

Sokolov, E.N. 1960. Neuronal models and the orienting reflex. In M.A.B. Brazier (ed.), *The central nervous system and behavior: transactions of third conference*. New York: Macy Foundation, pp. 187–276.

Solley, C.M., and G. Murphy 1960. *Development of the perceptual world*. New York: Basic Books.

_____ 1952. The effects of verbal instruction of speed and accuracy upon the learning of a motor skill. *Res. Quart.* **23**: 231–240.

Sorge, R.W. 1960. *The effects of levels of intense activity on total body reaction time*. Unpublished doctoral dissertation. Greeley, Colo.: University of Northern Colorado.

Sperry, R.W. 1964. The great cerebral commissure. *Sci. Am.* **210** (January): 42–52.

Spielberger, C.D., R.L. Gorsuch, and R.E. Lushene 1970. *State-trait anxiety inventory*. Palo Alto, Calif.: Consulting Psychologists Press.

_____ 1966. Theory and research on anxiety. In C.D. Spielberger (ed.), *Anxiety and behavior*. New York: Academic Press, pp. 3–20.

Sprague, J.M., W.W. Chambers, and E. Stellar 1961. Attentive, affective, and adaptive behavior in the cat. *Sci.* **133**: 165–173.

Stabler, J.R., and J.A. Dyal 1963. Discriminative reaction-time as a joint function of manifest anxiety and intelligence. *Am. J. Psychol.* **76**: 484–487.

Stallings, L.M. 1968. The role of visual-spatial abilities in the performance of certain motor skills. *Res. Quart.* **39**: 708–713.

Stebbins, R.J. 1968. A comparison of the effects of physical and mental practice in learning a motor skill. *Res. Quart.* **39**: 714–720.

Stelmach, G.E. 1974. Retention of motor skills. In J.H. Wilmore (ed.), *Exercise and sport science reviews*. (Vol. 2.) New York: Academic Press, pp. 1–31.

_____, and M. Wilson 1970. Kinesthetic retention, movement extent, and information processing. *J. Exp. Psychol.* **85**: 425–430.

_____ 1969. Efficiency of motor learning as a function of intertrial rest. *Res. Quart.* **40**: 198–202.

Stennett, R.G. 1957. The relationship of performance level to level of arousal. *J. Exp. Psychol.* **54**: 54–61.

Sternback, R.A., and B. Tursky 1965. Ethnic differences among housewives in psychophysical and skin potential responses to electric shock. *Psychophysiol.* **1**: 241–246.

Stevens, C.F. 1966. *Neurophysiology: a primer*. New York: Wiley.

Stockfelt, T. 1970. Mental performance during varied physiological exertion. In G.S. Kenyon (ed.), *Contemporary psychology of sport*. Chicago: The Athletic Institute, pp. 197–204.

Stockholm, A.J., and R. Nelson 1965. The immediate aftereffects of increased resistance upon physical performance. *Res. Quart.* **36**: 337–341.

Stolurow, L.M. 1966. *Psychological and education factors in transfer of training.* Section I. Final report. Urbana, Ill.: Training Research Laboratory.

Stratton, G.M. 1897. Vision without inversion of the retinal image. *Psychol. Rev.* **4**: 341-360, 463-481.

Straub, W.F. 1968. Effect of overload training procedures upon velocity and accuracy of the overarm throw. *Res. Quart.* **39**: 370-379.

Strong, C.H. 1963. Motivation related to performance of physical fitness tests. *Res. Quart.* **34**: 497-507.

Stroup, F. 1957. Relationship between measurements of field of motion perception and basketball ability in college men. *Res. Quart.* **28**: 72-76.

Suzuki, T., K. Otsuka, H. Matsui, S. Ohukuzi, K. Sakai, and Y. Harada 1967. Effects of muscular exercise on adrenal 17-hydroxycorticosteroid secretion in the dog. *Endocrin.* **80**: 1148-1151.

Swift, E.J. 1903. Studies in the psychology and physiology of learning. *Am. J. Psychol.* **14**: 201-251.

Szekely, A., G. Czeh, and G. Voros 1969. The activity pattern of limb muscles in freely moving normal and deafferented newts. *Exper. Brain Res.* **9**: 53-72.

Taub, E., P. Perrella, and G. Barro 1973. Behavioral development after forelimb deafferentation on day of birth in monkeys with and without blinding. *Sci.* **181**: 959-960.

_____, and A.J. Berman 1968. Movement and learning in the absence of sensory feedback. In S.J. Freedman (ed.), *The neuropsychology of spatially oriented behavior.* Homewood, Ill.: The Dorsey Press, pp. 173-192.

Tauber, H.L. 1964. Comment on E.H. Lenneberg's paper: speech as a motor skill with special reference to nonaphasic disorders. *Acquisition of Language Monographs of the Society for Research in Child Development* **29**: 131-138.

Taylor, A., and C.E. Noble 1962. Acquisition and extinction phenomena in human trial-and-error learning under different schedules of reinforcing feedback. *Percept. and Motor Skills* **15**: 31-44.

Taylor, J.C. 1972. *The quality of working life: an annotated bibliography.* Center for Organizational Studies, Graduate School of Management. Los Angeles: University of California.

Taylor, W.J. 1933. *The relationship between kinesthetic judgment and success in basketball.* Unpublished master's thesis. University Park, Pa.: Pennsylvania State University.

Teichner, W.H. 1954. Recent studies of simple reaction time. *Psychol. Bull.* **51**: 128-149.

Telford, C.W. 1931. The refractory phase of voluntary and associative responses. *J. Exp. Psychol.* **14**: 1-36.

Tharp, G.D., and R.J. Buuck 1974. Adrenal adaptation to chronic exercise. *J. Appl. Physiol.* **37**: 720-722.

Thayer, R.E. 1970. Activation states as assessed by verbal report and four psychophysiological variables. *Psychophysiology* **7**: 86–94.

_____ 1967. Measurement of activation through self-report. *Psychol. Reports* **20**: 663–678. Monograph Suppl. 1-V20.

Thomas, J.R., B.S. Chissom, C. Stewart, and F. Shelley 1974. Effects of perceptual-motor training on preschool children: a multivariate approach. Presented at the AAHPER Convention, Anaheim.

Thompson, W.R., and R. Melzack 1956. Early environment. *Sci. Am.* **194** (January): 38–42.

Thorndike, E.L. 1911. *Animal intelligence.* New York: Macmillan.

_____ 1903. *Educational psychology.* New York: Lemcke and Buechner.

Tolman, E.C. 1948. Cognitive maps in rats and men. *Psychol. Rev.* **55**: 189–208.

Tomlin, F.A. 1966. *A study of the relationship between depth perception of moving objects and sports skill.* Unpublished master's thesis. Greensboro, N.C.: University of North Carolina.

Towe, A.L., and S.J. Jabbur 1961. Cortical inhibition of neurons in dorsal column of cat. *J. Neurophysiol.* **24**: 488–498.

Trexler, J.T., and A.J. Schuh 1971. Personality dynamics in a military training command and its relationship to Maslow's motivation hierarchy. *J. Voc. Behav.* **1**: 245–254.

Trowbridge, M.H., and H. Cason 1932. An experimental study of Thorndike's theory of learning. *J. Gen. Psychol.* **7**: 245–260.

Tulving, E. 1966. Subjective organization and effects of repetition in multitrial free-recall learning. *J. Verb. Learn. and Verb. Behav.* **5**: 193–197.

Tutko, T.A., and B.C. Ogilvie 1967. The role of the coach in the motivation of athletes. In R. Slovenko and J.A. Knight (eds.), *Motivation in play, games, and sports.* Springfield, Ill.: Charles C. Thomas, pp. 355–361.

Twining, W.E. 1949. Mental practice and physical practice in learning a motor skill. *Res. Quart.* **20**: 432–435.

Vallerga, J.M. 1958. Influence of perceptual stimulus intensity on speed of movement and force of muscular contraction. *Res. Quart.* **29**: 93–101.

Vandell, R.A., R.A. Davis, and H.A. Clugston 1943. The function of mental practice in the acquisition of motor skills. *J. Gen. Psychol.* **29**: 243–250.

Vander, A.J., J.H. Sherman, and D.S. Luciano 1970. *Human physiology: the mechanisms of body function.* New York: McGraw-Hill.

Van Huss, W.D., L. Albrecht, R. Nelson, and R. Hagerman 1962. Effect of overload warm-up on the velocity and accuracy of throwing. *Res. Quart.* **33**: 472–475.

Vincent, W.J. 1968. Transfer effects between motor skills judged similar in perceptual components. *Res. Quart.* **39**: 380–388.

Vogel-Sprott, M. 1963. Influence of peripheral visual distraction on perceptual motor performance. *Percept. and Motor Skills* **16**: 765–772.

Volkmar, F.R., and W.T. Greenough 1972. Rearing complexity affects branching of dendrites in the visual cortex of the rat. *Sci.* **176**: 1445–1447.

Von Holst, E. 1954. Relations between the central nervous system and the peripheral organs. *Brit. J. Animal Behav.* **2**: 89–94.

Voor, J.H., A.J. Lloyd, and R.J. Cole 1969. The influence of competition on the efficiency of an isometric muscle contraction. *J. Motor Behav.* **1**: 210–219.

Wallace, R.K., and H. Benson 1972. The physiology of meditation. *Sci. Am.* **226** (February): 85–90.

Walker, E.L., and R.D. Tarte 1963. Memory storage as a function of arousal and time with homogeneous and heterogeneous lists. *J. Verb. Learn. and Verb. Behav.* **2**: 113–119.

Walker, J. 1971. Pain and distraction in athletes and nonathletes. *Percept. and Motor Skills* **33**: 1187–1190.

Walter, L.M., and S.S. Marzolf 1951. The relation of sex, age, and school achievement to levels of aspiration. *J. Educ. Psychol.* **42**: 285–292.

Waterland, J.C. 1956. *The effect of mental practice combined with kinesthetic perception when practice precedes each overt performance of a motor skill.* Unpublished master's thesis. Madison, Wisc.: University of Wisconsin.

Weiner, B. 1967. Motivational factors in short-term retention: II. Rehearsal or arousal? *Psychol. Rept.* **20**: 1203–1208.

_____ 1966. Motivation and memory. *Psychol. Monogr.* **80** (18, Whole No. 626).

_____, and E.L. Walker 1966. Motivational factors in short-term retention. *J. Exp. Psychol.* **71**: 190–193.

Weingarten, G. 1973. Mental performance during physical exertion: the benefit of being physically fit. *Int. J. Sport Psychol.* **4**: 16–26.

_____ 1970. *Effect of cardiorespiratory conditioning increase upon mental performance under physiological stress and on personality variables.* Unpublished doctoral dissertation. Minneapolis: University of Minnesota.

_____, and J.P. Alexander 1970. Effects of physical exertion on mental performance of college males of different physical fitness levels. *Percept. and Motor Skills* **31**: 371–378.

Weintraub, D.J., and E.L. Walker 1968. *Perception.* Belmont, Calif.: Brooks/Cole.

Weissman, S., and C.M. Freeburne 1965. Relationship between static and dynamic visual acuity. *J. Exp. Psychol.* **70**: 141–146.

Welford, A.T. 1968a. *Aging and human skill.* London: Methuen.

_____ 1968b. *Fundamentals of skill.* London: Methuen.

_____ 1959. Evidence of a single channel decision mechanism limiting performance in a serial reaction task. *Quart. J. Exp. Psychol.* **11**: 193–210.

_____ 1952. The "psychological refractory period" and the timing of high-speed performance: a review and a theory. *Brit. J. Psychol.* **43**: 2–19.

Weltman, G., and G.H. Egstrom 1966. Perceptual narrowing in novice divers. *Human Factors* **8**: 499–506.

Werner, P. 1972. Integration of physical education skills with the concept of levers at intermediate grade levels. *Res. Quart.* **43**: 423–428.

Wertheimer, M., and C.M. Leventhal 1958. Permanent satiation phenomena with kinesthetic figural aftereffects. *J. Exp. Psychol.* **55**: 255–257.

Westerland, J.H., and W.W. Tuttle 1931. The relationship between running events in track and reaction time. *Res. Quart.* **2**: 95–100.

Wettstone, E. 1938. Tests for predicting potential ability in gymnastics and tumbling. *Res. Quart.* **9** (Dec.): 115–125.

Weymouth, F.W. 1963. Visual acuity in children. In M.J. Hirsch and R.E. Wick (eds.), *Vision of children*. Philadelphia: Chilton.

White, B., and R. Held 1966. Plasticity of sensorimotor development. In J.f. Rosenblith and W. Allinsmith (eds.), *The causes of behavior: readings in child development and educational psychology*. (2nd ed.) Boston: Allyn and Bacon.

_____, P. Castle, and R. Held 1964. Observations on the development of visually directed reaching. *Child Dev.* **35**: 349–364.

White, J.C., and W.H. Sweet 1969. *Pain and the neurosurgeon*. Springfield, Ill.: Charles C. Thomas.

Whiting, H.T.A., G.J.K. Alderson, and F.H. Sanderson 1973. Critical time intervals for viewing and individual differences in performance of a ball-catching task. *Int. J. Sport Psychol.* **4**: 155–164.

_____, and F.H. Sanderson 1972. The effect of exercise on the visual and auditory acuity of table-tennis players. *J. Motor Behav.* **4**: 163–170.

_____ 1972. Overview of the skill learning process. *Res. Quart.* **43**: 266–294.

_____, E.B. Gill, and J. Stephenson 1970. Critical time intervals for taking in-flight information in a ball-catching task. *Ergonomics* **13**: 265–272.

_____ 1969. *Acquiring ball skill: a psychological interpretation*. Philadelphia: Lea and Febiger.

_____ 1968. Training in a continuous ball-throwing and catching task. *Ergonomics* **11**: 375–382.

Whitley, J.D. 1970. Effects of practice distribution on learning a fine motor task. *Res. Quart.* **41**: 576–583.

Whorf, B.L. 1961. Science and linguistics. In S. Saporta (ed.), *Psycholinguistics*. New York: Holt, pp. 460–468.

Wickelgren, W.A. 1966. Consolidation and retroactive interference in short-term recognition memory for pitch. *J. Exp. Psychol.* **72**: 250–259.

Wiebe, V.R. 1954. A study of tests of kinesthesis. *Res. Quart.* **25**: 222–230.

Wilkinson, J.J. 1959. A study of reaction-time measures to a kinesthetic and a visual stimulus for selected groups of athletes and nonathletes. *Proceedings of the 26th NCPEAM Convention*, pp. 158–161.

Williams, F.I. 1960. *Specificity of motor pattern learning as determined by performance of cursive writing by head, jaw, elbow, knee, and foot muscles.* Unpublished master of education problem. College of Health and Physical Education. University Park, Pa.: The Pennsylvania State University.

Williams, H.G. 1973a. The perception of moving objects by children. In C.B. Corbin, *A textbook of motor development*. Dubuque, Iowa: Wm. C. Brown, pp. 130–139.

_____ 1973b. Perceptual-motor development in children. In C.B. Corbin (ed.), *A textbook of motor development*. Dubuque, Iowa: Wm. C. Brown, pp. 109–148.

Williams, H.L., W.S. Beaver, M.T. Spence, and O.H. Rundell 1969. Digital and kinesthetic memory with interpolated information processing. *J. Exp. Psychol.* **80**: 530–536.

Williams, J.M., and J. Thirer 1975. Vertical and horizontal peripheral vision in male and female athletes and nonathletes. *Res. Quart.* **46**: 200–205.

Williams, L.R.T. 1971. Refractoriness of an extended movement to directional change. *J. Motor Behav.* **3**: 289–300.

Wilson, D.M. 1968. Inherent asymmetry and reflex modulation of the locust flight motor pattern. *J. Exp. Bio.* **48**: 631–641.

_____ 1964. The origin of the flight-motor command in grasshoppers. In R.R. Reiss (ed.), *The neural theory and modeling*. Palo Alto: Stanford University Press, pp. 331–345.

_____ 1961. The central nervous control of flight in a locust. *J. Exp. Bio.* **38**: 471–490.

Winningham, S.N. 1966. *Effect of training with ankel weights on runing skill.* Unpublished doctoral dissertation. University of Southern California.

Witkin, H.A., H.B. Lewis, M. Hertzman, K. Machover, P.B. Meissner, and S. Wapner 1954. *Personality through perception*. New York: Harper.

_____ 1950. Individual differences in the ease of perception of embedded figures. *J. Personality* **19**: 1–15.

Witte, F. 1962. Relation of kinesthetic perception to a selected motor skill for elementary school children. *Res. Quart.* **33**: 476–484.

Wober, M. 1966. Sensotypes. *J. of Soc. Psychol.* **70**: 181–189.

Woodburne, L.S. 1967. *The neural basis of behavior*. Columbus, Ohio: Charles E. Merrill.

Woods, J.B. 1967. The effect of varied instructional emphasis upon the development of a motor skill. *Res. Quart.* **38**: 132–142.

Woodworth, R.S., and H. Schlosberg 1954. *Experimental psychology*. (Rev. ed.) New York: Holt, Rinehart and Winston.

_____ 1938. *Experimental psychology*. New York: Holt, Rinehart and Winston.

_____ 1918. *Dynamic psychology*. New York: Columbia University Press.

_____ 1899. The accuracy of voluntary movement. *Psychol. Rev.* **3** (2, Whole No. 13).

Worell, L. 1959. Level of aspiration and academic success. *J. Educ. Psychol.* **50**: 47–54.

Yerkes, R.M., and J.D. Dodson 1908. The relation of strength of stimulus to rapidity of habit formation. *J. Comp. Neurol. Psychol.* **18**: 459–482.

Young, J., and M. Skemp 1955. *A comparison of peripheral vision reaction time of athletes and nonathletes in relationship to the colors of red and green.* Unpublished master's thesis. Madison, Wisc.: University of Wisconsin.

Young, O.G. 1954. Rate of learning in relation to spacing of practice periods in archery and badminton. *Res. Quart.* **25**: 231–243.

_____ 1945. A study of kinesthesis in relation to selected movements. *Res. Quart.* **16**: 277–287.

Youngen, L.A. 1959. A comparison of reaction and movement times of women athletes and nonathletes. *Res. Quart.* **30**: 349–355.

Zagora, E. 1959. Observations on the evolution and neurophysiology of eye-limb coordination. *Ophthalmol.* **138**: 241–254.

Zajonc, R.B. 1966. *Social psychology: an experimental approach.* Belmont, Calif.: Brooks/Cole.

_____ 1965. Social facilitation. *Sci.* **149**: 269–274.

Zander, A.F. 1971. *Motives and goals in groups.* New York: Academic Press.

Zeigarnik, B. 1927. Uber das Behalten von erledigten und unerledigten Handlungen. *Psychol. Forsch.* **9**: 1–85. Translated 1938 by W.D. Ellis, *A source book of Gestalt psychology.* London: Routledge.

Index

Index